Handbook of Gastrointestinal Surgery

Handbook of Gastrointestinal Surgery

Editor: Diana Pollard

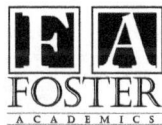

FA

FOSTER
ACADEMICS

www.fosteracademics.com

www.fosteracademics.com

FA
FOSTER
ACADEMICS

Cataloging-in-Publication Data

Handbook of gastrointestinal surgery / edited by Diana Pollard.
    p. cm.
Includes bibliographical references and index.
ISBN 978-1-63242-652-9
1. Gastrointestinal system--Surgery. 2. Alimentary canal--Surgery.
3. Digestive organs--Surgery. I. Pollard, Diana.
RD540 .H36 2019
61743--dc23

Foster Academics,
118-35 Queens Blvd., Suite 400,
Forest Hills, NY 11375, USA

ISBN 978-1-63242-652-9 (Hardback)

Contents

Preface

Surgeries related to the upper gastrointestinal tract as well as the lower gastrointestinal tract are under the scope of gastrointestinal surgery. The practice of surgery whose focus of study is on the upper parts of the gastrointestinal tract is called upper gastrointestinal surgery or upper GI surgery. Lower gastrointestinal surgery or lower GI surgery is the type of surgery which is concerned with colorectal surgery and the surgery of the small intestine. The main operations performed by upper GI surgeons include liver resection, pancreaticoduodenectomy and esophagectomy, whereas, lower GI surgeons perform operations like colectomy and low or ultralow resections for rectal cancer. This book provides comprehensive insights into the field of gastrointestinal surgery. It includes some of the vital pieces of work being conducted across the world, on various topics related to gastrointestinal surgery. Those in search of information to further their knowledge will be greatly assisted by this book.

The information contained in this book is the result of intensive hard work done by researchers in this field. All due efforts have been made to make this book serve as a complete guiding source for students and researchers. The topics in this book have been comprehensively explained to help readers understand the growing trends in the field.

I would like to thank the entire group of writers who made sincere efforts in this book and my family who supported me in my efforts of working on this book. I take this opportunity to thank all those who have been a guiding force throughout my life.

Editor

Conservative Management of an Iatrogenic Esophageal Tear in Kenya

Peter Waweru[1] and David Mwaniki[2]

[1]Department of Surgery, St. Mary's Mission Hospital, P.O. Box 3409, Nairobi 00506, Kenya
[2]Department of Surgery, The Karen Hospital, P.O. Box 74240, Nairobi 00200, Kenya

Correspondence should be addressed to Peter Waweru; pwaweru09@gmail.com

Academic Editor: Steve de Castro

Since its description over 250 years ago, diagnosis of esophageal perforation remains challenging, its management controversial, and its mortality high. This rare, devastating, mostly iatrogenic, condition can quickly lead to severe complications and death due to an overwhelming inflammatory response to gastric contents in the mediastinum. Diagnosis is made with the help of esophagograms and although such tears have traditionally been managed via aggressive surgical approach, recent reports emphasize a shift in favor of nonoperative care which unfortunately remains controversial. We here present a case of an iatrogenic esophageal tear resulting from a routine esophagoscopy in a 50-year-old lady presenting with dysphagia. The esophageal tear, almost missed, was eventually successfully managed conservatively, thanks to a relatively early diagnosis.

1. Introduction

Esophageal perforation is a rare, devastating, and often life-threatening clinical condition [1] typically resulting from endoscopic procedures [2]. This condition remains difficult to diagnose and manage and can quickly cause death without alarm [3], owing to its nonspecific and varied clinical symptomatology [1]. While surgery has been the mainstay of treatment, nonoperative management approaches for this condition are becoming more and more common [4], but they remain controversial.

We present a case of an iatrogenic esophageal perforation that developed after a diagnostic esophagoscopy in a female patient with odynophagia and the subsequent conservative treatment after an almost missed diagnosis. In view of the recent but controversial emphasis on nonoperative treatment, this case has been presented to add to the repertoire of success stories, thus encouraging nonoperative care, even in developing countries.

2. Case Report

A 50-year-old lady presented with dysphagia, odynophagia, and regurgitation of foods. Although an esophagogastroduodenoscopy (OGD) done previously had shown gastroesophageal reflux disease (GERD), resolving esophagitis and gastritis, this new onset dysphagia warranted further examination. A barium swallow, postnasal space and chest computed tomography (CT) scans were all normal. An indirect laryngoscopy was attempted but unsuccessful due to a strong gag reflex and consequently a direct laryngoscopy and esophagoscopy were done. The investigations revealed laryngeal erythema and gastric fundal erosion with no other abnormalities. After esophagoscopy, she was successfully reversed, observed in the postanesthetic care unit, and eventually discharged to the ward in stable conditions.

In the ward, she suddenly developed severe epigastric pains, respiratory distress, and difficulty in speaking, for which she was given intravenous (IV) Esomeprazole 80 mg and Buscopan (hyoscine butylbromide) 40 mg for what appeared like acute exacerbation of gastritis. She was also started on oxygen. There being minimal improvement, she was immediately transferred to the intensive care unit, where close monitoring and oxygen therapy were continued. Further investigations included an electrocardiogram (ECG) and echocardiogram which were both normal and a CT scan of the chest which revealed severe basal pneumonia. A gastrografin swallow was finally done (Figure 1) and showed

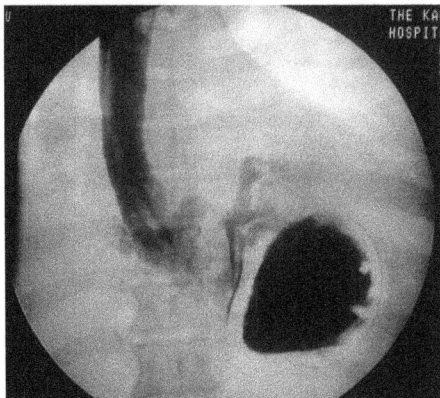

FIGURE 1: Gastrografin swallow showing leak of contrast into the left mediastinum and left pleural cavity.

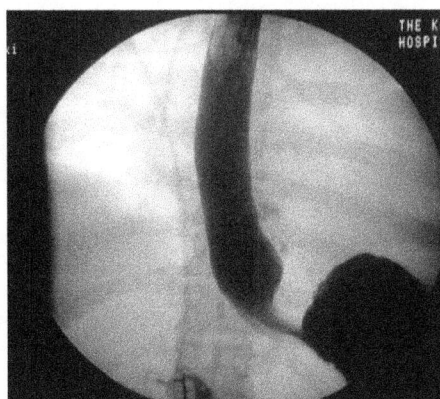

FIGURE 2: Follow-up gastrografin swallow showing reduced leakage.

leakage of the contrast into the mediastinum and left pleural cavity.

Following the diagnosis of an esophageal perforation, a decision was made to manage the patient nonoperatively considering the relatively early diagnosis (few hours after esophagoscopy). A chest drain was inserted percutaneously and a nasogastric tube (NGT) inserted to rest the esophagus and drain the gastric contents. She was kept *nil per oral (NPO)* and was started on broad-spectrum IV antibiotics, oxygen, IV proton pump inhibitors, IV fluids, and analgesics.

A follow-up gastrografin swallow done on day 12 after esophagoscopy showed notable reduced leakage (Figure 2).

Later, a repeat OGD was carefully performed on day 14 to review the status of the injury and showed a 2 cm tear at 30 cm in the posterior wall that was contracting. The patient showed good progress on conservative management and was transferred to the ward on day 15. Feeding was gradually advanced from total parenteral to feeding via NGT to oral sips and finally solid meals before she was discharged home after about one month in stable conditions.

3. Discussion

Esophageal perforation, reported as early as the 18th century (Hermann Boerhaave, 1724) [5], is a rare and often grave clinical condition [4] with high mortality rates over 40%, especially in septic patients [6]. While the true incidence is unclear [4], the majority of esophageal rupture cases (up to 59%) are iatrogenic [1] resulting from esophagoscopy [2] despite the actual risk of esophageal perforation during endoscopy being low [2, 7]. Boerhaave syndrome, a spontaneous esophageal rupture with no preexisting pathology, accounts for about 15% of the cases [8]. Foreign-body ingestion accounts for 12% of the cases, trauma 9%, operative injury 2%, tumors 1%, and other causes 2% [8].

Thoracic esophageal perforations occur frequently [1, 8] and can lead to serious complications and death without alarm [3, 9], owing to the mediastinal contamination that ensues soon after the perforation [7]. This contamination, which is exacerbated by the negative intrathoracic pressure that draws esophageal contents into the mediastinum [10], evokes an overwhelming inflammatory response [11] leading to mediastinitis, initially chemical mediastinitis, followed by bacterial invasion and severe mediastinal necrosis [7]. Eventually, sepsis ensues leading to multiple-organ failure and death [3, 4]. The extent of this inflammation (mediastinitis), and thus the morbidity and mortality of esophageal perforation, depends not only on the cause and location of the perforation but also on the time interval between onset and access to appropriate treatment [3, 12]. It has been shown that early detection reduces mortality by over 50% [11] and treatment delays over 24 hours increase mortality significantly [13]. Unfortunately, prompt diagnosis continues to be exigent for most clinicians [5].

Diagnosis of esophageal perforation is challenging owing to a nonspecific and varied clinical presentation [1] that mimics a myriad of other disorders such as myocardial infarction and peptic ulcer perforation [14]. Patients may present with any combination of nonspecific signs and symptoms including fever, tachycardia, tachypnea, acute onset chest pain, dysphagia, vomiting, and shortness of breath [4, 6, 15]. A high index of suspicion is therefore needed for recognition of esophageal perforation [5]. Once suspected, patients should be evaluated quickly with a combination of radiographs and esophagograms [8, 14]. Accurate diagnosis may however require added investigations including computed tomography and flexible esophagoscopy [7, 12].

Treatment of esophageal perforations remains a challenge [13] and the appropriate management is controversial [9]. Traditionally, surgery has been the mainstay of treatment [14], but recent reports emphasize a shift in treatment strategies with nonoperative approaches becoming more common [4, 9]. It has been shown that, with careful patient selection, nonoperative management can be the treatment of choice for esophageal perforations [6] with good outcomes [9, 12, 15, 16]. Altorjay et al. [17] and others have suggested criteria for selection of nonoperative treatment including early perforations (or contained leak if diagnosis delayed); leak draining back to the esophagus; nonseptic patients; perforation not involving a neoplasm, abdominal esophagus, or distal obstruction; and availability of an experienced thoracic surgeon and contrast. When these established guidelines are followed, survival rates of up to 100% have been reported [7, 9, 15].

Patients selected for nonoperative treatment are started on broad-spectrum antibiotics, intravenous fluids, oxygen therapy, adequate analgesia, and gastric acid suppression and kept nil by mouth in an intensive care unit [4, 18]. A nasogastric tube is placed to clear gastric contents and limit further contamination [9] and mediastinal contamination drained percutaneously/radiologically [18] via the chest tubes, thereby converting the esophageal perforations to esophagocutaneous fistulae that heal similar to gastrointestinal fistulae [6]. Apart from observation, the range of conservative management is growing, with the increasing use of endoscopic stents, clips, vacuum sponge therapy, and fibrin glue application [8, 12] for the selected patients. Notably though, even with meticulous patient selection, up to 20% develop multiple complications within 24 hours and require surgical intervention [2, 7].

In our patient, the diagnosis of an iatrogenic esophageal perforation was made relatively early and a multidisciplinary team chose conservative treatment as the treatment of choice given that the patient was not septic and had no contraindications to the treatment. This was instituted without complications, achieving good results. While there are few such reports in resource-limited settings, conservative management should be considered in the few hospitals with institutional capacities.

References

[1] H. Vidarsdottir, S. Blondal, H. Alfredsson, A. Geirsson, and T. Gudbjartsson, "Oesophageal perforations in Iceland: a whole population study on incidence, aetiology and surgical outcome," *Thoracic and Cardiovascular Surgeon*, vol. 58, no. 8, pp. 476–480, 2010.

[2] A. Merchea, D. C. Cullinane, M. D. Sawyer et al., "Esophagogastroduodenoscopy-associated gastrointestinal perforations: a single-center experience," *Surgery*, vol. 148, no. 4, pp. 876–882, 2010.

[3] A. Khaleghnejad Tabari, A. Mirshemirani, M. Rouzrokh, L. Mohajerzadeh, N. Khaleghnejad Tabari, and P. Ghaffari, "Acute mediastinitis in children: a nine-year experience," *Tanaffos*, vol. 12, no. 2, pp. 48–52, 2013.

[4] J. A. Søreide and A. Viste, "Esophageal perforation: diagnostic work-up and clinical decision-making in the first 24 hours," *Scandinavian Journal of Trauma, Resuscitation and Emergency Medicine*, vol. 19, article 66, 2011.

[5] E. L. Hoover, "The diagnosis and management of esophageal perforations," *Journal of the National Medical Association*, vol. 83, no. 3, pp. 246–248, 1991.

[6] S. B. Vogel, W. R. Rout, T. D. Martin et al., "Esophageal perforation in adults: aggressive, conservative treatment lowers morbidity and mortality," *Annals of Surgery*, vol. 241, no. 6, pp. 1016–1023, 2005.

[7] C. J. Brinster, S. Singhal, L. Lee, M. B. Marshall, L. R. Kaiser, and J. C. Kucharczuk, "Evolving options in the management of

esophageal perforation," *Annals of Thoracic Surgery*, vol. 77, no. 4, pp. 1475–1483, 2004.

[8] K. Mantzoukis, K. Kpadimitriou, I. Kouvelis et al., "Endoscopic closure of an iatrogenic rupture of upper esophagus (Lannier's triangle) with the use of endoclips—case report and review of the literature," *Annals of Gastroenterology*, vol. 24, no. 1, pp. 55–58, 2011.

[9] L. Kaman, J. Iqbal, B. Kundil, and R. Kochhar, "Management of esophageal perforation in adults," *Gastroenterology Research*, vol. 3, no. 6, pp. 235–244, 2010.

[10] J. A. Salo, J. O. Isolauri, L. J. Heikkila et al., "Management of delayed esophageal perforation with mediastinal sepsis. Esophagectomy or primary repair?" *Journal of Thoracic and Cardiovascular Surgery*, vol. 106, no. 6, pp. 1088–1091, 1993.

[11] E. Ko and A. H. O-Yurvati, "Iatrogenic esophageal injuries: evidence-based management for diagnosis and timing of contrast studies after repair," *International Surgery*, vol. 97, no. 1, pp. 1–5, 2012.

[12] A. Troja, P. Käse, N. El-Sourani, S. Miftode, H. R. Raab, and D. Antolovic, "Treatment of esophageal perforation: a single-center expertise," *Scandinavian Journal of Surgery*, 2014.

[13] S. Persson, P. Elbe, I. Rouvelas et al., "Predictors for failure of stent treatment for benign esophageal perforations—a single center 10-year experience," *World Journal of Gastroenterology*, vol. 20, no. 30, pp. 10613–10619, 2014.

[14] E. Razi, A. Davoodabadi, and A. Razi, "Spontaneous esophageal perforation presenting as a right-sided pleural effusion: a case report," *Tanaffos*, vol. 12, no. 4, pp. 53–57, 2013.

[15] R. Addas, J. Berjaud, C. Renaud, P. Berthoumieu, M. Dahan, and L. Brouchet, "Esophageal perforation management: a single-center experience," *Open Journal of Thoracic Surgery*, vol. 2, no. 4, pp. 111–117, 2012.

[16] W. B. Keeling, D. L. Miller, G. T. Lam et al., "Low mortality after treatment for esophageal perforation: a single-center experience," *Annals of Thoracic Surgery*, vol. 90, no. 5, pp. 1669–1673, 2010.

[17] Á. Altorjay, J. Kiss, A. Vörös, and Á. Bohák, "Nonoperative management of esophageal perforations. Is it justified?" *Annals of Surgery*, vol. 225, no. 4, pp. 415–421, 1997.

[18] J. M. Petersen, "The use of a self-expandable plastic stent for an iatrogenic esophageal perforation," *Gastroenterology and Hepatology*, vol. 6, no. 6, pp. 389–391, 2010.

Early Rupture of an Ultralow Duodenal Stump after Extended Surgery for Gastric Cancer with Duodenal Invasion Managed by Tube Duodenostomy and Cholangiostomy

Konstantinos Blouhos, Konstantinos A. Boulas, Anna Konstantinidou, Ilias I. Salpigktidis, Stavroula P. Katsaouni, Konstantinos Ioannidis, and Anestis Hatzigeorgiadis

Department of General Surgery, General Hospital of Drama, End of Hippokratous Street, 66100 Drama, Greece

Correspondence should be addressed to Konstantinos A. Boulas; katerinantwna@hotmail.com

Academic Editors: T. Hotta and S.-I. Kosugi

When dealing with gastric cancer with duodenal invasion, gastrectomy with distal resection of the duodenum is necessary to achieve negative distal margin. However, rupture of an ultralow duodenal stump necessitates advanced surgical skills and close postoperative observation. The present study reports a case of an early duodenal stump rupture after subtotal gastrectomy with resection of the whole first part of the duodenum, complete omentectomy, bursectomy, and D2+ lymphadenectomy performed for a pT3pN2pM1 (+ number 13 lymph nodes) adenocarcinoma of the antrum. Duodenal stump rupture was managed successfully by end tube duodenostomy, without omental patching, and tube cholangiostomy. Close assessment of clinical, physical, and radiological signs, output volume, and enzyme concentration of the tube duodenostomy, T-tube, and closed suction drain, which was placed near the tube duodenostomy site to drain the leak around the catheter, dictated postoperative management of the external duodenal fistula.

1. Introduction

When dealing with gastric cancer with duodenal invasion, gastrectomy with distal resection of the duodenum is necessary to achieve negative distal margin; however, closure of an ultralow duodenal stump may be difficult. Duodenal stump closure carries a leak rate of 1–3% and a mortality rate of 0–2% in recent series [1]. Early recognition of stump leakage and prompt surgical drainage are essential to a lowering of mortality and morbidity. Duodenal drainage can be obtained with either tube duodenostomy (TD) along with tube cholangiostomy (TC) or tube duodenocholangiostomy [2]. In parallel with duodenal drainage, biliary diversion, gastric diversion with Roux-en-Y reconstruction, secondary suture of the duodenal leak, although usually not feasible, and close postoperative observation are paramount requirements to provide a consummate approach to duodenal stump dehiscence [3].

The present paper describes a case of an ultralow duodenal stump rupture after an extended gastrectomy in a patient with gastric cancer of the antrum and duodenal invasion; the rupture occurred on postoperative day 1, which is an extremely rare event. Following stump rupture, hemoperitoneum occurred due to erosion of the unsheathed transverse mesocolon vessels from duodenal contents. After ligation of the bleeding vessels, duodenal drainage was accomplished by TD and TC.

2. Case Presentation

A 62-year-old male patient presented to our surgical department after observing the passage of black, tarry stools per rectum. Esophagogastroduodenoscopy identified an advanced type 3 60×30 mm tumor of the lower part of the stomach and at least 15 mm extension into the duodenum. Endoscopic biopsy revealed a poorly differentiated adenocarcinoma. An abdominal and thoracic CT obtained showing thickening of the gastric wall of the antrum and the first part of

Early Rupture of an Ultralow Duodenal Stump after Extended Surgery for Gastric Cancer with Duodenal Invasion...

5

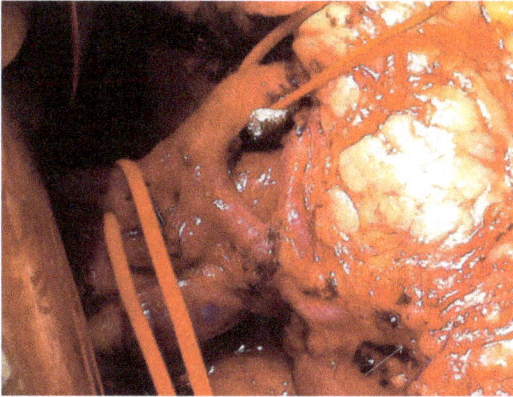

FIGURE 1: During initial laparotomy, the lateral aspect of the surgical bed after completion of bursectomy and the closed ultralow duodenal stump (arrow) can be seen.

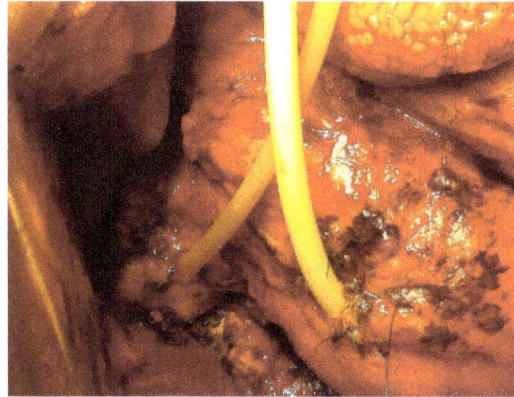

FIGURE 2: During relaparotomy, the ruptured ultralow duodenal stump was managed by tube duodenostomy and cholangiostomy.

the duodenum, absence of serosa invasion, associated regional lymph nodes, and absence of distant metastasis.

An extended gastrectomy was decided for a resectable cT3cN+cM0 tumor; however, pancreaticoduodenectomy was in mind if a clear distal margin could not be ensured. In our case, extended surgery consisted of (a) distal gastrectomy and at least 45 mm resection of the first part of the duodenum. Frozen section examination of the resection line showed no microinvasion of the carcinoma; consequently, an ultralow duodenal stump was left behind in the surgical bed (Figure 1) and closed after mobilization of 10 mm of the posterior duodenal wall from the pancreas using a 45 mm linear cutting stapler and interrupted seromuscular layer sutures; (b) complete omentectomy and bursectomy; (c) D2 plus number 11d, 12b, 12p, 13, 14v, 16a2, 16b1, 17, and 18 lymphadenectomy; (d) Roux-en-Y gastrojejunostomy in an antecolic way. Histology of the surgical specimen revealed a type 3, 60×30 mm, PM0, DM0, R0, CY(0), UL(+), ly(+), v(+), and poorly differentiated solid type pT3pN2pM1 and stage IV adenocarcinoma with 6/68 metastatic lymph node ratio [4]. The tumor was characterized as M1 due to involvement of number 13 nodes (1/3 metastatic ratio).

The patient was convalescing satisfactory; until suddenly on postoperative day 1 severe pain, abdominal rigidity, and fever developed. Bile-stained fluid was observed at the drain near the duodenal stump. Few hours after the onset of pain the patient exhibited a shock-like state and became hemodynamically unstable. Red blood was withdrawn from the drain near the gastrojejunal anastomosis. Relaparotomy was performed; dehiscence of the corner of the medial wall of the duodenal stump and hemoperitoneum due to erosion of vessels from the duodenal content at the left side of the transverse mesocolon, which left skeletalized due to bursectomy, were observed. After thorough peritoneal lavage and ligation of the bleeding mesenteric vessels, duodenal drainage and biliary diversion were performed (Figure 2). A 22 French Foley catheter was introduced through the open end of the duodenal stump. A pursestring of 3-0 absorbable suture was placed near the open edge of the duodenum and tied so that it gently held the tube in place. A second

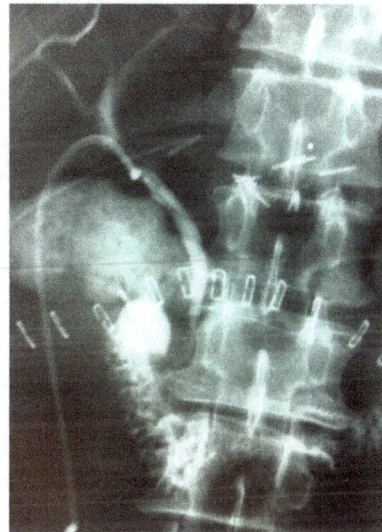

FIGURE 3: Contrast graph through tube duodenostomy. The tube duodenostomy, the closed suction drain, and the T-tube can be seen.

pursestring of 3-0 nonabsorbable suture was placed around the tube in the seromuscular layer and tied so that the first pursestring was invaginated into the lumen of the duodenum. Unfortunately, due to complete omentectomy, an omental pedicle was not available to secure the junction of the tube and the duodenum. The tube was then brought out through the abdominal wall leaving the intraperitoneal portion of the tube as short as possible. A closed suction drain was left near TD site to drain the leak around the catheter, and T-tube drainage of the common bile duct was added.

After the primary postoperative period, total parenteral nutrition and ocreotide at a dose of 100 mcg subcutaneously 3 times per day were administered; enteral diet was instituted on postoperative day 15. Assessment of clinical, physical, and radiological signs (Figure 3), output volume, and enzyme concentration of TD, T-tube, and closed suction drain (Figure 4) was employed in the overall management of the duodenocutaneous fistula (Figure 5). During hospitalization, the patient did not develop symptoms and signs of peritonitis

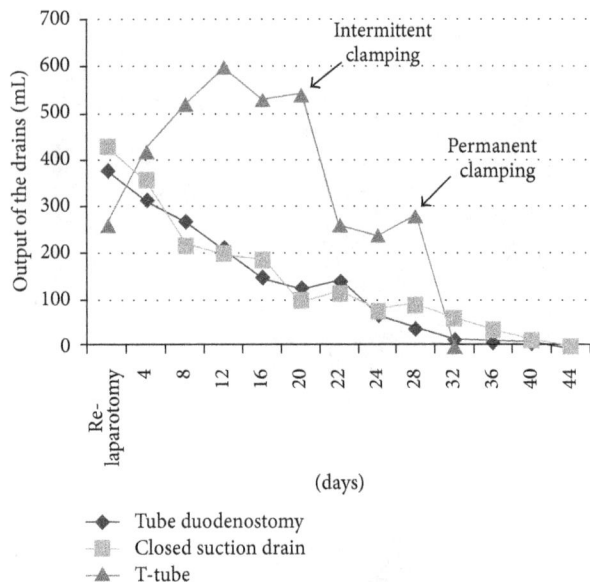

FIGURE 4: Comparison of mean daily outputs of the tube duodenostomy, T-tube, and closed suction drain near the tube duodenostomy. The lack of omental patch is depicted by the high output of the closed suction drain which reflects duodenal leak from the side of the tube duodenostomy.

or sepsis. The TD was removed on postoperative day 28, when (a) the output of the TD was minimum; (b) a contrast study did not reveal leak around the TD catheter; and (c) the closed suction catheter drainage did not fulfill pancreatic fistula criteria regarding output and amylase concentration [5]. The T-tube catheter was removed on postoperative day 32 with intermittent clamping 7 days before TD removal and permanent clamping after TD removal, when despite clamping, the output of the closed suction drain remained low. Finally, on postoperative day 36, the closed drain catheter was removed, and the patient was discharged home; the external duodenal fistula ceased spontaneously on postoperative day 45.

3. Discussion

Gastric cancer with duodenal invasion has been reported with an incidence of 15–40% [6]. Kakeji et al. analyzed 95 patients with duodenal invasion by gastric cancer and found that tumor spread into the duodenum was limited to within 2 cm in 76% of the patients and to within 3 cm in 81% of the patients. Therefore, he suggested gastrectomy with resection of 3-4 cm of the duodenum for patients with advanced gastric cancer and duodenal invasion [7]. However, closure of an ultralow duodenal stump may be difficult, and today's surgeons should be familiar with the procedures that have been developed for dealing with this problem, such as standard duodenal closures, Nissen's closure, Bancroft's closure, and primary TD [8]. However, when facing duodenal stump rupture, there it is one way to provide adequate duodenal drainage which isby secondary TD.

The most successful method of managing duodenal stump rupture has been TD; however, published series about TD have either few patients or insufficient information related to indication, technique, and postoperative care [9]. When performing TD for duodenal stump rupture, questions about technical details arise: (a) end or lateral duodenostomy? We chose end duodenostomy in an effort to create a controlled duodenal fistula; lateral duodenostomy is primarily used for intraluminal decompression and is not employed when technical factors prevent adequate closure of the duodenal stump [10]; (b) TD with or without TC? By draining the common bile duct, we accomplish to decrease the output of the TD by draining out the bile from the upper duodenum, we managed to decrease duodenal leak from the side of the TD, which was expressed by decreased closed suction drain output, and we gain time for relaxation of partial obstruction from edema in the distal common bile duct caused by the sutures placed around the tube in the seromuscular layer of the duodenum, as a result of the close anatomic relationship [11]; (c) what about TD without omental patch? In our case, a viable omental pedicle was not secured around the junction of the tube and the duodenum due to complete omentectomy; consequently, the output of the closed suction drain was higher and the time interval for closure of the external duodenal fistula was longer than previously reported by other studies in the literature [12].

What is interesting in our case is that duodenal stump rupture occurred on postoperative day 1. Technical failure such as malfunction of the linear stapler or overzealous closure and avascularization of the distal duodenal stump due to the radicality of the procedure that we performed are implicated for duodenal stump rupture [13]. Avascularization of the distal duodenal stump can be attributed to (a) duodenal skeletalization due to Kocher maneuver and separation of the gastrocolic omentum from the first and second parts of the duodenum by ligating small vessels which pass between them; (b) bursectomy; (c) although the trunk of the gastroduodenal artery preserved, other more peripheral branches, like the supraduodenal, retroduodenal, right gastroepiploic, and anterior superior pancreaticoduodenal arteries were divided; (d) wide dissection of the posterior and anterior surface of the pancreatic head (numbers 13 and 17 lymph nodes dissection), which disturbed the already deteriorated blood supply to the second portion of the duodenum.

Another remarkable fact is intra-abdominal hemorrhage due to erosion of vessels from the duodenal content at the left side of the transverse mesocolon whichoriginated few hours after duodenal stump rupture. Bursectomy definitely played a role as the superior layer of the peritoneum of the transverse mesocolon was dissected along with the posterior layer of the peritoneum of the greater omentum leaving the anterior leaf of the transverse mesocolon unsheathed. Another point we should highlight in our case is that histopathology revealed involvement of number 13 lymph nodes. The Japanese gastric cancer treatment guidelines suggest dissection of number 13 lymph nodes for tumors invading the duodenum [14]; indeed, our decision changed adjuvant therapy strategy as the disease was classified as pM1 and prevented early obstructive jaundice resulting from retropancreatic nodes metastasis.

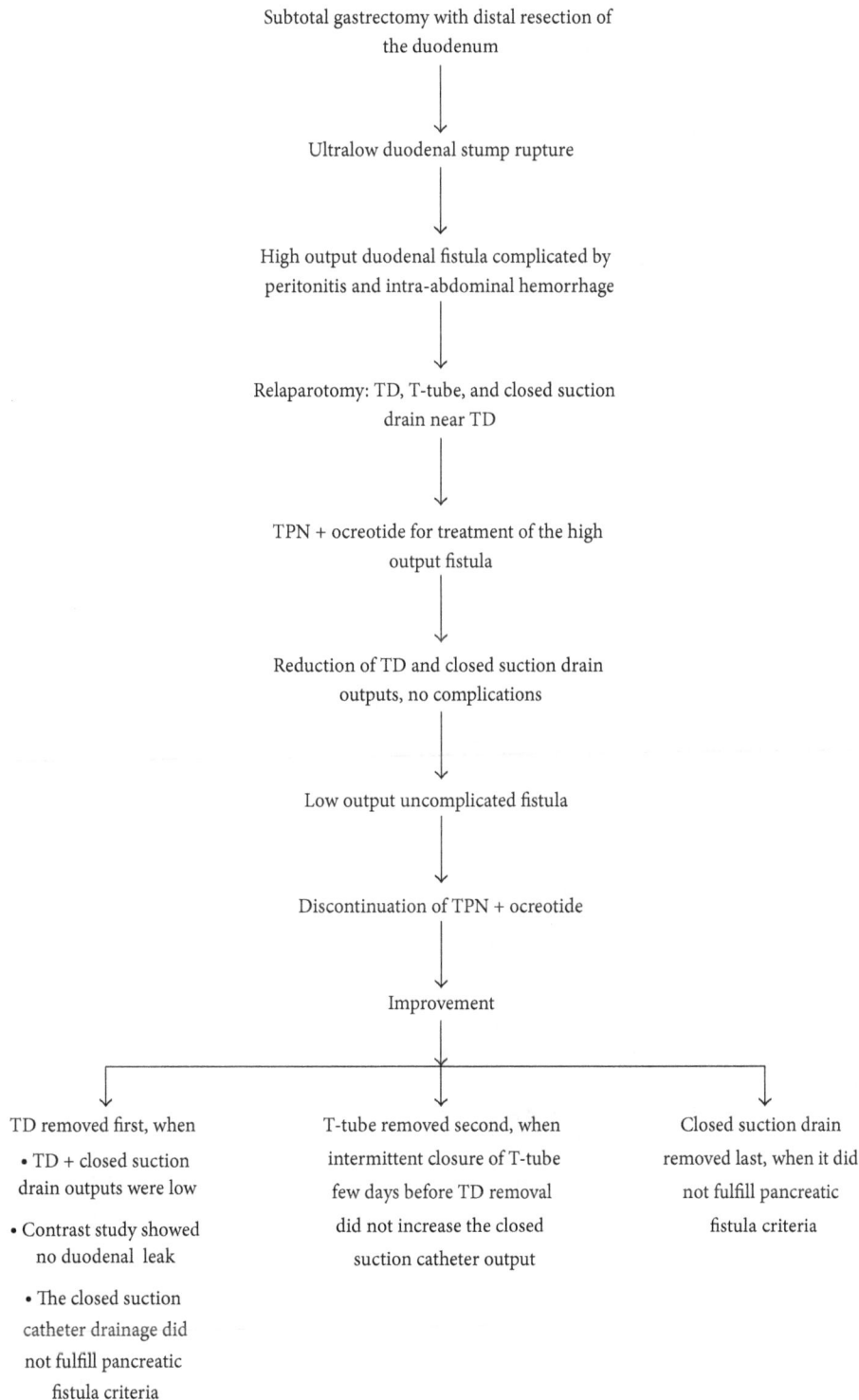

Subtotal gastrectomy with distal resection of
the duodenum

↓

Ultralow duodenal stump rupture

↓

High output duodenal fistula complicated by
peritonitis and intra-abdominal hemorrhage

↓

Relaparotomy: TD, T-tube, and closed suction
drain near TD

↓

TPN + ocreotide for treatment of the high
output fistula

↓

Reduction of TD and closed suction drain
outputs, no complications

↓

Low output uncomplicated fistula

↓

Discontinuation of TPN + ocreotide

↓

Improvement

↓

TD removed first, when	T-tube removed second, when	Closed suction drain
• TD + closed suction drain outputs were low	intermittent closure of T-tube few days before TD removal did not increase the closed suction catheter output	removed last, when it did not fulfill pancreatic fistula criteria
• Contrast study showed no duodenal leak		
• The closed suction catheter drainage did not fulfill pancreatic fistula criteria		

FIGURE 5

In conclusion, rupture of the ultralow duodenal stump due to extensive avascularization of the second part of the duodenum and intra-abdominal hemorrhage due to erosion of small vessels from the unsheathed transverse mesocolon are potential complications after extended surgery for gastric cancer with duodenal invasion. End TD, even without an omental patch, and TC along with close postoperative observation are a successful method to manage the leakage.

References

[1] B. J. Tsuei and R. W. Schwartz, "Management of the difficult duodenum," *Current Surgery*, vol. 61, no. 2, pp. 166–171, 2004.

[2] P. Paluszkiewicz, W. Dudek, N. Daulatzai, A. Stanislawek, and C. Hart, "T-tube duodenocholangiostomy for the management of duodenal fistulae," *World Journal of Surgery*, vol. 34, no. 4, pp. 791–796, 2010.

[3] N. M. A. Williams, N. A. Scott, and M. H. Irving, "Successful management of external duodenal fistula in a specialized unit," *American Journal of Surgery*, vol. 173, no. 3, pp. 240–241, 1997.

[4] Japanese Gastric Cancer Association, "Japanese classification of gastric carcinoma: 3rd English edition," *Gastric Cancer*, vol. 14, no. 2, pp. 101–112, 2011.

[5] I. González-Pinto and E. M. González, "Optimising the treatment of upper gastrointestinal fistulae," *Gut*, vol. 49, supplement 4, pp. iv21–iv28, 2001.

[6] T. Namikawa and K. Hanazaki, "Clinicopathological features of early gastric cancer with duodenal invasion," *World Journal of Gastroenterology*, vol. 15, no. 19, pp. 2309–2313, 2009.

[7] Y. Kakeji, D. Korenaga, H. Baba et al., "Surgical treatment of patients with gastric carcinoma and duodenal invasion," *Journal of Surgical Oncology*, vol. 59, no. 4, pp. 215–219, 1995.

[8] H. Merhav, H. Rothstein, D. Simon, and R. Pfeffermann, "Duodenostomy revisited," *International Surgery*, vol. 73, no. 4, pp. 254–256, 1988.

[9] J. M. Burch, C. L. Cox, D. V. Feliciano, R. J. Richardson, and R. R. Martin, "Management of the difficult duodenal stump," *American Journal of Surgery*, vol. 162, no. 6, pp. 522–526, 1991.

[10] K. S. Woodman, "Management of the difficult duodenal stump," *American Journal of Surgery*, vol. 167, no. 4, article 460, 1994.

[11] P. Paluszkiewicz, "Should the tube cholangiostomy be performed as a supplement procedure to duodenostomy for treatment or prevention of duodenal fistula?" *World Journal of Surgery*, vol. 32, no. 8, article 1905, 2008.

[12] B. Isik, S. Yilmaz, V. Kirimlioglu, G. Sogutlu, M. Yilmaz, and D. Katz, "A life-saving but inadequately discussed procedure: tube duodenostomy. Known and unknown aspects," *World Journal of Surgery*, vol. 31, no. 8, pp. 1616–1624, 2007.

[13] E. J. Zivic, "Duodenal stump blow-out in the Billroth II gastric resection," *Journal of the National Medical Association*, vol. 61, no. 1, pp. 17–19, 1969.

[14] Japanese Gastric Cancer Association, "Japanese gastric cancer treatment guidelines 2010 (ver. 3)," *Gastric Cancer*, vol. 14, no. 2, pp. 113–123, 2011.

A Case Report and Review of the Literature of Adult Gastric Duplication Cyst

Scott Samona and Richard Berri

General Surgery Department, St. John Hospital and Medical Center, Detroit, MI 48236, USA

Correspondence should be addressed to Scott Samona; ssamonamd@gmail.com

Academic Editor: Alexander R. Novotny

Gastrointestinal (GI) duplication cysts are a rare congenital disease. They may involve any level of the alimentary tract, but they most commonly involve the ileum, esophagus, and jejunum. Gastric duplication cysts represent approximately 4–8% of GI duplication cysts, the majority of which present in early childhood. We present a rare case of adult gastric duplication cyst in a 25-year-old female found to have abdominal mass on computed tomography imaging. There are several potential methods to diagnose gastric duplication cyst and treatment of choice is complete surgical resection.

1. Introduction

Gastrointestinal duplication cysts are a rare congenital disease. They tend to be hollow, spherical, or tubular structures, with well-developed smooth muscle coats, lined by mucosal epithelium. These structures tend to develop prior to complete differentiation of gastrointestinal epithelium and as such are often named after their organ of association [1, 2]. The most common gastrointestinal duplication cysts are those that involve the ileum, esophagus, and jejunum [3, 4]. Being highly uncommon, gastric duplication cysts represent approximately 4–8% of all gastrointestinal duplication cysts [5]. The majority of gastric duplication cysts present in early childhood with 67% identified within the first year of life [6]. We report an adult case of gastric duplication cyst in a 25-year-old female.

2. Case Presentation

The patient is a 25-year-old female, with no significant previous medical or surgical history, who presented to an outside facility after experiencing approximately one week of abdominal pain of acute onset. Pain was described as primarily mid-abdominal in origin with sharp quality but gradually became diffuse and colicky in nature. The patient also experienced associated nausea and bilious vomiting. There were no changes in bowel habits. Patient denied coffee ground emesis, hematemesis, melena, or hematochezia. She also denied any recent history of weight loss or weight gain. Differential diagnoses at this time included gallbladder disease, reflux esophagitis, gastritis, peptic ulcer disease, acute pancreatitis, and partial bowel obstruction. The patient underwent diagnostic evaluation by computed tomography (CT), which demonstrated a cystic-appearing lesion near the splenic flexure measuring 7.6 cm cranial-caudal × 4.1 cm transverse × 4.3 cm anterior-posterior (Figures 1 and 2). CT-guided fine needle aspiration was performed, of which pathology demonstrated mucinous fluid with mucus epithelium, concerning potential mucinous neoplasm of either gastrointestinal or gynecologic origin. The patient's CT scan demonstrated normal architecture of the colon, appendix, uterus, and ovaries; however additional diagnostic evaluation was performed. The patient underwent transvaginal ultrasonography of the uterus and ovaries, which was unremarkable. She also underwent total colonoscopy without any evidence of malignancy. CA 19-9, CA-125, and CEA levels were all found to be within normal limits.

The patient subsequently underwent diagnostic laparoscopy demonstrating evidence of dense adhesions within the left upper quadrant; however they appeared inflammatory versus malignant in nature. There was no evidence of carcinomatosis, ascites, or liver metastases. There was evidence

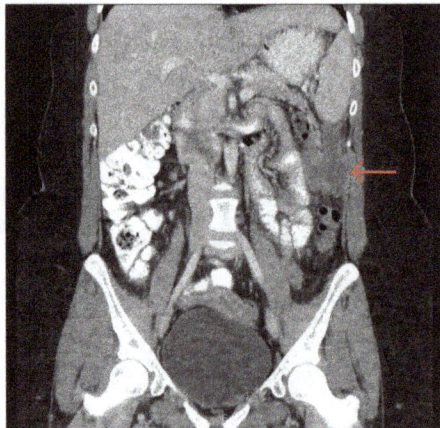

FIGURE 1

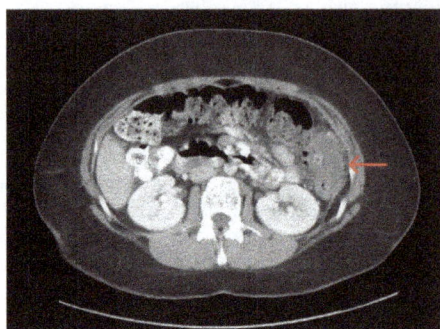

FIGURE 2

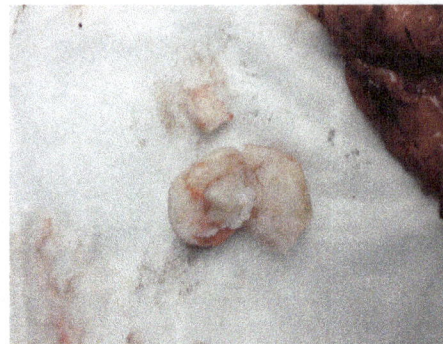

FIGURE 3

of a localized mass versus inflammatory reaction within the omentum in the left upper quadrant near the spleen and tail of the pancreas. Conversion to open exploratory laparotomy was performed and the patient underwent debulking of tumor with omentectomy and partial pancreatectomy. The gross specimen (Figure 3) with omental adhesions was closely examined. The specimen was evaluated under frozen section by our institution's pathology team; however no evidence of malignancy was identified by histologic examination. At this time the operation was completed and the specimen was sent to an outside facility for further analysis by expert gastrointestinal pathologist. Final pathology of the specimen demonstrated a $3.1 \times 2.7 \times 2.6$ cm cyst with mucinous epithelial lining (foveolar type) and prominent smooth muscle with evidence of inflammation. Further examination established diagnosis of gastric duplication cyst.

The patient was seen at one-month follow-up and had an uncomplicated postoperative course. She was found to be doing well with no complaints. Abdominal pain had completely resolved and she was able to tolerate a regular diet without nausea or vomiting. She continued to do well and was instructed to follow up in one year's time.

3. Discussion

Duplication cysts of the gastrointestinal tract are relatively rare phenomena with the majority occurring in the ileum

[3, 4] and rarely involving the stomach [5]. Established criteria for diagnosis of gastric duplication cyst include the wall of the cyst being contiguous with the stomach wall, the presence of smooth muscle surrounding the cyst and in continuation with the gastric musculature, and lining of the cyst wall by epithelial, gastric, or gut mucosa of any type [1, 2, 6, 7]. These lesions are thought to be congenital in nature and develop prior to complete differentiation of the gastrointestinal epithelium. As such they are named after the organ of association [1, 2, 8].

Because of the potential for neoplastic transformation, it is recommended that duplication cysts be surgically excised when found [9]. These malformations have been associated with development of carcinoma and adenomyoma [6]. As most of these lesions remain asymptomatic until becoming large enough to cause compressive symptoms, most present after significant associated inflammatory reaction has taken place. Although preoperative diagnosis may be difficult, various diagnostic techniques may be utilized. CT imaging as well as endoscopic ultrasound may be of use for establishing location, size, and local tissue involvement. Specific radiographic features may aid in diagnosis. Gastric duplication cysts typically appear as cystic lesions with thick walls and often exhibit contrast enhancement of the inner lining on CT examination. These lesions may also demonstrate calcifications; however this may mimic pancreatic cystic tumors if in close proximity to the pancreas [10]. Endoscopic ultrasound may also provide some aid in diagnosis. Features of gastric duplication cysts include cystic lesion with hypoechoic muscle layer and echogenic internal mucosal layer [2, 10]. Additional radiographic techniques, such as magnetic resonance imaging, may also be of use in select patients.

In conclusion, although rare, gastrointestinal duplication cysts are unique entities that are often detected after significant growth with development of compressive symptoms. They are often diagnosed postoperatively by careful pathologic examination, and treatment of choice is complete surgical resection.

References

[1] K. Kuraoka, H. Nakayama, T. Kagawa, T. Ichikawa, and W. Yasui, "Adenocarcinoma arising from a gastric duplication cyst with invasion to the stomach: a case report with literature review," *Journal of Clinical Pathology*, vol. 57, no. 4, pp. 428–431, 2004.

[2] J. P. Singh, H. Rajdeo, K. Bhuta, and J. A. Savino, "Gastric duplication cyst: two case reports and review of the literature," *Case Reports in Surgery*, vol. 2013, Article ID 605059, 4 pages, 2013.

[3] J. Falleti, E. Vigliar, P. Zeppa, P. Schettino, V. Napolitano, and M. D'Armiento, "Gastric duplication cyst: a rare congenital disease often misdiagnosed in adults," *Case Reports in Gastrointestinal Medicine*, vol. 2013, Article ID 850967, 3 pages, 2013.

[4] M. Scatizzi, M. Calistri, F. Feroci et al., "Gastric duplication cyst in an adult: case report," *In Vivo*, vol. 19, no. 6, pp. 975–978, 2005.

[5] S. S. Ríos, J. L. Noia, I. A. Nallib et al., "Adult gastric duplication cyst: diagnosis by endoscopic ultrasound-guided fine-needle aspiration (EUS-FNA)," *Revista Espanola de Enfermedades Digestivas*, vol. 100, no. 9, pp. 586–590, 2008.

[6] J. Johnston, G. H. Wheatley III, H. F. El Sayed, W. B. Marsh, E. C. Ellison, and M. Bloomston, "Gastric duplication cysts expressing carcinoembryonic antigen mimicking cystic pancreatic neoplasms in two adults," *The American Surgeon*, vol. 74, no. 1, pp. 91–94, 2008.

[7] G. Horne, C. Ming-Lum, A. W. Kirkpatrick, and R. L. Parker, "High-grade neuroendocrine carcinoma arising in a gastric duplication cyst: a case report with literature review," *International Journal of Surgical Pathology*, vol. 15, no. 2, pp. 187–191, 2007.

[8] K. Mardi, V. Kaushal, and S. Gupta, "Foregut duplication cysts of stomach masquerading as leiomyoma," *Indian Journal of Pathology and Microbiology*, vol. 53, no. 1, pp. 160–161, 2010.

[9] X. B. D'Journo, V. Moutardier, O. Turrini et al., "Gastric duplication in an adult mimicking mucinous cystadenoma of the pancreas," *The Journal of Clinical Pathology*, vol. 57, no. 11, pp. 1215–1218, 2004.

[10] H. Maeda, T. Okabayashi, I. Nishimori et al., "Diagnostic challenge to distinguish gastric duplication cyst from pancreatic cystic lesions in adult," *Internal Medicine*, vol. 46, no. 14, pp. 1101–1104, 2007.

Small Bowel Perforation as a Postoperative Complication from a Laminectomy

Robert H. Krieger,[1] Katherine M. Wojcicki,[1] Andrew C. Berry,[2]
Warren L. Reuther III,[3] and Kendrick D. McArthur[4]

[1]Kansas City University of Medicine and Biosciences (KCU), 1750 E. Independence Avenue, Kansas City, MO 64106, USA
[2]Department of Internal Medicine, University of South Alabama, Mobile, AL 36608, USA
[3]Department of Radiology, West Palm Hospital, West Palm Beach, FL 33407, USA
[4]Department of Surgery, West Palm Hospital, West Palm Beach, FL 33407, USA

Correspondence should be addressed to Robert H. Krieger; rkrieger@kcumb.edu

Academic Editor: Yoshiharu Kawaguchi

Chronic low back pain is one of the leading chief complaints affecting adults in the United States. As a result, this increases the percentage of patients that will eventually undergo surgical intervention to alleviate debilitating, chronic symptoms. A 37-year-old woman presented ten hours postoperatively after a lumbar laminectomy with an acute abdomen due to the extraordinarily rare complication of small bowel injury secondary to deep surgical penetration.

1. Introduction

In the United States, back pain remains the second most common reason why patients visit a clinician and up to 84 percent of adults will eventually endure low back pain [1, 2]. Approximately 250,000–500,000 people in the United States have symptoms of spinal stenosis, and although many patients remain asymptomatic to mildly symptomatic, the prevalence of symptomatic back pain is significant enough to warrant neurosurgical intervention and case volume will remain steady [3]. Cohort studies of individuals with lumbar spinal stenosis (LSS) demonstrated that 30 percent of the patients subsequently requested surgical treatment after initially choosing nonsurgical, medical management [4, 5]. As one would expect, surgery to the vertebral column is not without risk and although ventral perforation is rare, injury to the retroperitoneal vessels is the most common, serious, complication in this scenario [6]. However, this case illustrates one of the rare instances where the small bowel was injured during a lumbar laminectomy and highlights the importance of recognizing the acute abdomen as a potentially lethal complication of a laminectomy or discectomy. Furthermore,

a review of the literature revealed that this uncommon complication is more likely during a discectomy when compared to a laminectomy, which makes our reported case an exceptionally rare report [7].

2. Case Report

A 37-year-old female, postlaminectomy status for the treatment of lumbar back pain, presented with unrelenting abdominal pain 10 hours after the procedure. The patient denied any nausea, vomiting, diarrhea, fevers, or chills at that time, but due to the acute nature of the pain it was evident to her that she had either developed some type of postoperative complication or was experiencing a nascent abdominal pathology that would require immediate medical attention. The patient's past medical history was significant for chronic back pain and lumbar disc disease, with no significant surgical history prior to the laminectomy. Vital signs upon admission and consultation were stable and the patient was afebrile. Physical exam revealed a well-nourished, well-developed female that was alert and oriented albeit in obvious discomfort. The patient's physical exam was unremarkable except

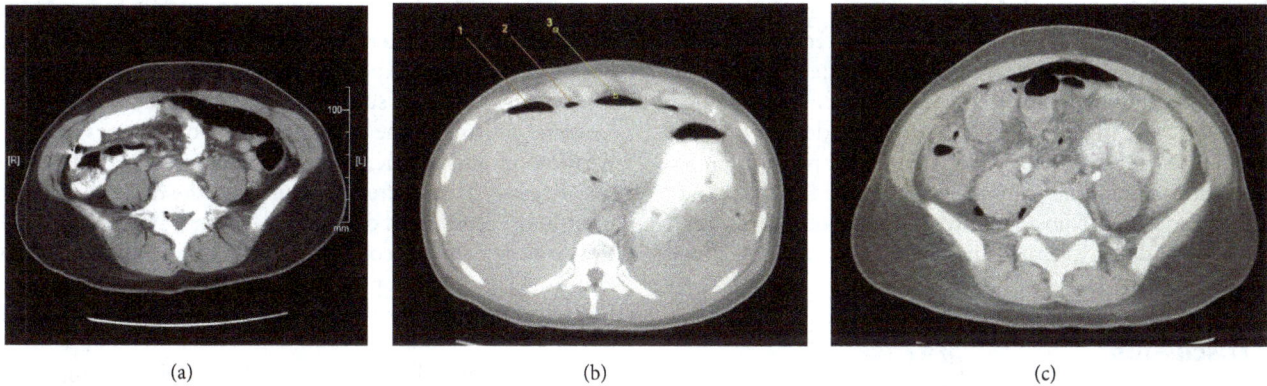

FIGURE 1: Computed tomography (CT) of the abdomen/pelvis demonstrates the progression of intra-abdominal injury and free air accumulation. (a) Transaxial view highlighting the accumulation of air in the spinal canal, psoas muscles, and the retroperitoneum, secondary to deep penetration and injury of the small bowel during the laminectomy. (b) This axial view demonstrates three distinct locations (labeled 1, 2, and 3) of intra-abdominal free air found on a follow-up CT of the abdomen/pelvis. (c) Axial view depicting extraluminal air anterior to the bowel, as well as air within the mesentery and posterior to the right psoas muscle.

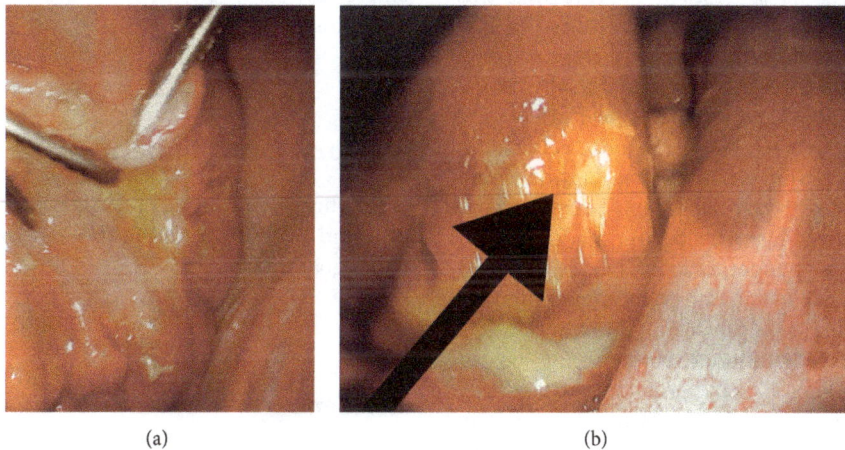

FIGURE 2: Laparoscopic views of the inflamed and perforated small bowel photographed prior to the conversion to laparotomy. (a) The photograph demonstrates a highly erythematous, inflamed segment of small bowel with fibrinous exudation and inflammation adjacent to the instrument. (b) The arrow pointing to the site of perforation located at the approximate jejunal-ileal junction.

that her abdomen was exquisitely tender to palpation without any distension and there was significant tympany upon percussion. The electrolyte profile was essentially normal, but total bilirubin was elevated at 2.1 mg/dL. Urine pregnancy test was negative and the complete blood count showed an elevated white blood cell count of $15.4 \times 10^3/\mu L$, with a hemoglobin and hematocrit of 12 g/dL and 34%, respectively.

Computed tomography (CT) of the abdomen and pelvis showed evidence of retroperitoneal air, which seemingly tracked back into the spinal canal (Figure 1(a)). In addition, there was free air seen intraperitoneally without an obvious source or evidence of an inflammatory process in her abdomen at that time (Figure 1(b)). It was suspected that the retroperitoneal air may be secondary to deep surgical penetration into the small bowel during the laminectomy and the patient was initially treated expectantly with intravenous antibiotics and observation. On hospital course days two and three the patient began to spike and maintain fevers, with air

continuing to appear in the psoas muscles and significant air within the peritoneal cavity. The follow-up CT showed that the patient had developed ascites suggesting a small bowel perforation until proven otherwise (Figure 1(c)). The patient was taken to the operating room for emergent laparoscopic exploration.

After dissecting through the subcutaneous tissue and the anterior rectus fascia in a standard fashion, the Hassan trocar was inserted and a laparoscopic view of the abdomen was undertaken. There was a marked amount of seropurulent fluid extending from the right and left colic gutters down to the Pouch of Douglas. The appendix was visualized and appeared normal; however, while running the small bowel, beginning at the terminal ileum, a significant amount of inflammatory and fibrinous exudate was discovered (Figure 2(a)). Upon approaching the proximal ileum and jejunum, an area of perforation was identified as evidenced by where the omentum had adhered to the small bowel

(Figure 2(b)). With very light manipulation, enteric contents exuded from the small bowel and the procedure was converted to an open exploratory laparotomy. After repairing the enterotomy with interrupted Vicryl sutures and reinforcing it with silk suture in a Lembert fashion, the abdomen was irrigated copiously. Other than the jejunal-ileal perforation, no other intra-abdominal pathologies were noted during exploration. The patient's postoperative hospital course was unremarkable and she tolerated the small bowel repair without complication.

3. Discussion

When considering the supportive anatomy of the vertebral column, specifically the annulus fibrosus and the anterior longitudinal ligament, it is not inconceivable that ventral perforation is a rather rare complication of laminectomy. In a study of 30,000 lumbar discectomies, there was a reported ventral perforation rate of 0.016% [8] and when reviewing another study of documented cases it appears that this would be even less common during a laminectomy [7]. This seems logical that laminectomies would be a rarer cause of anterior perforation as the lamina is located dorsally on the vertebral body and the bowel and retroperitoneal vasculature lies anterior to the vertebral body. The most acute, life-threatening complication from an anterior perforation would be due to an intraoperative vascular injury, which may be evident by brisk bleeding, hypotension, or shock. In fact, hemorrhage of the large retroperitoneal vessels is the most common complication due to anterior perforation of the vertebral column [9–11]. Due to the pressure in the common iliac arteries, the most commonly injured vessels during lumbar laminectomy or discectomy, an acute vascular injury is likely to be quickly recognized by the surgical team. However, in the few reported cases of small bowel injury, the patients will typically begin experiencing severe abdominal pain by the second postoperative day, which was consistent with our patient's hospital course [12]. Therefore, it is imperative to have a high index of suspicion for bowel perforation when a postoperative laminectomy or discectomy patient develops peritoneal signs.

The incidence of intestinal injury following lumbar discectomy was reported, in a large-scale study with 68,329 patients, to be 0.0015% by the German Society of Neurological Surgery [8]. Thorough literature search identified this as the 16th reported case of small bowel injury occurring after a discectomy or laminectomy, dating back to the first reported case by Harbison in 1954 [7, 13, 14]. Of all of the cases discovered in the review of the literature, we believe that this is the 2nd reported case of small bowel injury after a laminectomy [7]. The most likely mechanism by which the small bowel may be penetrated is due to the root of the mesentery arising from the anterior vertebral column at approximately L2, traveling obliquely and terminating at the right sacroiliac joint. When the patient is prone during the operation, segments of the small bowel may appear anterior to the lumbar vertebral column [6]. This mechanism, along with deep surgical penetration during laminectomy, is precisely the means by which our patient had her jejunal-ileal junction perforated.

A delay in diagnosis is associated with high morbidity and mortality rate after bowel injury, especially with small bowel perforation. Exploratory laparoscopy or laparotomy followed by repair via suture or resection and anastomosis is essential [13, 15]. In one of the earlier reported cases of bowel perforation during microscopic discectomy, the patient was not diagnosed until after 48 hours and the delay resulted in peritonitis, sepsis, and death of the patient [16]. In our case, the surgical team was consulted within one postoperative day and the patient was rapidly diagnosed which prevented her from developing septic shock and a potentially fatal outcome.

Neurosurgical intervention in the vertebral column will remain common as long as chronic low back pain is a leading chief complaint in the United States. While it is not a typical complication, perforation of the viscus is associated with a high mortality rate; therefore, the surgeon must maintain a high index of suspicion when a patient presents with an acute abdomen after lumbar spinal surgery and be prepared to emergently surgically diagnose and correct the injury in the operating room.

Authors' Contribution

All authors contributed to evaluating and/or managing the case and to writing/editing the paper. R. H. Krieger is the paper guarantor.

References

[1] R. A. Deyo and Y. J. Tsui-Wu, "Descriptive epidemiology of low-back pain and its related medical care in the United States," *Spine*, vol. 12, no. 3, pp. 264–268, 1987.

[2] J. D. Cassidy, L. J. Carroll, and P. Côté, "The Saskatchewan health and back pain survey: the prevalence of low back pain and related disability in Saskatchewan adults," *Spine*, vol. 23, no. 17, pp. 1860–1866, 1998.

[3] L. Kalichman, R. Cole, D. H. Kim et al., "Spinal stenosis prevalence and association with symptoms: the Framingham Study," *Spine Journal*, vol. 9, no. 7, pp. 545–550, 2009.

[4] T. Amundsen, H. Weber, H. J. Nordal, B. Magnaes, M. Abdelnoor, and F. Lilleås, "Lumbar spinal stenosis: conservative or surgical management? A prospective 10-year study," *Spine*, vol. 25, no. 11, pp. 1424–1436, 2000.

[5] Y. Chang, D. E. Singer, Y. A. Wu, R. B. Keller, and S. J. Atlas, "The effect of surgical and nonsurgical treatment on longitudinal outcomes of lumbar spinal stenosis over 10 years," *Journal of the American Geriatrics Society*, vol. 53, no. 5, pp. 785–792, 2005.

[6] P. Hoff-Olsen and J. Wiberg, "Small bowel perforation as a complication of microsurgical lumbar diskectomy: a case report and brief review of the literature," *The American Journal of Forensic Medicine & Pathology*, vol. 22, no. 3, pp. 319–321, 2001.

[7] M. J. Cases-Baldó, V. Soria-Aledo, J. A. Miguel-Perello, J. L. Aguayo-Albasini, and M. R. Hernández, "Unnoticed small bowel perforation as a complication of lumbar discectomy," *Spine Journal*, vol. 11, no. 1, pp. e5–e8, 2011.

[8] L. F. Ramirez, R. Thisted, G. W. Sypert, and N. Horwitz, "Complications and demographic characteristics of patients undergoing lumbar discectomy in community hospitals," *Neurosurgery*, vol. 25, no. 2, pp. 226–231, 1989.

[9] R. Goodkin and L. L. Laska, "Vascular and visceral injuries associated with lumbar disc surgery: medicolegal implications," *Surgical Neurology*, vol. 49, no. 4, pp. 358–372, 1998.

[10] Y.-D. Tsai, P.-C. Yu, T.-C. Lee, H.-S. Chen, S.-H. Wang, and Y.-L. Kuo, "Superior rectal artery injury following lumbar disc surgery," *Journal of Neurosurgery*, vol. 95, no. 1, pp. 108–110, 2001.

[11] S. Papadoulas, D. Konstantinou, H. P. Kourea, N. Kritikos, N. Haftouras, and J. A. Tsolakis, "Vascular injury complicating lumbar disc surgery. A systematic review," *European Journal of Vascular and Endovascular Surgery*, vol. 24, no. 3, pp. 189–195, 2002.

[12] J. K. Houten, A. K. Frempong-Boadu, and M. S. Arkovitz, "Bowel injury as a complication of microdiscectomy: case report and literature review," *Journal of Spinal Disorders and Techniques*, vol. 17, no. 3, pp. 248–250, 2004.

[13] D.-S. Kim, J.-K. Lee, K.-S. Moon, J.-K. Ju, and S.-H. Kim, "Small bowel injury as a complication of lumbar microdiscectomy: case report and literature review," *Journal of Korean Neurosurgical Society*, vol. 47, no. 3, pp. 224–227, 2010.

[14] S. P. Harbison, "Major vascular complications of intervertebral disc surgery," *Annals of Surgery*, vol. 140, no. 3, pp. 342–348, 1954.

[15] J. M. Dixon, A. B. Lumsden, and J. Piris, "Small bowel perforation," *The Journal of the Royal College of Surgeons of Edinburgh*, vol. 30, no. 1, pp. 43–46, 1985.

[16] I. W. Birkeland Jr. and T. K. F. Taylor, "Bowel injuries coincident to lumbar disk surgery: a report of four cases and a review of the literature," *Journal of Trauma*, vol. 10, no. 2, pp. 163–168, 1970.

An Option of Conservative Management of a Duodenal Injury Following Laparoscopic Cholecystectomy

MA Modi, SS Deolekar, and AK Gvalani

Department of General Surgery, King Edward Memorial Hospital and Seth Gordhandas Sunderdas Medical College, Parel, Mumbai 400012, India

Correspondence should be addressed to MA Modi; malavm25@gmail.com

Academic Editor: Boris Kirshtein

Duodenal injury following laparoscopic cholecystectomy is rare complications with catastrophic sequelae. Most injuries are attributed to thermal burns with electrocautery following adhesiolysis and have a delayed presentation requiring surgical intervention. We present a case of a 47-year-old gentleman operated on for laparoscopic cholecystectomy with a bilious drain postoperatively; for which an ERC was done showing choledocholithiasis with cystic duct stump blow-out and a drain in the duodenum suggestive of an iatrogenic duodenal injury. He was managed conservatively like a duodenal fistula and recovered without undergoing any intervention.

1. Introduction

Bowel injuries are an uncommon complication after laparoscopic cholecystectomy but are an extremely serious complication when they do occur. Although the reported incidence rate of bowel injury is between 0.05% and 0.14% [1, 2], a large number of cases do not get reported. Most of these cases are due to injury caused while thermal injury and insertion of trocar and rarely due to dissection or adhesiolysis [3]. Most of these duodenal injuries are managed surgically, either laparoscopic or laparotomy. We present a case of an iatrogenic duodenal injury postlaparoscopic cholecystectomy managed conservatively.

2. Case Presentation

A 47-year-old gentleman had a 10-day history of painful obstructive jaundice. Ultrasonography revealed chronic cholecystitis with choledocholithiasis. EUS revealed a slightly dilated common bile duct (CBD) 9 mm with multiple stones impacted just above the ampulla in the lower CBD with multiple gall stones. ERC with sphincterotomy, stone extraction, and stent placement was done; complete clearance was achieved. A month later, he underwent laparoscopic cholecystectomy at a community hospital; intraoperatively he had dense omental adhesions around Calot's triangle which were separated and the wide cystic duct was identified and clipped. In view of bleeding, while adhesiolysis a drain was placed postoperatively. On the second postoperative day, the drain was bilious in nature and was referred to our centre for further management. On arrival he was vitally stable with minimal epigastric tenderness and had a bilious drain. A CT scan done revealed a drain in the second part of the duodenum (Figure 1). We sent the patient for ERC in view of suspected duodenal and biliary injury (Figure 2). Duodenoscopy revealed the tip of the drain at the junction of D1-D2, previous stent was removed, and cholangiogram revealed mid-CBD calculi with cystic duct stump blow-out (Figure 3). Stone extraction was done and another stent was placed. The patient did not show any signs of sepsis; hence we managed him conservatively with the drain behaving like a tube duodenostomy with a daily output of around 200 mL. He was started on orals which he tolerated well. A conray gram done after 3 weeks, through the drain, showed no intraperitoneal leak and free flow of contrast into the duodenum (Figure 4). The drain was clamped and removed and this was followed by CBD stent removal (Figure 5). On 6-month follow-up, he is doing well.

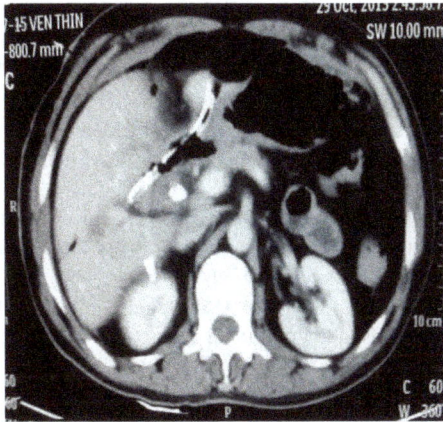

FIGURE 1: CT scan showing the drain in the 2nd part of duodenum.

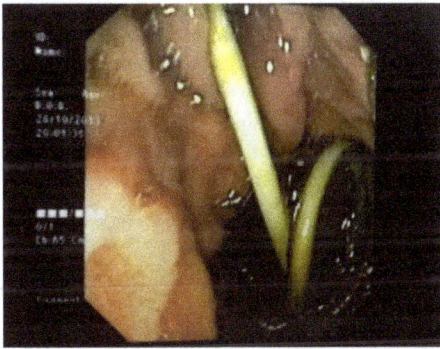

FIGURE 2: Postoperative ERCP showing a coiled drain in the duodenum.

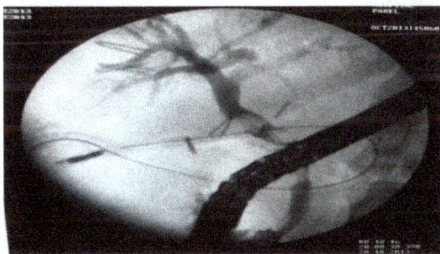

FIGURE 3: Postoperative ERCP showing a mid-CBD calculi and cystic duct stump blow-out. A drain (ryles tube) is seen in the region of duodenum.

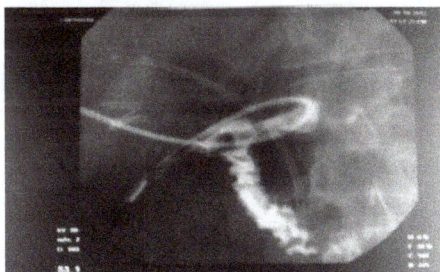

FIGURE 4: Tube conray gram showing the dye filling up in the duodenum without evidence of any intraperitoneal leak.

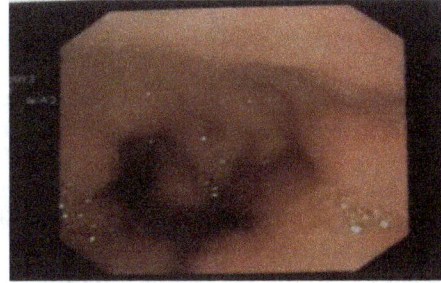

FIGURE 5: Duodenum at stent removal after removal of drain.

3. Discussion

Duodenal injuries are infrequent complications of laparoscopic cholecystectomy mostly seen due to dense adhesions. Acute and chronic inflammation of gallbladder causes dense adhesions around Calot's triangle and duodenal wall, thus rendering laparoscopic dissection more difficult and sometimes unsafe. In these cases, injury to duodenum may be difficult to appreciate, especially in patients in whom the apex of the duodenal bulb is tented up in front of the neck of the gallbladder [4, 5]. The reason for duodenal injury could be ascribed to the use of cautery during dissection. Thermal bowel injuries usually are not seen at the time of laparoscopic procedures and are diagnosed much later, when transmural necrosis progresses to perforation [2, 4, 6, 7]. The time of injury to onset of symptoms can vary from 18 hours to 14 days [7]. Only in 2 published cases of duodenal perforation due to electrocautery burns during LC injury was observed during surgery [6, 8]. In the other cases, focal thermal injury was unrecognized during the procedure and was presented much later until perforation of duodenal wall developed (1st to 16th postoperative day) [9–13]. Drains eroding into bowel are very well known. Trocar insertion is an early cause of duodenal injuries especially in an inflammatory condition. We do not know the exact reason for the duodenal perforation. Trocar related injury, thermal injury, and drain fistulising into the duodenum are possible hypothesis, the latter two theoretically being less likely on postoperative day two.

The late recognition of these injuries in patients leads to peritonitis and sepsis which contributes to the relatively high associated mortality. Deziel et al. [2] reported an 8.3% mortality rate among 12 patients with duodenal injuries in their analysis of 77,604 cases. El-Banna et al. [6] noted that three of four duodenal thermal injuries complicating laparoscopic cholecystectomy were fatal. Huang et al. [1] reported that 4 out of 19 (21.05%) patients with duodenal injury expired in their study of 39,238 LC cases.

Despite reports of the successful laparoscopic repair of duodenal perforation [14] during laparoscopic cholecystectomy discovered during surgery [8] or diagnosed after surgery [15], most authorities managed this dangerous complication by immediate laparotomy to assess the abdomen and secure a safe repair [2, 6, 9, 16–18].

The site of duodenal injury is important in the surgical management and prognosis. Injuries to duodenal bulb or superior flexure (as in our case) have a better prognosis than descending duodenal injuries around the ampulla of Vater which invariably require complex surgical management and have a high mortality rate [19].

Duodenal injury is a rare but a dangerous complication of laparoscopic cholecystectomy and is associated with a high mortality. In most cases, these injuries are attributed to careless adhesiolysis with electrocautery, remain unrecognized during the procedure, and present later as peritonitis. The authors advocate placement of a drain in all patients with dense adhesions and suspicion of injury in cases of difficult laparoscopic cholecystectomy. At the end of the procedure an accurate control of the abdomen is absolutely necessary.

In conclusion, the authors wish to stress that the general practise for duodenal injuries should be to repair either laparoscopically or surgically and nonoperative management of duodenal injury in selective patients with controlled drainage.

Authors' Contribution

MA Modi, SS Deolekar, and AK Gvalani participated in writing the paper and revising the draft. MA Modi took the photos. All authors read and approved the final paper.

Acknowledgment

The authors would like to thank the patient for his written consent and permission to present this paper.

References

[1] X. Huang, Y. Feng, and Z. Huang, "Complications of laparoscopic cholecystectomy in China: an analysis of 39 238 cases," *Chinese Medical Journal*, vol. 110, no. 9, pp. 704–706, 1997.

[2] D. J. Deziel, K. W. Millikan, S. G. Economou, A. Doolas, S.-T. Ko, and M. C. Airan, "Complications of laparoscopic cholecystectomy: a national survey of 4,292 hospitals and an analysis of 77,604 cases," *The American Journal of Surgery*, vol. 165, no. 1, pp. 9–14, 1993.

[3] A. Shamiyeh and W. Wayand, "Laparoscopic cholecystectomy: early and late complications and their treatment," *Langenbeck's Archives of Surgery*, vol. 389, no. 3, pp. 164–171, 2004.

[4] C. C. Nduka, P. A. Super, J. R. T. Manson, and A. W. Darzi, "Cause and prevention of electrosurgical injuries in laparoscopy," *Journal of the American College of Surgeons*, vol. 179, no. 2, pp. 161–170, 1994.

[5] C.-M. Lo, C.-L. Liu, S.-T. Fan, E. C. S. Lai, and J. Wong, "Prospective randomized study of early versus delayed laparoscopic cholecystectomy for acute cholecystitis," *Annals of Surgery*, vol. 227, no. 4, pp. 461–467, 1998.

[6] M. El-Banna, M. Abdel-Atty, M. El-Meteini, and S. Aly, "Management of laparoscopic-related bowel injuries," *Surgical Endoscopy*, vol. 14, no. 9, pp. 779–782, 2000.

[7] F. D. Loffer and D. Pent, "Indications, contraindications and complications of laparoscopy," *Obstetrical and Gynecological Survey*, vol. 30, no. 7, pp. 407–427, 1975.

[8] C.-K. Kum, E. Eypasch, A. Aljaziri, and H. Troidl, "Randomized comparison of pulmonary function after the "French" and "American" techniques of laparoscopic cholecystectomy," *British Journal of Surgery*, vol. 83, no. 7, pp. 938–941, 1996.

[9] A. M. Ress, M. G. Sarr, D. M. Nagorney, M. B. Farnell, J. H. Donohue, and D. C. McIlrath, "Spectrum and management of major complications of laparoscopic cholecystectomy," *American Journal of Surgery*, vol. 165, no. 6, pp. 655–662, 1993.

[10] X. R. Chen, D. Lou, S. H. Li et al., "Avoiding serious complications in laparoscopic cholecystectomy—lessons learned from an experience of 2428 cases," *Annals of the Academy of Medicine Singapore*, vol. 25, no. 5, pp. 635–639, 1996.

[11] D. Hebebrand, R. Menningen, H. Sommer, S. P. Roehr, and H. Troidl, "Small-bowel necrosis following laparoscopic cholecystectomy: a clinically relevant complication?" *Endoscopy*, vol. 27, no. 3, p. 281, 1995.

[12] Z. Cala, D. Velnic, B. Cvitanovic et al., "Laparoscopic cholecystectomy: results after 1,000 procedures," *Acta Medica Croatica*, vol. 50, pp. 147–149, 1996.

[13] S. Baev, T. Pozarliev, and G. T. Todorov, "Laparoscopic cholecystectomy: 700 consecutive cases," *International Surgery*, vol. 80, no. 4, pp. 296–298, 1995.

[14] A.-H. Kwon, H. Inui, and Y. Kamiyama, "Laparoscopic management of bile duct and bowel injury during laparoscopic cholecystectomy," *World Journal of Surgery*, vol. 25, no. 7, pp. 856–861, 2001.

[15] A. M. Taylor and M. K. W. Li, "Laparoscopic management of complications following laparoscopic cholecystectomy," *Australian and New Zealand Journal of Surgery*, vol. 64, no. 12, pp. 827–829, 1994.

[16] C. G. Eden and T. G. Williams, "Duodenal perforation after laparoscopic cholecystectomy," *Endoscopy*, vol. 24, no. 9, pp. 790–792, 1992.

[17] Y. Yamashita, T. Kurohiji, T. Kakegawa, and T. L. Dent, "Evaluation of two training programs for laparoscopic cholecystectomy: Incidence of major complications," *World Journal of Surgery*, vol. 18, no. 2, pp. 279–285, 1994.

[18] S. M. Berry, K. J. Ose, R. H. Bell, and A. S. Fink, "Thermal injury of the posterior duodenum during laparoscopic cholecystectomy," *Surgical Endoscopy*, vol. 8, no. 3, pp. 197–200, 1994.

[19] M. Testini, G. Piccinni, G. Lissidini et al., "Management of descending duodenal injuries secondary to laparoscopic cholecystectomy," *Digestive Surgery*, vol. 25, no. 1, pp. 12–15, 2008.

Simultaneous Gastric and Duodenal Erosions due to Adjustable Gastric Banding for Morbid Obesity

Dimitrios K. Manatakis, Ioannis Terzis, Ioannis D. Kyriazanos, Ioannis D. Dontas, Christos N. Stoidis, Nikolaos Stamos, and Demetrios Davides

1st Surgical Department, Athens Naval and Veterans Hospital, 70 Deinokratous Street, 11521 Athens, Greece

Correspondence should be addressed to Dimitrios K. Manatakis; dmanatak@yahoo.gr

Academic Editor: Boris Kirshtein

Erosion is an uncommon but feared late complication of adjustable gastric banding for morbid obesity. A high index of clinical suspicion is required, since symptoms are usually vague and nonspecific. Diagnosis is confirmed on upper gastrointestinal endoscopy and band removal is the mainstay of treatment, with band revision or conversion to other bariatric modalities at a later stage. Duodenal erosion is a much rarer complication, caused by the connection tubing of the band. We present our experience with a case of simultaneous gastric and duodenal erosions, managed by laparoscopic explantation of the band, primary suture repair of the duodenum, and omentopexy.

1. Introduction

Laparoscopic adjustable gastric banding (LAGB) is a well-established restrictive procedure, still popular among many bariatric surgeons, because of its adjustability, reversibility, and preservation of gastrointestinal tract continuity [1–4]. While perioperative complications are minimal, compared to other bariatric modalities, it has a relatively high reoperation rate. Recent reviews, studying long-term results and complications, reveal a failure rate between 10 and 20% in the short run and 40% in the long run and an incidence of 12–48% of device-related complications [3]. These include early (band obstruction, gastric perforation, wound infection, and bleeding) and late (band slippage, pouch enlargement, port/tubing complications, and gastric erosion) complications, leading generally to unacceptable weight loss rates and requiring revision or conversion to other modalities [3].

With a reported incidence of 1–3%, gastric erosion is a relatively rare but potentially life-threatening complication [3–5]. We present our experience with a case of simultaneous gastric and duodenal erosions, caused by the band and the connection tubing, respectively.

2. Case Presentation

A 34-year-old female Caucasian patient presented at the emergency department with a 5-day history of protracted vomiting and epigastric pain. She had undergone LAGB (Bioring, Cousin Biotech, France) for morbid obesity 4 years before (height: 165 cm, weight: 100 kg, BMI: 36.7, and comorbidities: arterial hypertension, dyslipidemia, and low back pain) resulting in a weight loss of 30 kg (85% EBWL). The original band had been replaced laparoscopically 3 years after initial surgery, due to connection tubing failure.

Clinical examination revealed tachycardia, mild tenderness over the epigastrium, and signs of dehydration. Laboratory tests and plain abdominal radiographs were within normal range. Abdominal ultrasonography and CT scans were inconclusive; however the band was visible on upper GI endoscopy (Figure 1), protruding partially into the gastric lumen (stage 2 according to Nocca classification, >50% of the band free in the gastric lumen [6]). Endoscopy of the duodenum revealed concurrent erosion of the first part by the connection tubing (Figure 2).

The patient consented to surgical treatment and removal of the band. On laparoscopy, adhesions were taken down

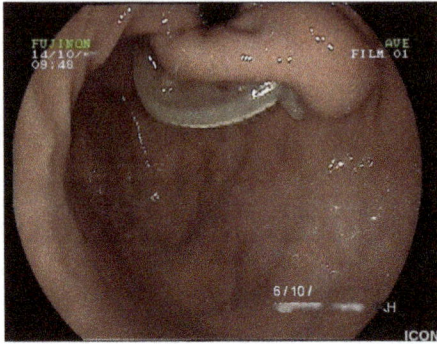

FIGURE 1: Retroflexed inspection of the gastric fundus and gastric erosion by the band.

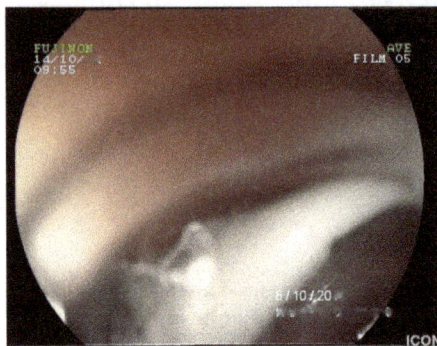

FIGURE 2: Duodenal erosion by the connection tubing.

and the band was dissected free, cut near the buckle, and extracted. The duodenal erosion, about 1 cm in length, was repaired primarily by interrupted, absorbable polyglactin (Vicryl, Ethicon, Somerville, NJ, USA) 2/0 sutures, while a vascularized omental pedicle was fashioned and inserted into the gastric tunnel, to close the gastric defect. A vacuum-assisted drain was placed alongside the gastric repair and a Penrose drain at the duodenal repair. The band was sent for culture, which grew a multiresistant strain of *Klebsiella pneumoniae* and a sensitive strain of *Pseudomonas aeruginosa*.

Postoperatively the nasogastric tube was removed on the 4th day, and the patient was started on clear fluids, after gastrografin swallow test showed no leakage. On the 8th postoperative day she developed pneumonia, for which she received appropriate antibiotics. She was discharged on the 12th postoperative day. Gradually she regained weight (height: 165 cm, weight: 110 kgr, and BMI: 40.4) and two years later she underwent open Roux-en-Y gastric bypass.

3. Discussion

LAGB is generally considered a safe procedure, with less postoperative complications compared to other bariatric operations, which require more extensive dissections and anastomoses. Erosion is a relatively uncommon complication, where the band slowly erodes through the gastric wall and into the gastric lumen and becomes visible at endoscopy [5]. It is considered the most dangerous of all

LAGB complications, due to its potentially life-threatening character. While the stomach is the commonest site, erosion of neighboring structures by the connecting tubing has also been reported (transverse colon, jejunum, celiac axis, and renal hilum) [7–10]. Duodenal erosion by the connecting tubing has been recently described and is a much rarer complication [11].

Most authors report erosion rates of 1–3%; however incidence varies greatly between different centers (0,23%–32%) and may reflect not only level of surgical experience and volume of patients but also length and method of followup [4, 12]. The complication presents usually late in the postoperative course, with a median time of 12–24 months from banding to erosion but can even be seen more than 10 years postoperatively [12, 13]. Erosions in the early postoperative period are usually associated with undetected intraoperative gastric wall injury [14].

The pathophysiology of erosion is still not completely understood. Early erosions are thought to be the result of microinjury to the gastric serosa, band infection, or too tight band placement [1, 5, 15, 16]. Late erosions are secondary to chronic band pressure on the stomach and local ischemia of the gastric wall [1, 5, 15, 16].

A variety of risk factors have been implicated, but no single factor can cause erosion. Although it has not been definitely proven, newer band designs (high-volume, low-pressure systems) tend to be associated less frequently with gastric erosions than older designs (low-volume, high-pressure systems), due to improved geometry and more even distribution of pressure on the gastric wall [3, 13, 17]. The surgical technique has also evolved. The perigastric approach involved more dissection around the stomach and was prone to gastric wall injuries, which could lead to erosion over time. The pars flaccida technique requires less dissection and is associated with a significantly lower erosion incidence [3, 18]. Potential risk factors may also include overfilling of the band, tension by the gastrogastric sutures, excessive vomiting, NSAIDs and other ulcerogenic drugs, smoking, alcohol, and surgeon's level of experience [3, 5, 12, 13, 15, 16]. As far as duodenal erosions are concerned, both free-floating tubing tips and attached tubing have been shown to cause erosions [11]. One may speculate that length of excess tubing could be a predisposing factor, as tubing loops may exert chronic pressure on neighboring organs.

Most cases of LAGB erosion develop gradually over time and thus are nonurgent and non-life-threatening [13]. Therefore a high index of clinical suspicion is required especially in patients with ambiguous symptomatology [19]. Almost half of the patients with erosion remain asymptomatic [3, 4, 19, 20]. Symptomatic patients present with a variety of complaints, ranging from nonspecific epigastric pain, nausea, and vomiting, as in our case, to intraabdominal abscess and generalized peritonitis [12, 15]. Unexplained weight regain and loss of satiety could be early signs of loss of restriction, due to intragastric migration of the band. Late or recurrent portsite wound infections could also point towards gastric, colonic, or duodenal erosion, with cultures typically revealing gastrointestinal, and not skin, microbial flora [11, 15]. Intraabdominal catastrophes are rare and include septic complications (abscess, peritonitis) due to free perforation or massive upper gastrointestinal hemorrhage due to erosion of adjacent vessels [9, 21].

Clinical suspicion of band erosion mandates further diagnostic workup. Contrast medium swallow test may reveal gastrografin passing from the upper to the lower gastric pouch outside the band but is usually inconclusive [15]. Abdominal CT scans can only be suggestive of erosions, showing free air or localized abscess formation around the band [15]. The cornerstone of diagnosis is upper gastrointestinal endoscopy, with retroflexed inspection of the gastric fundus [5, 12, 13, 15]. Based on endoscopic findings, erosions are classified according to Nocca as stage 1, small part of the band visible through a hole in the gastric mucosa; stage 2, partial migration (>50% of the band free in the gastric lumen); and stage 3, complete intragastric migration [6].

Management of erosions is a matter of debate. Band removal is the sine qua non of treatment, yet there is no consensus regarding timing of removal and type of future intervention. Surgical explantation can be performed as laparotomy or laparoscopy [12]. Yoon et al. advocate a 4-step procedure for repair of the gastric wall, with primary suture repair to close the defect, omental plugging into the gastric tunnel, 2 drains, and nasogastric tube for decompression [15]. Endoscopy is the least invasive modality but requires specific instruments, skilled endoscopists, and total or near-total erosion (Nocca stage 3), while it carries a relatively high risk of esophageal tearing [12]. Only asymptomatic, well-informed patients can be regularly followed, on a wait-and-watch basis, until complete erosion, thus allowing for delayed endoscopic removal [6, 20].

The majority of duodenal perforations can be effectively managed by simple repair [22]. Disruption of the suture line however is a universally feared complication and is aggravated by high intraluminal pressures and the autodigestive action of bile and pancreatic enzymes [23]. Omentopexy has comparable results, especially in perforations up to 3 cm [23]. Simultaneous gastric and duodenal erosions may contribute to higher morbidity and leakage rates.

Prognosis of gastric erosions is usually good. Evidence on LAGB-related duodenal erosions however is limited. Gastric banding causes a 360-degree sheath of reactive tissue around the band [24]. We hypothesize that this fibrosclerotic tissue may act protectively against free perforation and leakage, whereas this may not occur with duodenal erosions, which involve only the anterior wall of the first part.

In the long run, band explantation leads almost inevitably to weight regain; therefore another bariatric intervention is warranted. Selection of patients depends on local factors and the efficacy of banding on weight control. Immediate band replacement in cases without serious infection has been described but leads generally to unacceptably high reerosion rates of up to 40% [13, 20]. In cases with technical LAGB problems but good weight control, a 2-stage revision procedure, with delayed rebanding at 4–6 months, is safe and efficient and should be among the surgeon's options [13, 25–27]. On the other hand, patients with poor weight loss or noncompliance are candidates for more radical solutions and conversion to different bariatric modalities (sleeve gastrectomy, Roux-en-Y gastric bypass, and biliopancreatic diversion) [26–30].

4. Conclusion

Gastric erosion is an uncommon but feared complication of adjustable gastric banding for morbid obesity. Symptoms are nonspecific and diagnosis is confirmed on upper gastrointestinal endoscopy. The mainstay of treatment is surgical or endoscopic band removal, with revision or conversion to other bariatric modalities at a later stage. Erosion of the connecting tubing into the duodenum is a much rarer complication, managed adequately by primary suture repair, omentopexy, and drainage.

References

[1] B. Kirshtein, L. Lantsberg, S. Mizrahi, and E. Avinoach, "Bariatric emergencies for non-bariatric surgeons: complications of laparoscopic gastric banding," *Obesity Surgery*, vol. 20, no. 11, pp. 1468–1478, 2010.

[2] C. Stroh, U. Hohmann, H. Schramm, F. Meyer, and T. Manger, "Fourteen-year long-term results after gastric banding," *Journal of Obesity*, vol. 2011, Article ID 128451, 6 pages, 2011.

[3] B. Snyder, T. Wilson, S. Mehta et al., "Past, present, and future: critical analysis of use of gastric bands in obese patients," *Diabetes, Metabolic Syndrome and Obesity: Targets and Therapy*, vol. 3, pp. 55–65, 2010.

[4] C. Owers and R. Ackroyd, "A study examining the complications associated with gastric banding," *Obesity Surgery*, vol. 23, no. 1, pp. 56–59, 2013.

[5] J. Chisholm, N. Kitan, J. Toouli, and L. Kow, "Gastric band erosion in 63 cases: endoscopic removal and rebanding evaluated," *Obesity Surgery*, vol. 21, no. 11, pp. 1676–1681, 2011.

[6] D. Nocca, V. Frering, B. Gallix et al., "Migration of adjustable gastric banding from a cohort study of 4,236 patients," *Surgical Endoscopy and Other Interventional Techniques*, vol. 19, no. 7, pp. 947–950, 2005.

[7] L. B. K. Tan, J. B. Y. So, and A. Shabbir, "Connection tubing causing small bowel obstruction and colonic erosion as a rare complication after laparoscopic gastric banding: a case report," *Journal of Medical Case Reports*, vol. 6, article 9, 2012.

[8] A. Tekin, "Migration of the connecting tube into small bowel after adjustable gastric banding," *Obesity Surgery*, vol. 20, no. 4, pp. 526–529, 2010.

[9] M. Iqbal, S. Manjunath, M. Seenath, and A. Khan, "Massive upper gastrointestinal hemorrhage: an unusual presentation after laparoscopic adjustable gastric banding due to erosion into the celiac axis," *Obesity Surgery*, vol. 18, no. 6, pp. 759–760, 2008.

[10] R. Sneijder, H. A. Cense, M. Hunfeld, and R. S. Breederveld, "A rare complication after laparoscopic gastric banding: connecting-tube penetration into the hilus of the kidney," *Obesity Surgery*, vol. 19, no. 4, pp. 531–533, 2009.

[11] J. A. Cintolo, M. S. Levine, S. Huang, and K. Dumon, "Intraluminal erosion of laparoscopic gastric band tubing into duodenum with recurrent port-site infections," *Journal of Laparoendoscopic and Advanced Surgical Techniques*, vol. 22, no. 6, pp. 591–594, 2012.

[12] K. Egberts, W. A. Brown, and P. E. O'Brien, "Systematic review of erosion after laparoscopic adjustable gastric banding," *Obesity Surgery*, vol. 21, no. 8, pp. 1272–1279, 2011.

[13] W. A. Brown, K. J. Egberts, D. Franke-Richard, P. Thodiyil, M. L. Anderson, and P. E. O'Brien, "Erosions after laparoscopic adjustable gastric banding: diagnosis and management," *Annals of Surgery*, vol. 257, no. 6, pp. 1047–1052, 2013.

[14] S. Abu-Abeid, A. Keidar, N. Gavert, A. Blanc, and A. Szold, "The clinical spectrum of band erosion following laparoscopic adjustable silicone gastric banding for morbid obesity," *Surgical Endoscopy and Other Interventional Techniques*, vol. 17, no. 6, pp. 861–863, 2003.

[15] C. I. Yoon, K. H. Pak, and S. M. Kim, "Early experience with diagnosis and management of eroded gastric bands," *Journal of the Korean Surgical Society*, vol. 82, no. 1, pp. 18–27, 2012.

[16] R. Singhal, C. Bryant, M. Kitchen et al., "Band slippage and erosion after laparoscopic gastric banding: a meta-analysis," *Surgical Endoscopy and Other Interventional Techniques*, vol. 24, no. 12, pp. 2980–2986, 2010.

[17] G. P. Kohn, C. A. Hansen, R. W. Gilhome, R. C. McHenry, D. C. Spilias, and C. Hensman, "Laparoscopic management of gastric band erosions: a 10-year series of 49 cases," *Surgical Endoscopy and Other Interventional Techniques*, vol. 26, no. 2, pp. 541–545, 2012.

[18] N. di Lorenzo, F. Furbetta, F. Favretti et al., "Laparoscopic adjustable gastric banding via pars flaccida versus perigastric positioning: technique, complications, and results in 2,549 patients," *Surgical Endoscopy and Other Interventional Techniques*, vol. 24, no. 7, pp. 1519–1523, 2010.

[19] I. Eid, D. W. Birch, A. M. Sharma, V. Sherman, and K. Shahzeer, "Complications associated with adjustable gastric banding for morbid obesity: a surgeon's guide," *Canadian Journal of Surgery*, vol. 54, no. 1, pp. 61–66, 2011.

[20] S. Abu-Abeid, D. B. Zohar, B. Sagie, and J. Klausner, "Treatment of intra-gastric band migration following laparoscopic banding: safety and feasibility of simultaneous laparoscopic band removal and replacement," *Obesity Surgery*, vol. 15, no. 6, pp. 849–852, 2005.

[21] C. Lum, J. Small, L. Dimarco, and S. Currie, "A rare complication: laparoscopically placed gastric band erosion into splenic artery," *ANZ Journal of Surgery*, vol. 81, no. 4, p. 303, 2011.

[22] O. C. Kutlu, S. Garcia, and S. Dissanaike, "The successful use of simple tube duodenostomy in large duodenal perforations from varied etiologies," *International Journal of Surgery Case Reports*, vol. 4, no. 3, pp. 279–282, 2013.

[23] S. Gupta, R. Kaushik, R. Sharma, and A. Attri, "The management of large perforations of duodenal ulcers," *BMC Surgery*, vol. 5, no. 15, 2005.

[24] E. Lattuada, M. A. Zappa, E. Mozzi et al., "Histologic study of tissue reaction to the gastric band: does it contribute to the problem of band erosion?" *Obesity Surgery*, vol. 16, no. 9, pp. 1155–1159, 2006.

[25] E. Niville, A. Dams, K. van der Speeten, and H. Verhelst, "Results of lap rebanding procedures after Lap-Band® removal for band erosion—a mid-term evaluation," *Obesity Surgery*, vol. 15, no. 5, pp. 630–633, 2005.

[26] G. H. E. J. Vijgen, R. Schouten, L. Pelzers, J. W. Greve, S. H. van Helden, and N. D. Bouvy, "Revision of laparoscopic adjustable gastric banding: success or failure?" *Obesity Surgery*, vol. 22, no. 2, pp. 287–292, 2012.

[27] R. Schouten, D. Japink, B. Meesters, P. J. Nelemans, and J. W. M. Greve, "Systematic literature review of reoperations after gastric banding: is a stepwise approach justified?" *Surgery for Obesity and Related Diseases*, vol. 7, no. 1, pp. 99–109, 2011.

[28] C. A. S. Berende, J.-P. de Zoete, J. F. Smulders, and S. W. Nienhuijs, "Laparoscopic sleeve gastrectomy feasible for bariatric revision surgery," *Obesity Surgery*, vol. 22, no. 2, pp. 330–334, 2012.

[29] M. Weber, M. K. Müller, J.-M. Michel et al., "Laparoscopic Roux-en-Y gastric bypass, but not rebanding, should be proposed as rescue procedure for patients with failed laparoscopic gastric banding," *Annals of Surgery*, vol. 238, no. 6, pp. 827–834, 2003.

[30] M. Suter, V. Giusti, E. Héraief, and J.-M. Calmes, "Band erosion after laparoscopic gastric banding: occurrence and results after conversion to Roux-en-Y gastric bypass," *Obesity Surgery*, vol. 14, no. 3, pp. 381–386, 2004.

Small Bowel Injury in Peritoneal Encapsulation following Penetrating Abdominal Trauma

K. Naidoo, S. Mewa Kinoo, and B. Singh

Department of Surgery, Nelson R Mandela School of Medicine, University of KwaZulu-Natal,
719 Umbilo Road, Congella 4013, South Africa

Correspondence should be addressed to S. Mewa Kinoo; smewakinoo@gmail.com

Academic Editors: T. Çolak, N. D. Merrett, and A. A. Saber

Small bowel encapsulation is a rare entity which is usually found incidentally at autopsy. We report the first case of peritoneal encapsulation encountered serendipitously at laparotomy undertaken for penetrating abdominal trauma and review the literature on peritoneal encapsulation. We also compare this phenomenon to abdominal cocoon and sclerosing encapsulating peritonitis.

1. Introduction

The terms peritoneal encapsulation (PE), abdominal cocoon, and sclerosing encapsulating peritonitis (SEP) are used interchangeably to describe the rare conditions of small bowel encapsulation. The literature on this subject is dominated by case reports. Presently there is no consensus on the classification of these 3 distinct pathological entities that effectively constitute small bowel encapsulation [1]. Whereas PE is an embryological disorder and abdominal cocoon is an idiopathic condition, SEP is today increasingly associated with peritoneal dialysis as well as a variety of other conditions [2].

2. Case Presentation

A 40-year-old male patient presented to our surgical unit following an isolated stab wound to the abdomen in the region of the epigastrium. The patient had no medical history of note.

On examination, the patient was noted to be haemodynamically stable. Abdominal examination revealed peritonitis. The admission chest and abdominal radiographs were noted to be normal.

At laparotomy the entire small bowel was encapsulated in a peritoneal sac. The peritoneal sac was noted to be attached to the ascending and descending colon laterally, to the transverse colon superiorly, and to the pelvic peritoneum inferiorly. The peritoneal sac was transparent and was noted to contain blood. The sac was not attached to the underlying small bowel and neither to the abdominal wall parietes nor to the greater omentum (Figure 1).

A perforation in the peritoneal sac was noted at the site of the stab. On opening the peritoneal sac the small bowel was noted to be freely mobile. Multiple small bowel perforations were evident, probably due to the concertina effect of the bowel layered within the peritoneal sac (Figure 2).

The sac was excised after the repair of the small bowel perforations (Figure 3). The patient made an eventual recovery and was discharged on the 5th postoperative day.

3. Discussion

PE is a congenital abnormality in which the small bowel is contained in an accessory peritoneal sac derived from the yolk sac. This condition is considered to develop in the 12th embryological week following the abnormal return of the physiological umbilical hernia containing the midgut into the abdominal cavity. The accessory peritoneal sac is attached laterally to the ascending and descending colon, superiorly to the transverse colon, and to the parietal peritoneum inferiorly. A segment or entire small bowel extending from the duodenojejunal flexure to the ileocaecal junction (as in the case presented) may be contained in the accessory

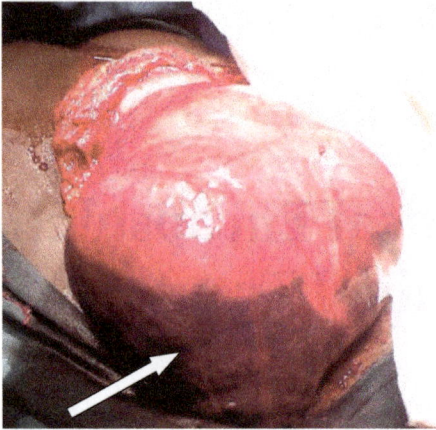

FIGURE 1: Peritoneal sac encountered at laparotomy; note free blood pooled at the bottom of the peritoneal sac (indicated by arrow).

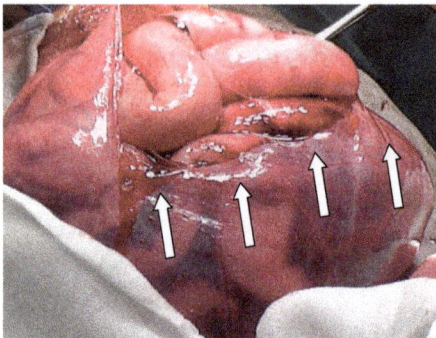

FIGURE 2: Multiple small bowel perforations (indicated by arrows).

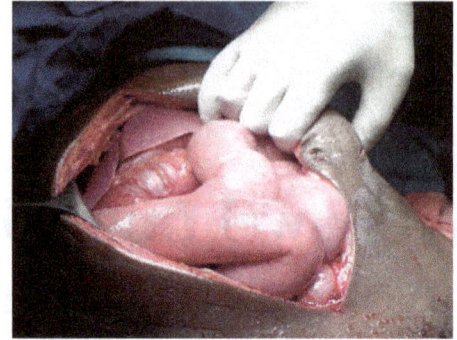

FIGURE 3: On opening the peritoneal sac the small bowel was noted to be free of adhesions and fully mobile.

peritoneal sac. As evident in this paper, the greater omentum covers the sac but is not attached to it [3].

PE was first reported by Cleland in 1868. Defining the true incidence of PE has been hampered by the failure to distinguish this condition from abdominal cocoon and SEP. The literature suggests that incidence of PE ranges between 20 and 40 cases [4–6]. PE is usually an incidental finding noted at autopsy or at laparotomy, as in this paper [7]. Rarely, PE may present with either complete or incomplete small bowel obstruction in patients who usually have a long history of abdominal pain [8, 9]. Small bowel gangrene and aortic occlusion have each been reported once [10, 11].

The literature supports the excision of the peritoneal sac when encountered incidentally at laparotomy with lysis of interloop adhesions, if present, in symptomatic patients. Histological examination of the excised peritoneal sac invariably demonstrates normal peritoneum without signs of inflammation [12].

PE must be differentiated from SEP and the abdominal cocoon phenomenon. These are distinctly different entities.

SEP was first described by Owtschinnkow in 1907 as "peritonitis chronic fibrosa incapsulata." SEP is an acquired condition characterized by the covering of the small bowel with a thick grayish white fibr collagenous membrane. SEP

is associated with chronic ambulatory peritoneal dialysis, the beta-blocker protocol (now withdrawn from use), recurrent peritonitis, ventriculoperitoeal and peritoneovenous shunts, sarcoidosis, tuberculosis, Mediterranean fever, protein-S deficiency, following liver transplantation, systemic lupus erythematosus, and fibrogenic foreign material [13].

The abdominal cocoon was first described by Foo et al. in 1978 [14]. Classically, this condition was described as occurring in young adolescent females from the tropical and subtropical countries. However, case reports from temperate zones have been reported in all age groups regardless of gender [15–17].

The etiology of the abdominal cocoon is poorly understood. Various theories have been proffered, including retrograde menstruation with a superimposed viral infection, retrograde peritonitis, and cell-mediated immunological tissue damage incited by gynecological infection.

It is probable that the abdominal cocoon is the result of "subclinical" peritonitis. The abdominal cocoon has been described as "idiopathic SEP". The small bowel is encapsulated by a fibrocollagenous membrane in a manner not dissimilar to that encountered in SEP. The association with embryologic abnormalities such as greater omentum hypoplasia and mesenteric vessel malformation suggests that developmental abnormality may be a probable etiology [18].

Notwithstanding the reported differentiation of SEP and abdominal cocoon on the basis of etiology, it is reasonable to assume that these conditions belong to a similar pathological process resulting in the fibrous encapsulation of the small bowel.

In patients presenting with small bowel obstruction associated with the fibrous encapsulation of the small bowel, 2 clinical signs have been described. The first is a fixed, asymmetrical distension of the abdomen, which does not vary with peristaltic activity due to the unvarying position of the fibrous capsule. The second is the difference in the consistency of the abdominal wall to palpation. The bowel proximal to the capsule can distend and is soft to palpation, as opposed to the flat area that is firm, due to the dense fibrous capsule that encases the underlying small bowel [19].

Although standard radiographic studies are usually normal, it has been suggested that a combination of barium meal will follow through studies, and abdominal computed tomography may contribute to making a preoperative diagnosis. In abdominal cocoon, barium studies may demonstrate a serpentine-or concertina-like configuration of dilated small bowel loops in a fixed U-shaped cluster and delayed transit of the contrast medium [20].

Computed tomography of the abdomen may demonstrate congregation of small bowel loops to the center of the abdomen encased by a soft-tissue density mantle representing the peritoneal membrane; other features include signs of obstruction, fixation of intestinal loops, bowel wall thickening, ascites, and localized fluid collections [21–23].

Despite anecdotal reports of a preoperative diagnosis of peritoneal encapsulation being established, in the majority of cases this is fortuitous particularly in the absence of discerning clinical signs. However, a better awareness of this condition with appropriate use of imaging techniques may facilitate preoperative diagnosis [18].

References

[1] O. Lifschitz, J. Tiu, and R. A. Sumeruk, "Peritoneal encapsulation of small intestine. A case report," South African Medical Journal, vol. 71, no. 7, p. 452, 1987.

[2] J. N. Tannoury and B. N. Abboud, "Idiopathic sclerosing encapsulating peritonitis: abdominal cocoon," World Journal of Gastroenterology, vol. 18, no. 17, pp. 1999–2004, 2012.

[3] J. M. Sherigar, B. McFall, and J. Wali, "Peritoneal encapsulation: presenting as small bowel obstruction in an elderly woman," Ulster Medical Journal, vol. 76, no. 1, pp. 42–44, 2007.

[4] J. Cleland, "On an abnormal arrangement of peritoneum with remarks on development of the mesocolon," Journal of Anatomy and Physiology, vol. 2, pp. 201–206, 1868.

[5] J. Mordehai, O. Kleiner, B. Kirshtein, Y. Barki, and A. J. Mares, "Peritoneal encapsulation: a rare cause of bowel obstruction in children," Journal of Pediatric Surgery, vol. 36, no. 7, pp. 1059–1061, 2001.

[6] E. Ibrahim Bassiouny IE and T. O. Abbas, "Small Bowel Cocoon: a distinct disease with a new developmental etiology," Case Reports in Surgery, vol. 2011, Article ID 940515, 5 pages, 2011.

[7] S. Jaber, K. Dulaijan, M. Sadoun, K. Moghazy, and M. El-Said, "Post-traumatic intra-cocoon mesenteric tear: a case report," Case Reports in Gastroenterology, vol. 5, no. 1, pp. 206–211, 2011.

[8] S. Awasthi, V. A. Saraswat, and V. K. Kapoor, "Peritoneal encapsulation of the small bowel: a rare cause of intestinal obstruction," American Journal of Gastroenterology, vol. 86, no. 3, p. 383, 1991.

[9] O. A. Adedeji and W. A. F. McAdam, "Small bowel obstruction due to encapsulation and abnormal artery," Postgraduate Medical Journal, vol. 70, no. 820, pp. 132–133, 1994.

[10] I. Akhtar, "Small bowel gangrene secondary to peritoneal encapsulation," The Professional Medical Journal, vol. 5, no. 2, pp. 231–232, 1998.

[11] M. B. Silva Jr., M. M. Connolly, A. Burford-Foggs, and W. R. Flinn, "Acute aortic occlusion as a result of extrinsic compression from peritoneal encapsulation," Journal of Vascular Surgery, vol. 16, no. 2, pp. 286–289, 1992.

[12] J. D. Casas, A. Mariscal, and M. Martinez, "Peritoneal encapsulation: CT appearance," American Journal of Roentgenology, vol. 171, pp. 1017–1019, 1998.

[13] S. B. Jenkins, B. L. Leng, J. R. Shortland, P. W. Brown, and M. E. Wilkie, "Sclerosing encapsulating peritonitis: a case series from a single U.K. center during a 10-year period," Advances in Peritoneal Dialysis, vol. 17, pp. 191–195, 2001.

[14] K. T. Foo, K. C. Ng, and A. Rauff, "Unusual small intestinal obstruction in adolescent girls: the abdominal cocoon," British Journal of Surgery, vol. 65, no. 6, pp. 427–430, 1978.

[15] P. Xu, L. H. Chen, and Y. M. Li, "Idiopathic sclerosing encapsulating peritonitis (or abdominal cocoon): a report of 5 cases," World Journal of Gastroenterology, vol. 13, no. 26, pp. 3649–3651, 2007.

[16] B. Cleffken, G. Sie, R. Riedl, and E. Heineman, "Idiopathic sclerosing encapsulating peritonitis in a young female-diagnosis of abdominal cocoon," Journal of Pediatric Surgery, vol. 43, no. 2, pp. e27–e30, 2008.

[17] N. A. Ibrahim and M. A. Oludara, "Abdominal cocoon in an adolescent male patient," Tropical Doctor, vol. 39, no. 4, pp. 254–256, 2009.

[18] A. S. Rajagopal and R. Rajagopal, "Conundrum of the cocoon: report of a case and review of the literature," Diseases of the Colon and Rectum, vol. 46, no. 8, pp. 1141–1143, 2003.

[19] V. Naraynsingh, D. Maharaj, M. Singh, and M. J. Ramdass, "Peritoneal encapsulation: a preoperative diagnosis is possible," Postgraduate Medical Journal, vol. 77, no. 913, pp. 725–726, 2001.

[20] J. O. Sieck, R. Cowgill, and W. Larkworthy, "Peritoneal encapsulation and abdominal cocoon. Case reports and a review of the literature," Gastroenterology, vol. 84, no. 6, pp. 1597–1601, 1983.

[21] H. Nakamoto, "Encapsulating peritoneal sclerosis—a clinician's approach to diagnosis and medical treatment," Peritoneal Dialysis International, vol. 25, supplement 4, pp. S30–S38, 2005.

[22] B. Wei, H. B. Wei, W. P. Guo et al., "Diagnosis and treatment of abdominal cocoon: a report of 24 cases," American Journal of Surgery, vol. 198, no. 3, pp. 348–353, 2009.

[23] D. Mohanty, B. K. Jain, J. Agrawal, A. Gupta, and V. Agrawal, "Abdominal cocoon: clinical presentation, diagnosis, and management," Journal of Gastrointestinal Surgery, vol. 13, no. 6, pp. 1160–1162, 2009.

8

Transabdominal Approach for Chylorrhea after Esophagectomy by Using Fluorescence Navigation with Indocyanine Green

Takeshi Matsutani,[1] Atsushi Hirakata,[2] Tsutomu Nomura,[1] Nobutoshi Hagiwara,[1] Akihisa Matsuda,[1] Hiroshi Yoshida,[2] and Eiji Uchida[1]

[1] Department of Gastrointestinal and Hepato-Biliary-Pancreatic Surgery, Nippon Medical School, 1-1-5 Sendagi, Bunkyo-ku, Tokyo 113-8603, Japan
[2] Department of Surgery, Nippon Medical School Tama-Nagayama Hospital, 1-7-1 Nagayama, Tama, Tokyo 206-8512, Japan

Correspondence should be addressed to Takeshi Matsutani; matsutani@nms.ac.jp

Academic Editor: Shin-ichi Kosugi

A 70-year-old man who underwent two sessions of thoracoscopy-assisted ligation of the thoracic duct to treat refractory chylorrhea after radical esophagectomy for advanced esophageal cancer received conservative therapy. However, there was no improvement in chylorrhea. Then, transabdominal ligation of the lymphatic/thoracic duct at the level of the right crus of the diaphragm was performed using fluorescence navigation with indocyanine green (ICG). The procedure successfully reduced chylorrhea. This procedure provides a valid option for persistent chylothorax/chylous ascites accompanied by chylorrhea with no response to conservative treatment, transthoracic ligation, or both.

1. Introduction

Chylorrhea including chylothorax is uncommon after esophagectomy, with an incidence of 1% to 4% [1–3]. When conservative treatments fail to stop the leakage of chyle, surgical treatment is necessary to avoid increased morbidity and mortality. Current surgical options for ligation of the lymphatic/thoracic duct include the transthoracic approach [4–7] and the transabdominal approach [8–11]. However, the site of a chyle fistula is often difficult to detect intraoperatively because of inflammation and edema. Recently, intraoperative indocyanine green (ICG) fluorescence lymphography was introduced to exactly define the site of a fistula causing chylorrhea [4]. We report the usefulness of lymphatic/thoracic duct ligation by intraoperative ICG fluorescence navigation via a transabdominal approach.

2. Case Report

A 70-year-old man was referred to the hospital because of an advanced squamous cell carcinoma of the lower thoracic esophagus (T3N1M0, stage III). The patient received one course of neoadjuvant chemotherapy with 5-fluorouracil, docetaxel, and cisplatin. After a partial response was confirmed on repeated endoscopy and CT scan, the patient underwent a thoracoscopic subtotal esophagectomy with lymph node dissection in the prone position. Laparoscopy-assisted reconstruction was done using a gastric tube through the posterior mediastinal route with the patient in the supine position, combined with a jejunostomy. The thoracic duct from superior mediastinum to the diaphragm was resected with the esophagus, and the stump of the residual thoracic duct was clipped twice. Although the postoperative vital signs were stable, the chest-drain output continued to exceed 1500 mL/day on postoperative day (POD) 5. When elemental nutrition was started through the jejunostomy, the fluid from the chest drain turned milky white, confirming the diagnosis of chylorrhea. Conservative therapy with octreotide (intermittent subcutaneous injection 100 μg × 3/day) and total parental nutrition for 5 days failed to reduce chylorrhea. We decided to perform repeated thoracoscopy-assisted ligation of the thoracic duct with the patient in the prone position on POD 10. However, reconstructed gastric tube occupied the space to search the thoracic duct in the right thoracic

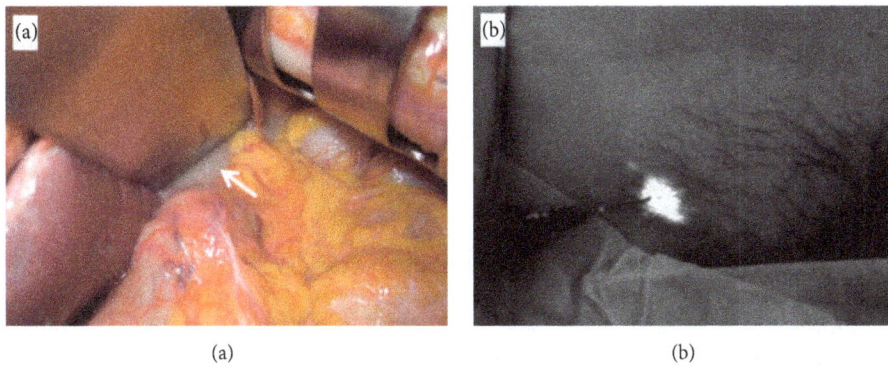

FIGURE 1: (a) The cisterna chili in the retroabdominal space below the diaphragm. (b) Indocyanine green is bilaterally injected subcutaneously into the inguinal region.

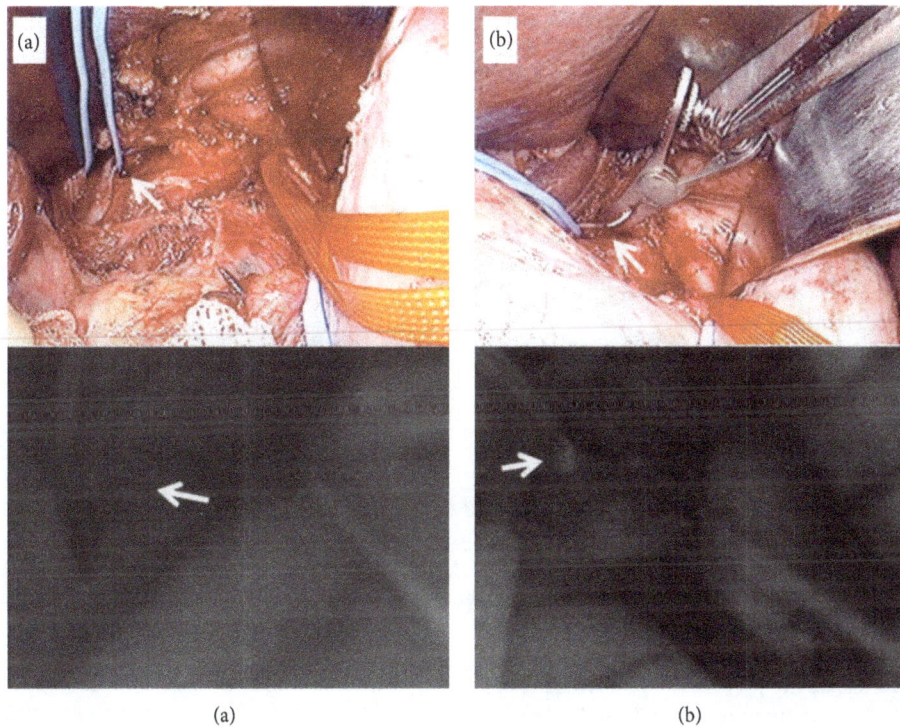

FIGURE 2: Intraoperative view and indocyanine green fluorescence lymphography. (a) The thoracic duct is seen on the right side of gastric tube (arrow). (b) A bulldog clamp is placed around the thoracic duct and the dilated thoracic duct is confirmed (arrow).

cavity. Then, the thoracic duct was not detected and ligated successfully. On POD 28, we performed an open laparotomy to ligate the thoracic duct at the level of the aortic hiatus after the administration of milk cream through the feeding jejunostomy tube. On the exploration of the upper abdomen, a milky effusion, chylous ascites, was found in the retroperitoneal space below the diaphragm (Figure 1(a)). The gastric tube was mobilized to the left side, but the exact site of the lymph fistula could not be identified. Approximately 10 min after a bilateral subcutaneous injection of 1.5 mL ICG (Diagnogreen 0.5%, Daiichi Sankyo Co., Tokyo, Japan) into the inguinal region (Figure 1(b)), the lymphatic duct was confirmed on fluorescence imaging performed with a near-infrared PDE camera system (Hamamatsu Photonics, Hamamatsu, Japan) at a 760 nm wavelength, filtering out

light with a wavelength below 820 nm. The lymphatic duct, communicating with the thoracic duct, was visible at the level of right crus of the diaphragm (Figure 2(a)). A bulldog clamp was placed around the lymphatic duct, thereby confirming the dilated lymphatic duct as cisterna chili (Figure 2(b)). The root of thoracic duct was clipped successfully and easily at the right side of the esophageal hiatus. The chylorrhea stopped completely on POD 30. The postoperative course was uneventful. After the patient was able to ingest a solid meal, he was discharged on POD 35.

3. Discussion

Despite careful ligation of the thoracic duct following esophagectomy for esophageal cancer, the patients who undergo an extended lymphadenectomy for positive lymph node metastases have increased risk of chylorrhea by secondary injury to the main thoracic duct. A meta-analysis of 44 studies showed that chylorrhea developed in 2.1% of patients after transhiatal esophagectomy and 3.4% after transthoracic esophagectomy [12]. Systemic review and institutional analysis showed that postoperative chylorrhea occurred significantly more frequently among patients who had surgery after neoadjuvant chemotherapy than among patients undergoing surgery alone [13]. Loss of chyle leads to impaired wound healing due to loss of protein, lack of weight gain due to loss of fat, or immunodeficiency due to loss of lymphocytes. Early diagnosis and effective management are therefore necessary for good outcomes. However, the treatment of chylorrhea is controversial, and the choice between conservative therapy and surgery remains a matter of debate. Conservative therapy includes pleural drainage, parenteral nutritional support, and measures that reduce chyle flow, such as administration of medium-chain triglycerides and somatostatin analogs [2, 5, 14]. Although such conservative methods can avoid the need for surgery, they usually require several weeks for complete resolution of chyle flow [2, 5]. Thus, early operative intervention remains a good alternative for some physicians [6, 9]. In our patient, extended lymphadenectomy might have damaged the lymphatic system and caused persistent chylorrhea, despite careful ligation of the thoracic duct at initial operation.

Lymphangiography has traditionally been considered the gold standard for the evaluation of chylorrhea. This imaging technique is useful for preoperatively estimating the extent of lymphadenectomy. However, lymphangiography is a difficult procedure that requires cannulation of lymphatic channels, which can cause adverse effects such as local tissue necrosis, fat embolism to the lungs, hypersensitivity reactions, or worsening of lymphedema due to the contrast medium. To intraoperatively detect chyle leakage points, the administration of cream containing methylene blue dye via the oral or nasogastric route can facilitate leak identification [2, 6, 13]. A recent study reported that the precise site of chyle leakage was successfully detected on imaging by ICG fluorescence [4]. ICG particles are small and easily taken into lymph ducts. In addition, ICG binds to blood lipoproteins and shows diffuse fluorescence after excitation by near-infrared light. The photodynamic eye and fluorescence detector used in our patient were equipped with a light-emitting diode (760 nm) and CCD camera. Intraoperative ICG injection has no known adverse effects. Our findings confirmed that intraoperative ICG fluorescence lymphography can help surgeons detect sites of lymphatic duct injury. However, surgeons should know that the side effects by ICG administration as anaphylactic reaction, hypotension, tachycardia, dyspnea, and urticaria only occurred in individual cases; the risk of severe side effects rises in patients with chronic renal dysfunction.

The ligation of the thoracic duct through a second right-sided thoracotomy may be difficult not to detect the thoracic duct above the diaphragm after radical lymph node dissection. Moreover, it is likely that chyle was not leaked from one injury of the thoracic duct, from multiple lymphatic injuries in the upper abdominal cavity. A recent study reported that laparotomy with ligation of the thoracic duct at the level of the aortic hiatus is a simple and safe method for the management of postthoracotomy chyle leakage [9]. The study found that this technique is an effective treatment for postoperative chylorrhea; an abdominal approach has lower morbidity than a second transthoracic approach. Another advantage of a transabdominal approach is that surgeons can easily identify the lymphatic duct at the level of the hiatus because there are few anatomical variations of the thoracic duct, which is relatively consistent in the lower part of its course.

4. Conclusion

Intraoperative ICG fluorescence lymphography was useful for detecting the precise site of a lymphatic/thoracic duct injury after esophagectomy.

References

[1] D. V. L. N. Rao, S. P. Chava, P. Sahni, and T. K. Chattopadhyay, "Thoracic duct injury during esophagectomy: 20 years experience at a tertiary care center in a developing country," *Diseases of the Esophagus*, vol. 17, no. 2, pp. 141–145, 2004.

[2] B. A. Merrigan, D. C. Winter, and G. C. O'Sullivan, "Chylothorax," *British Journal of Surgery*, vol. 84, no. 1, pp. 15–20, 1997.

[3] D. Dougenis, W. S. Walker, E. W. J. Cameron, and P. R. Walbaum, "Management of chylothorax complicating extensive esophageal resection," *Surgery Gynecology and Obstetrics*, vol. 174, no. 6, pp. 501–506, 1992.

[4] K. Kamiya, N. Unno, and H. Konno, "Intraoperative indocyanine green fluorescence lymphography, a novel imaging technique to detect a chyle fistula after an esophagectomy: report of a case," *Surgery Today*, vol. 39, no. 5, pp. 421–424, 2009.

[5] M. Haniuda, H. Nishimura, O. Kobayashi et al., "Management of chylothorax after pulmonary resection," *Journal of the American College of Surgeons*, vol. 180, no. 5, pp. 537–540, 1995.

[6] E. M. Sieczka and J. C. Harvey, "Early thoracic duct ligation for postoperative chylothorax," *Journal of Surgical Oncology*, vol. 61, pp. 56–60, 1996.

[7] G. L. Crosthwaite, B. V. Joypaul, and A. Cuschieri, "Thoracoscopic management of thoracic duct injury," *Journal of the Royal College of Surgeons of Edinburgh*, vol. 40, no. 5, pp. 303–304, 1995.

[8] O. J. Icaza Jr., K. Andrews, and M. Kuhnke, "Laparoscopic ligation of the thoracic duct in management of chylothorax," *Journal of Laparoendoscopic & Advanced Surgical Techniques A*, vol. 12, no. 2, pp. 129–133, 2002.

[9] P. F. Mason, R. H. Ragoowansi, and J. A. C. Thorpe, "Postthoracotomy chylothorax—a cure in the abdomen?" *European Journal of Cardio-Thoracic Surgery*, vol. 11, no. 3, pp. 567–570, 1997.

[10] G. Schumacher, H. Weidemann, J. M. Langrehr et al., "Transabdominal ligation of the thoracic duct as treatment of choice for postoperative chylothorax after esophagectomy," *Diseases of the Esophagus*, vol. 20, no. 1, pp. 19–23, 2007.

[11] B. C. Vassallo, D. Cavadas, E. Beveraggi, and E. Sivori, "Treatment of postoperative chylothorax through laparoscopic thoracic duct ligation," *European Journal of Cardiothoracic Surgery*, vol. 21, no. 3, pp. 556–557, 2002.

[12] R. Rindani, C. J. Martin, and M. R. Cox, "Transhiatal versus Ivor-Lewis oesophagectomy: is there a difference?" *Australian and New Zealand Journal of Surgery*, vol. 69, no. 3, pp. 187–194, 1999.

[13] M. Kranzfelder, R. Gertler, A. Hapfelmeier, H. Friess, and M. Feith, "Chylothorax after esophagectomy for cancer: impact of the surgical approach and neoadjuvant treatment: systematic review and institutional analysis," *Surgical Endoscopy*, vol. 27, no. 10, pp. 3530–3538, 2013.

[14] J. I. Miller Jr., "Diagnosis and management of chylothorax," *Chest Surgery Clinics of North America*, vol. 6, no. 1, pp. 139–148, 1996.

Diagnosis and Management of Perforated Duodenal Ulcers following Roux-En-Y Gastric Bypass: A Report of Two Cases and a Review of the Literature

Mazen E. Iskandar, Fiona M. Chory, Elliot R. Goodman, and Burton G. Surick

Department of Surgery, Mount Sinai Beth Israel Medical Center, New York, NY 10003, USA

Correspondence should be addressed to Mazen E. Iskandar; miskandar@chpnet.org

Academic Editor: Alexander R. Novotny

Perforated duodenal ulcers are rare complications seen after roux-en-Y gastric bypass (RYGP). They often present as a diagnostic dilemma as they rarely present with pneumoperitoneum on radiologic evaluation. There is no consensus as to the pathophysiology of these ulcers; however expeditious treatment is necessary. We present two patients with perforated duodenal ulcers and a distant history of RYGP who were successfully treated. Their individual surgical management is discussed as well as a literature review. We conclude that, in patients who present with acute abdominal pain and a history of RYGB, perforated ulcer needs to be very high in the differential diagnosis even in the absence of pneumoperitoneum. In these patients an early surgical exploration is paramount to help diagnose and treat these patients.

1. Introduction

Peptic ulcer disease and specifically a perforated duodenal ulcer in the excluded stomach or duodenum are a very rare occurrence in patients who have undergone RYGP. Well over one hundred thousand gastric bypass procedures are performed yearly in the USA [1], but only twenty-one cases of perforated duodenal ulcers have been reported in the literature (Table 1) [2–8]. Moreover, most of the reported cases correspond to the early days of gastric bypass when proton pump inhibitors (PPIs) were not as liberally used. The diagnosis of a perforated duodenal ulcer in a RYGP patient can be challenging, and there is variability in the surgical treatment, especially when it comes to the possible role of removing the gastric remnant. We present two cases of a perforated duodenal ulcer following roux-en-Y gastric bypass and discuss the management of these patients.

2. Case #1

A 59-year-old male tourist presented to the emergency room with a one-day history of acute onset epigastric pain radiating to the right side of his abdomen and to his back. He denied any other gastrointestinal symptoms and denied taking any nonsteroidal anti-inflammatory agents (NSAIDs). He gave a history of a laparoscopic roux-en-Y gastric bypass performed 10 years priorly at his home country without any short or long term complications. He weighed 125 kilograms before the RYGB (body mass index, BMI 37.7), and he suffered from hypertension and type 2 diabetes mellitus. Following RYGB, his weight nadir was ninety kilograms, and his comorbidities resolved. Physical examination revealed mild tachycardia and tenderness in the epigastrium without evidence of peritonitis. His weight was ninety-six kilograms, and laboratory tests were only significant for an elevated lipase level of 1,043 units/liter (normal range 23–300 units/liter). Chest and abdominal radiographs did not demonstrate free air. A computed tomography (CT) scan with oral and intravenous contrast was obtained that demonstrated a few foci of free air tracking along the falciform ligament, free fluid in the right paracolic gutter, and a distended and thickened gallbladder (Figure 1). There was no extravasation of contrast and the gastrojejunal anastomosis appeared intact. With the concern of a perforated viscus in the excluded segment of the stomach

TABLE 1: Summary of all reported cases with their treatment.

Author/year published	Number of patients	Urgent treatment	Definitive treatment
Moore et al./1979 [2]	2	Closure	Medical
Charuzi et al./1986 [3]	2	Closure	Medical
Bjorkman et al./1989 [4]	1	Medical	Closure/gastrectomy
Macgregor et al./1999 [5]	10	Closure in 9/duodenostomy/gastrostomy in 1	Gastrectomy in 9, medical in 1
Mittermair and Renz/2007 [6]	1	Closure	Medical
Snyder/2007 [7]	4	Closure in 1	Gastrectomy in 3 as initial treatment
Gypen et al./2008 [8]	1	Closure	Gastrectomy
This report	2	Closure in 1/duodenostomy	Medical

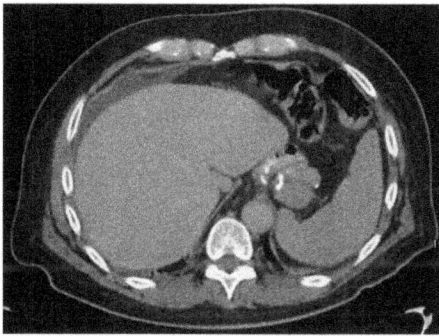

FIGURE 1: CT showing free fluid in the right paracolic gutter, no free air, and intact gastrojejunal anastomosis.

or duodenum, the decision was made for laparoscopic exploration.

Initial exploration revealed bilious ascites that was irrigated and suctioned. Careful inspection of the first portion of the duodenum revealed an 8 mm perforation that was partially sealed by the medial wall of the gallbladder. The defect was closed laparoscopically and primarily using nonabsorbable sutures and buttressed with omentum. Two closed suction drains were left in the subhepatic space next to the duodenum. *Helicobacter pylori* (*H. pylori*) serology was negative. A hepatobiliary iminodiacetic acid (HIDA) scan was obtained postoperatively to make sure that the perforation remained sealed. By the fourth postoperative day, the patient had completely recovered, and the drains were removed. He was seen 1 week after his discharge for a postoperative checkup after which he returned to his country.

3. Case #2

A 37-year-old male with history of laparoscopic roux-en-Y gastric bypass in 2002 at an outside institution presented to the emergency department with one week of progressively increasing, sharp epigastric abdominal pain, with a new diffuse quality. It was associated with radiation to the back and development of nausea and emesis in the 24 hours prior to presentation. He denied fever, constipation, obstipation, and NSAID use. His history was significant for peptic ulcer disease and gastrointestinal bleeding from anastomotic erosions. He consumed one bottle of wine daily and had two

negative upper endoscopies of his gastric pouch and jejunum, the last one being seven months prior to this admission.

On exam he remained morbidly obese BMI 47; he was afebrile and vital signs were within normal limits. He had a soft abdomen with mild epigastric tenderness and no peritoneal signs. His WBC was 9.3 with 79% neutrophils. *H. pylori* serology was negative. Chest and abdominal radiographs did not demonstrate pneumoperitoneum. A computed tomography (CT) scan revealed a markedly distended, fluid-filled excluded stomach and edema of the first portion of the duodenum, jejunum, and transverse colon. There was moderate ascites and no evidence of pneumoperitoneum, and the radiologic diagnosis was enteritis (Figure 2).

The patient became hypotensive, tachycardic, and diaphoretic and developed worsening abdominal tenderness with guarding shortly after the CT scan. The patient was rapidly optimized in the SICU with fluid resuscitation and vasopressor support and was taken emergently to surgery for an exploratory laparotomy for suspected perforation of the excluded stomach or duodenum. A laparoscopic approach was not considered due to the patient's hemodynamics. At surgery, a large amount of bilious ascites was encountered upon opening the abdomen. The excluded stomach was dilated, and there was a 2-centimeter, 50-percent circumferential duodenal defect in the proximal second portion of the duodenum (Figure 3). The surrounding tissue was very friable and the size of the defect made primary or patch closure impractical. The patient's hemodynamic status was labile intraoperatively and a decision was made to drain the excluded stomach. Two 28 F silicone catheters were placed through the perforation: one was advanced into the excluded stomach and the second into the third portion of the duodenum. The tubes were secured to the edge of the perforation to create a controlled duodenal-cutaneous fistula. A feeding jejunostomy tube was placed, as well as multiple closed suction drains.

By the third postoperative day, the patient was able to be extubated and weaned off vasopressors. His hospitalization was complicated by an upper extremity deep vein thrombosis requiring anticoagulation, acute renal failure which resolved without dialysis, and high output biliary drainage from the silicone catheters. By postoperative day 25 he was discharged tolerating a low fiber diet, on an oral proton-pump inhibitor, anticoagulation, and antibiotics. By the 8th postoperative week, the fistula output was negligible. Subsequently,

(a)

(b)

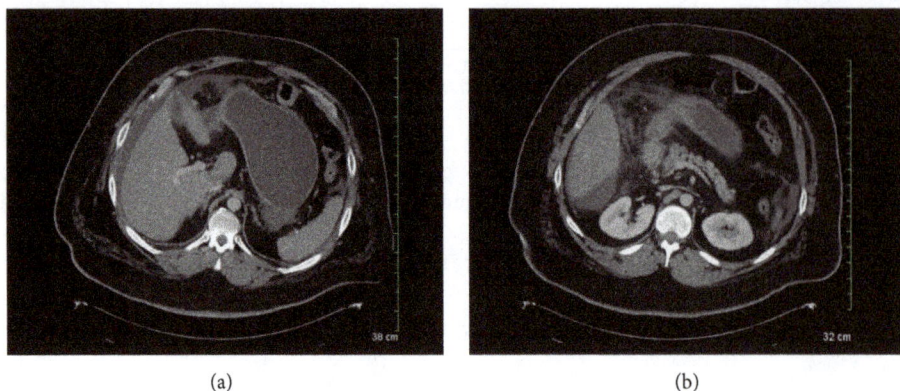

FIGURE 2: CT demonstrating a distended excluded stomach with perigastric and perihepatic ascites in the absence of pneumoperitoneum and an edematous duodenum with adjacent fat stranding.

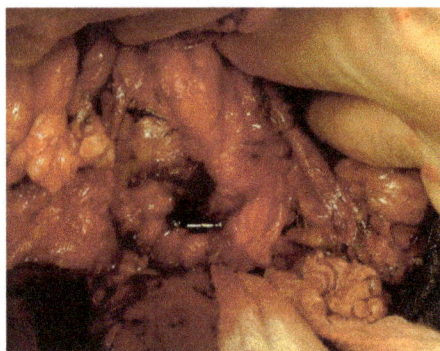

FIGURE 3: Duodenal defect with bile pooling within defect.

the tubes were clamped and a HIDA scan revealed preferential flow of bile into the duodenum and none into the fistula. The tubes were removed and the patient has been doing well since.

4. Discussion

Diagnosing a perforated duodenal ulcer in a patient following a gastric bypass procedure can be challenging. In a patient who had a prior gastric bypass with acute onset of pain and an acute abdomen, exploration is warranted. However, in a hemodynamically stable patient without peritonitis, imaging provides valuable information in planning operative or nonoperative management. Typically, pneumoperitoneum is absent on radiographs because ingested air would preferentially flow through the gastrojejunostomy rather than retrograde into the biliopancreatic limb. In reviewing the literature there is only one patient where pneumoperitoneum was found on radiologic assessment [3]. In all other patients, the radiographs failed to demonstrate free air. Computed tomography (CT) scan is the most accurate test in making the diagnosing of perforation of the excluded stomach or biliopancreatic limb. The CT scan images will demonstrate free peritoneal fluid, with an inflammatory process in the

right upper quadrant. Usually, there will not be any pneumoperitoneum or extravasation of oral contrast. In addition the CT scan will help identify other possible causes of the acute surgical abdomen in a patient after RYGB such as internal herniation (Figure 1).

Several mechanisms have been proposed to explain the pathophysiology of peptic ulcer disease in the excluded stomach and small bowel. *Helicobacter pylori* has been clearly implicated in the formation of ulcers in the gastric bypass population by weakening the mucosal protective barriers [9]. Mucosal injury could also result from the ingestion of nonsteroidal anti-inflammatory drugs (NSAIDs) or excessive alcohol consumption. In the current cases, both *H. Pylori* and NSAIDs were noncontributory but in the second case the consumption of excessive alcohol may have been a factor in the ulcer formation. Bjorkman suggested another mechanism of injury [4]. He postulated that acid produced in the excluded stomach is not neutralized by food as would usually happen in normal anatomy. Moreover, a delay in the release of pancreatic bicarbonate can allow the mucosa to be exposed to the gastric acid for a prolonged period of time. At the same time bile reflux can also damage the mucosa, compounding the effects of the unbuffered acid.

The surgical treatment of perforated duodenal ulcers consists of first the urgent treatment and potentially a more definitive surgical approach. The urgent treatment is usually closure of the defect with an omental patch either through an open or laparoscopic approach. The laparoscopic approach has been shown to be safe in the treatment of perforated marginal ulcers in RYGP patients [10]. A vital question in the treatment of perforated duodenal ulcers in RYGB patients is whether definitive surgery, with completion gastrectomy, is indicated. Resection of the bypassed stomach would lead to a decrease in acid production by eliminating antral gastric secretion. It can also avoid the formation of gastro-gastric fistulae and eliminates the difficult problems of having to access the gastric remnant such as in the case of a bleeding ulcer [8]. However, resection of the excluded stomach is not without consequences and prolongs the operative time. Short term sequelae include duodenal stump leakage and bleeding, and bacterial overgrowth in the biliopancreatic limb and metabolic derangements such as vitamin B 12 deficiency can be seen in the long term [8]. Because of the rarity of this complication and the consequent absence of adequate data, the decision to proceed with a definitive surgical treatment should be based on the particular risks and benefits for each patient. In patients with high operative risk such as case 2, long term PPI therapy is a reasonable alternative.

5. Conclusion

Perforated duodenal ulcers following RYGB are rare events and may present a diagnostic challenge as they almost never lead to the formation of free air. Even in the absence of laboratory abnormalities, a high index of suspicion should be maintained, as the presence of free fluid on CT scan may be the only radiologic finding. Surgical exploration remains the mainstay of diagnosis and treatment of acute abdominal pain in RYGB patients. Patients with perforated duodenal ulcers treated with closure in the emergency setting may benefit from resection of the gastric remnant to prevent recurrences but will need to stay on long term PPI therapy.

References

[1] M. Eidy, A. Pazouki, F. Raygan, Y. Ariyazand, M. Pishgahroudsari, and F. Jesmi, "Functional abdominal pain syndrome in morbidly obese patients following laparoscopic gastric bypass surgery," *Archives of Trauma Research*, vol. 3, no. 1, Article ID e13110, 2014.

[2] E. E. Moore, C. Buerk, and G. Moore, "Gastric bypass operation for the treatment of morbid obesity," *Surgery Gynecology & Obstetrics*, vol. 148, no. 5, pp. 764–765, 1979.

[3] I. Charuzi, A. Ovrat, J. Peiser, E. Avinoah, and J. Lichtman, "Perforation of duodenal ulcer following gastric exclusion operation for morbid obesity," *Journal of Clinical Gastroenterology*, vol. 8, no. 5, pp. 605–606, 1986.

[4] D. J. Bjorkman, J. R. Alexander, and M. A. Simons, "Perforated duodenal ulcer after gastric bypass surgery," *The American Journal of Gastroenterology*, vol. 84, no. 2, pp. 170–172, 1989.

[5] A. M. C. Macgregor, N. E. Pickens, and E. K. Thoburn, "Perforated peptic ulcer following gastric bypass for obesity," *The American Surgeon*, vol. 65, no. 3, pp. 222–225, 1999.

[6] R. Mittermair and O. Renz, "An unusual complication of gastric bypass: perforated duodenal ulcer," *Obesity Surgery*, vol. 17, no. 5, pp. 701–703, 2007.

[7] J. M. Snyder, "Peptic ulcer following gastric bypass," *Obesity Surgery*, vol. 17, no. 10, p. 1419, 2007.

[8] B. J. Gypen, G. J. A. Hubens, V. Hartman, L. Balliu, T. C. G. Chapelle, and W. Vaneerdeweg, "Perforated duodenal ulcer after laparoscopic gastric bypass," *Obesity Surgery*, vol. 18, no. 12, pp. 1644–1646, 2008.

[9] I. G. M. Cleator, A. Rae, C. L. Birmingham, and E. E. Mason, "Ulcerogenesis following gastric procedures for obesity," *Obesity Surgery*, vol. 6, no. 3, pp. 260–261, 1996.

[10] M. R. Wendling, J. G. Linn, K. M. Keplinger et al., "Omental patch repair effectively treats perforated marginal ulcer following Roux-en-Y gastric bypass," *Surgical Endoscopy and Other Interventional Techniques*, vol. 27, no. 2, pp. 384–389, 2013.

10

Developmentally Delayed Male with Mincer Blade Obstructing the Oesophagus for a Period of Time Suspected to Be 6 Months

Christian Grønhøj Larsen and Birgitte Charabi

Department of Otorhinolaryngology, Head and Neck Surgery and Audiology, Copenhagen University Hospital (Rigshospitalet), 2100 Copenhagen, Denmark

Correspondence should be addressed to Christian Grønhøj Larsen; c.gronhoj@gmail.com

Academic Editor: Marcello Picchio

Introduction. Sharp, retained foreign bodies in the oesophagus are associated with severe complications. Developmentally delayed patients are especially subject to foreign objects. We describe a 37-year-old, developmentally delayed male with a mincer blade obstructing the oesophagus. Six months prior to surgical intervention, the patient was hospitalized in a condition of sepsis and pneumonia where the thoracic X-ray reveals a foreign body in the proximal oesophagus. When rehospitalized 6 months later, a mincer blade of the type used in immersion blenders was surgically removed. During these 6 months the patient's main symptoms were dysphagia, weight loss, and diarrhoea. When developmentally delayed patients present with dysphagia, we strongly encourage the awareness of the possible presence of foreign bodies. To our knowledge this is the first reported case of a mincer blade in the oesophagus.

1. Introduction

Chronically retained foreign bodies (FBs) are common in children but rare in adults [1, 2]. For developmentally delayed adults, especially those in the subgroup with pica, FBs can not only be the cause of severe morbidity such as obstruction, bleeding, and perforation but also be lethal because the patient's inability to communicate the symptoms makes it difficult to arrive at an accurate diagnosis. Ingestion of a sharp FB is associated with a high risk of morbidity as a result of the possible perforation of the gastrointestinal tract. Early diagnosis and adequate management are imperative for the prevention of serious complications.

2. Case Report

A 37-year-old male with the mental age of a 1-year-old was referred to our department. Six months earlier, the patient had been admitted to a neighbouring hospital with aspiration pneumonia in a condition of sepsis and complaining of dysphagia. A chest X-ray was performed (Figure 1). The patient was treated with antibiotics and discharged on the 23th day, returning to his nursing home in good clinical condition, but with the dysphagia unchanged. During the 6 months following his initial hospitalization the patient's loss of 20 kilograms, persistent diarrhoea, and aversion to solid foods led to his readmittance. Because of the severe dysphagia the patient was referred to the local ear, nose, and throat department, where a cervical X-ray (Figure 2) visualized a FB. Oesophagoscopy revealed a shiny, asymmetric, metallic structure located in the proximal oesophagus. Despite several attempts, the object was not retractable. Therefore, open oesophagotomy was performed on level C4-C5, revealing severe inflammation and fibrosis in the tissue surrounding the oesophagus. After access to the oesophageal lumen was attained, a mincer blade of the type used in immersion blenders was surgically removed (Figure 3). The blades of the mincer had penetrated all layers of the oesophagus. After removal of the blade, direct suture without reinforcements was performed to close the oesophagus. The patient was treated with antibiotics, received parenteral nutrition for 7 days, and was discharged on the 10th day. Staff at the nursing home where the patient resides recalled that a mincer blade had gone missing.

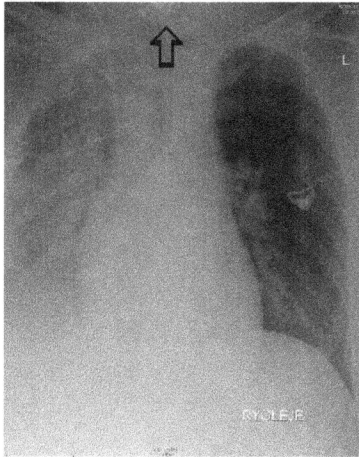

FIGURE 1: Chest X-ray 6 months prior to admittance to our department. Severe right-sided pneumonia and a suspected foreign object in the oesophagus.

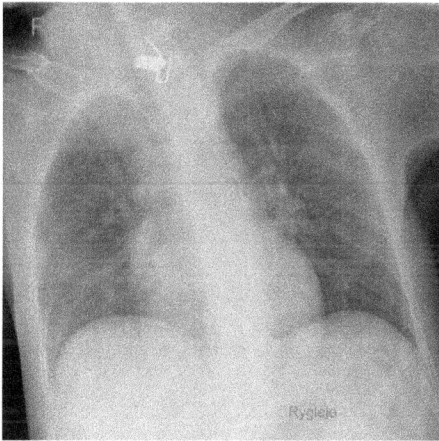

FIGURE 2: Chest X-ray.

3. Discussion

Developmentally delayed persons with pica are especially subject to FBs in the oesophagus [3]. Objects often impact here because of the passive, distensible, and accommodating nature of the organ. Our report documents the case of a developmentally delayed male with a mincer blade lodged in the proximal oesophagus. When assessing the thoracic X-ray 6 months prior to admittance it is likely that the object was visible in the top edge of the picture with the characteristic asymmetric sharp edges of the mincer pointing out (Figure 1). This might explain the patient's symptoms of prolonged dysphagia, weight loss, and diarrhoea.

Similar cases of chronically retained FBs have been reported with successful outcomes, [1, 4, 5] although most objects usually pass spontaneously, and less than 1% need surgical removal [4]. Early diagnosis and management might prevent the serious complications of penetration, infection, and necrosis [6]. When FBs are suspected, the appropriate diagnostic approach should be biplane X-rays, which reveal

the location, size, and shape of possible objects, alternatively a CT scan of the esophagus [5]. Direct vision such as oesophagoscopy or laryngoscopic-aided views are highly useful means of obtaining additional diagnostic information. Moreover, endoscopy may also provide the treatment as many objects can be extracted endoscopically [7]. Migratory oesophageal FBs are particularly rare [1].

Sharp objects most commonly lodge at the upper level of the oesophagus due to penetration into the upper oesophageal sphincter. Whenever possible, FBs in the oesophagus should be sought and removed endoscopically [5]; however, if surgical removal is unavoidable, it must be performed without delay, in order to avoid potentially severe complications, such as mediastinitis, fistula, pneumothorax, respiratory distress, retropharyngeal abscess, and stricture. Nonsharp objects lodged in the oesophagus for more than 24 hours should also be removed endoscopically. However, if they remain for more than a week, there is significant risk of erosion into surrounding structures, and surgical backup should always be available [1, 5].

When dealing with the severely mentally retarded group of patients, common symptoms such as dysphagia, odynophagia, coughing, choking, and haematemesis may be compromised. For this reason, information about the patient's general condition, appetite, and bowel habits is vital. If the general condition of a patient with these symptoms worsens and persists over a long period of time, FBs should always be considered and biplane X-rays of the upper oesophagus must be performed without delay [8].

Earlier cases of oesophageal FBs involving developmentally challenged individuals have included impacted dentures [3], coins [9], and food items, but this is the first reported case of a mincer blade from an immersion blender lodging in the oesophagus.

A thorough elucidation of developmentally delayed patients with dysphagia is imperative, and the presence of foreign objects in the pharynx, oesophagus, or intestine must always be considered when such patients present with a declining general condition, reduced appetite, abnormal bowel movements, or dysphagia. Biplane X-rays of the oesophagus and endoscopy should be performed initially and, particularly in cases involving sharp FBs, surgery must not be delayed.

4. Conclusion

We know the following:

(i) The elucidation of developmentally delayed patients is difficult.

(ii) This specific patient-population is especially subject to foreign bodies in the oesophagus.

This study adds the following:

(i) When developmentally delayed patients present with dysphagia, altered bowel movements, and declining general condition, foreign bodies must be considered.

(ii) Biplane X-rays and endoscopy are vital initial steps.

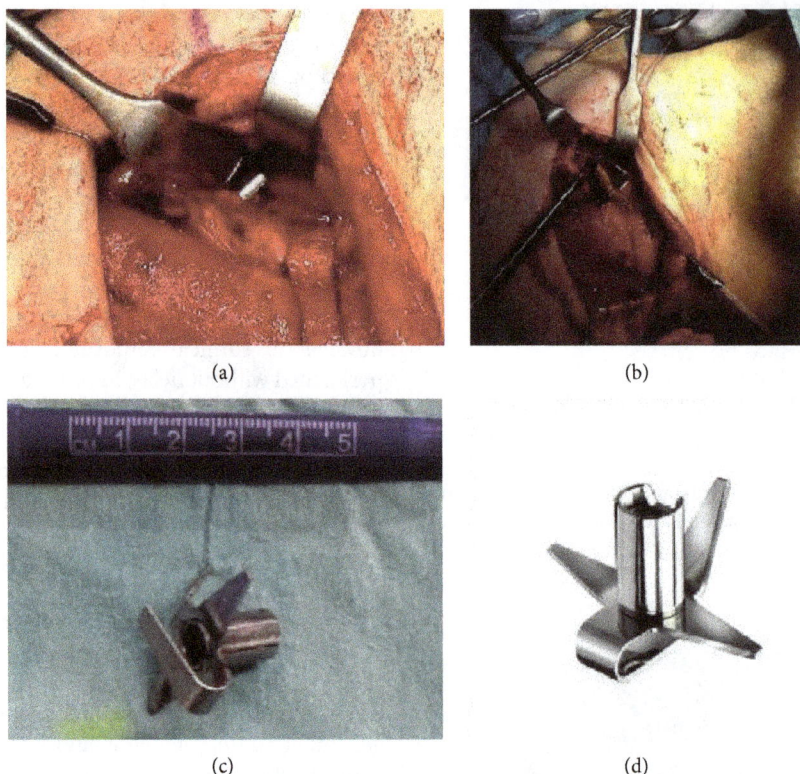

(a)

(b)

(c)

(d)

FIGURE 3: (a, b, c) Perioperative image, (d) Bamix, Mézières, Schweiz.

Authors' Contribution

All authors provided conceptual input and contributed in significant ways to the final paper.

Acknowledgments

Christian Grønhøj Larsen is funded by the Candy Foundation and Kræftfonden (Cancer Foundation).

References

[1] M. K. Chen and E. A. Beierle, "Gastrointestinal foreign bodies," *Pediatric Annals*, vol. 30, no. 12, pp. 736–742, 2001.

[2] R. Byaruhanga, E. Kakande, and T. Mwambu, "A rare case of a patient with a foreign body in the esophagus for two years which perforated into the mediastinum," *African Health Sciences*, vol. 12, no. 4, pp. 569–571, 2012.

[3] M. J. Lee, "Delayed diagnosis of impacted partial denture in a patient with mental retardation," *Singapore Medical Journal*, vol. 54, no. 9, pp. e190–e192, 2013.

[4] F. R. Mallick, R. S. Sahota, M. D. Elloy, and P. J. Conboy, "A rare case of foreign body impaction requiring oesophagotomy," *Annals of the Royal College of Surgeons of England*, vol. 96, no. 5, pp. e11–e13, 2014.

[5] H. Rodriguez, G. C. Passali, D. Gregori et al., "Management of foreign bodies in the airway and oesophagus," *International Journal of Pediatric Otorhinolaryngology*, vol. 76, supplement 1, pp. S84–S91, 2012.

[6] B. Sahn, P. Mamula, and C. A. Ford, "Review of foreign body ingestion and esophageal food impaction management in adolescents," *Journal of Adolescent Health*, vol. 55, no. 2, pp. 260–266, 2014.

[7] C. Sugawa, H. Ono, M. Taleb, and C. E. Lucas, "Endoscopic management of foreign bodies in the upper gastrointestinal tract: a review," *World Journal of Gastrointestinal Endoscopy*, vol. 6, pp. 475–481, 2014.

[8] G. M. Eisen, T. H. Baron, J. Dominitz et al., "Guideline for the management of ingested foreign bodies," *Gastrointestinal Endoscopy*, vol. 55, pp. 802–806, 2002.

[9] S. K. Dutta, S. N. Ghosh, D. M. Munsi, and P. S. Giri, "Growth retardation due to undiagnosed foreign body oesophagus," *Indian Journal of Otolaryngology and Head and Neck Surgery*, vol. 57, no. 2, pp. 162–163, 2005.

11

Laparoscopic Repair of a Large Duodenal Perforation Secondary to an Indwelling Nasogastric Tube in a Tracheotomized Adult

Sanoop Koshy Zachariah

Department of General, Laparoscopic and Gastrointestinal Surgery, MOSC Medical College Kolenchery, Cochin 682311, India

Correspondence should be addressed to Sanoop Koshy Zachariah; skzach@yahoo.com

Academic Editors: P. De Nardi, T. Hotta, and S.-i. Kosugi

Laparoscopic repair of perforated duodenal ulcers is safe and effective in centers with experience and increasingly performed by laparoscopic surgeons. However, the role of laparoscopy for the management of large duodenal perforations (>1 cm) is unclear. To date, no experience has been reported with emergency laparoscopic repair of large perforations for gastroduodenal ulcers. The commonest reason for conversion to open surgery is a perforation size of more than 1 cm. This paper reports a case of a large duodenal perforation due to a nasogastric tube in a 26-year-old male who had undergone a tracheostomy, following a cut-throat injury. This large perforation was successfully diagnosed and repaired laparoscopically. This is probably the first paper in the English literature to report duodenal perforation due to a nasogastric tube in an adult and also the first report of a successful laparoscopic repair of a large duodenal perforation.

1. Introduction

Laparoscopic repair of perforated duodenal ulcers is safe and effective in centers with experience and increasingly performed by laparoscopic surgeons. However, based on the existing literature, it is uncertain whether large duodenal perforations have been managed laparoscopically. Studies have shown that the commonest reasons for conversion from laparoscopic to open surgery is the finding of a large perforation (>1 cm) [1]. A consensus conference recently reported that laparoscopic repair of perforated gastric and duodenal ulcers is safe and effective in centers with experience, and to date no experience has been reported with emergency laparoscopic repair of large perforations [2]. In all these studies analyzed for the laparoscopic technique, the patients had small ulcers (mean diameter of 1 cm) and all the patients received simple suture, mostly with omental patch, or sutureless repair.

Duodenal perforations due to nasoenteral tubes are a recognized complication in pediatric patients [3, 4]. The present paper reports a case of a large duodenal perforation in a tracheotomiced adult, caused by an indwelling feeding nasogastric tube, which was managed laparoscopically. The

paper discusses the potential complications of gastrointestinal intubation and also diagnostic role of laparoscopy in such situations and its possibility in management of large duodenal perforations.

2. Case Report and Operative Technique

A 26-year-old male had sustained a partial transverse tracheal transection following a cut-throat assault using a knife. There were no other significant findings on clinical examination and the abdomen appeared to be normal. The patient was initially managed by the "otorhinolaryngology team." He underwent a neck exploration, followed by a primary suture repair of tracheal transection and a tracheostomy was also performed. A flexible polyvinyl nasogastric tube (14 Fr) was instituted for the purpose of enteral feeding. The patient also received intravenous antibiotics and proton pump inhibitors. The patient received feeds and seemed to be recuperating well until on the fifth POD (postoperative day) when he developed severe upper abdominal pain and distension with clinical features of peritonitis. The patient had no previous history suggestive of acid peptic disease. Laboratory investigations revealed borderline leucocytosis with elevated polymorphs, normal serum amylase, and lipase values. Plain erect abdominal radiograph was inconclusive. Ultrasonography revealed moderate intraperitoneal free fluid with dilated bowel loops. The patient was taken up for emergency diagnostic laparoscopy under general anesthesia.

The open technique of laparoscopic access was used. Three ports, namely, a 10 mm (umbilical port for the 30° videoscope) and two 5 mm ports in the right and left midclavicular line were used (working instruments). Laparoscopic evaluation revealed purulent peritonitis with the omentum localized over the first part of the duodenum and in the vicinity of the gall bladder. On lifting off the omentum, the nasogastric tube was seen perforating and protruding out from the first part of the duodenum and impacting on to the gall bladder (Figure 1). The perforation was 2 cm in diameter (Figure 2). Laparoscopic intracorporeal suturing and knotting was done for closure of the perforation using three interrupted 2-0 absorbable (polyglactin 910) sutures. The bites were taken 1 cm from the edge of the ulcer. The middle suture was tied first, followed successively by the upper and lower sutures and this was reinforced by an onlay omental pedicle (Figures 3(a) and 3(b)). The integrity of the repair was confirmed by the "tire test" (air insufflation via the NG tube). Blood loss was minimal. The operating time was 90 minutes. The postoperative period was uneventful. Bowel sounds were evident from the 2nd postoperative day and the patient was started on oral fluids by the 3rd POD and discharged on the 10th POD. An upper GI endoscopy 5 weeks later confirmed that perforation had healed well. The patient had been on regular followup for up to 10 months.

3. Discussion

3.1. Nasoenteral Tubes and Duodenal Perforation. The insertion of a nasogastric tube is a common clinical procedure which is relatively simple and safe. Nevertheless, various unexpected and potentially lethal complications have been reported [5]. The reported complication rates are between 0.3% and 15%. Duodenal perforations due to nasoenteral tubes have been reported to occur in the pediatric patients. It is postulated that the peristaltic activity propels the tube along the relatively rigid duodenal loop. In adults, endoscopic guided duodenal tube (postpyloric feeding) placements are known to be associated with complications such as bleeding and duodenal perforation [6]. This is probably the first case in the literature to report duodenal perforation due to nasogastric tube (NGT) in an adult. In this patient the NGT would have migrated further down beyond the pylorus. The initial clinical suspicion was the probability of perforated stress ulcer. Stress ulcers are known to occur in critically ill patients. Perforation due to stress ulcers is rare, occurring in less than 1% of surgical ICU patients [7]. The other possibility could be that the NG tube would have just found its way out through an already perforated stress/peptic ulcer. In either case if it had remained there for a longer time, it could have possibly migrated into the gall bladder, thereby making the situation even more hazardous. In order to prevent such serious complications, various methods of confirming proper placement of the nasogastric tube have been described and studied [8].

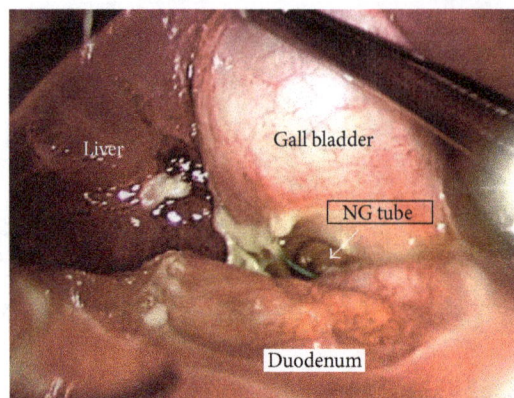

FIGURE 1: The nasogastric (NG) tube (white arrow) can be seen perforating the duodenum and impacting on the gall bladder.

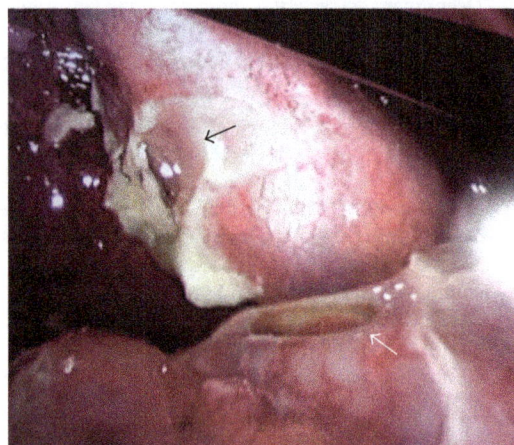

FIGURE 2: The large duodenal perforation (white arrow) is clearly seen after withdrawing the NG tube. The site of impaction of the NG tube on the gall bladder is also seen (black arrow).

3.2. Laparoscopic Repair of Duodenal Perforations. Laparoscopic repair of duodenal perforations has been studied extensively with respect to perforated duodenal ulcers. Various studies including the LAMA (*LAparoscopische MAagperforatie*) trial have shown that the laparoscopic repair of peptic ulcer perforations is feasible, safe and associated with lesser postoperative pain, lower median hospital stay, earlier return to normal activity, and better cosmesis [9, 10].

The commonly encountered duodenal ulcer perforations are 1 cm or smaller, and these perforations are the easiest to repair either by open or laparoscopic techniques when compared to larger perforations. The outcome in this subset is also better. However there has been some confusion regarding categorizing duodenal perforations based on their size. The term "giant perforations" has been randomly used by various authors to describe the size of perforations ranging anywhere between 0.5 cm to 2.5 cm. A more meaningful classification based on the size of perforations has been suggested by Gupta et al. [11]. Accordingly, duodenal perforations can be classified into three main groups: *small* perforations that are less than 1 cm in size, *large* perforations that have a size between 1 cm and 3 cm, and *giant* perforations that exceed 3 cm size.

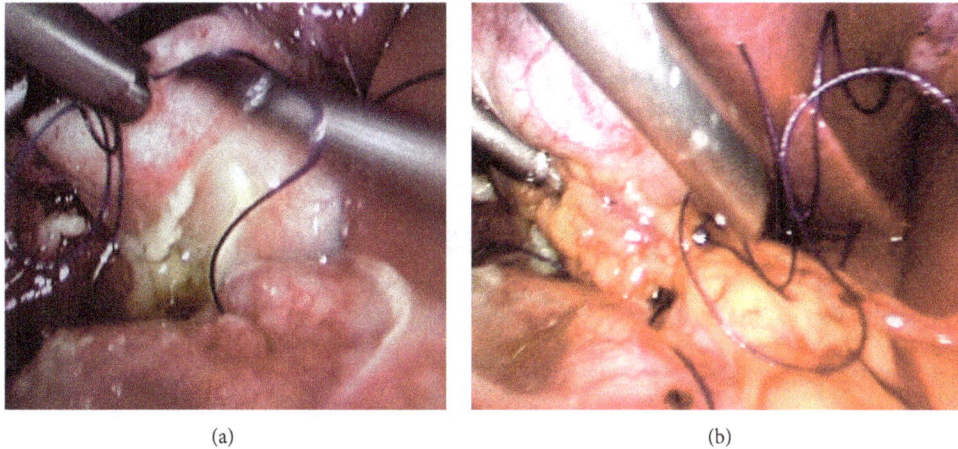

(a) (b)

FIGURE 3: Repair of the large ulcer by primary suture (a) followed by onlay pedicled omentoplasty (b).

Bertleff and Lange [1] in their review opined that in case of suspected perforated peptic ulcer, laparoscopy should be advocated as diagnostic and therapeutic tool as there is a notable difference in morbidity (14.35 in laparoscopic group versus 26.9% in open group) and mortality (3.6% versus 6.4%). The overall conversion rate is around 12.4% (range 0–28.5%). The most common reason for conversion was the size of the perforation (often >10 mm), but by using a pedicled omentoplasty, size of the perforation might not necessarily be a reason to convert any longer.

In the present case, laparoscopic primary suture closure followed by onlay pedicled omentoplasty was used to repair the large perforation. However certain aspects need mentioning. Here it is felt that the perforation was not due to a duodenal ulcer and that is probably the reason why the edges were not friable and the sutures could be easily placed without the risk of tearing or cutting through. Moreover this was a young patient (with no known previous major medical illness) and the surgical treatment was accomplished before 24 hours after the onset of symptoms. In the present case, the patient was already on antibiotics, and this would have reduced the local inflammation and sepsis thereby making the procedure simpler. Therefore it is not certain whether the same technique could be replicated in case of a large duodenal ulcer perforation with greatly inflamed and friable margins. In such cases it would probably make sense to use a laparoscopic omental plug or laparoscopic version of a Cellan-Jones repair (suturing pedicled omentum on top of perforation without primary suture closure) or even convert to an open procedure which would probably require resective gastroduodenal surgery based on the surgeon's decision at that time. The factors associated with adverse outcomes after peptic ulcer perforations include older age, associated major medical illness, perforations of >24 hours duration, and delay in surgery beyond >12 hours after onset of symptoms [12, 13]. The lack of these adverse factors probably worked in favor of this patient. Therefore at present there is no strong evidence to support the role of laparoscopic technique for closure of large duodenal perforations. The probable argument would be that even with open surgery larger ulcers are more difficult

to repair and the outcomes in this subset are poorer. Laparoscopic suture repair is more technically demanding and hence various novel methods are being developed to replace sutures for perforation closure. Nevertheless this paper illustrates the possibility of safe laparoscopic repair of large duodenal perforation.

4. Conclusions

Duodenal perforation secondary to nasogastric tubes is a rare complication in adults. Increasing awareness of potential complications associated with the insertion and maintenance of nasogastric tubes will facilitate early diagnosis and treatment. Laparoscopy is useful in the diagnosis and treatment of duodenal perforations and may be feasible for repairing large duodenal perforations. However, further research is needed to confirm the true benefits of laparoscopic repair for large or giant duodenal perforations.

References

[1] M. J. Bertleff and J. F. Lange, "Laparoscopic correction of perforated peptic ulcer: first choice? A review of literature," *Surgical Endoscopy and Other Interventional Techniques*, vol. 24, no. 6, pp. 1231–1239, 2010.

[2] M. Sartelli, P. Viale, K. Koike et al., "WSES consensus conference: guidelines for first-line management of intra-abdominal infections," *World Journal of Emergency Surgery*, vol. 6, no. 1, article 2, 2011.

[3] J. C. Flores, J. López-Herce, I. Sola, and A. Carrillo, "Duodenal perforation caused by a transpyloric tube in a critically ill infant," *Nutrition*, vol. 22, no. 2, pp. 209–212, 2006.

[4] S. Agarwala, S. Dave, A. K. Gupta, and D. K. Mitra, "Duodenorenal fistula due to a nasogastric tube in a neonate," *Pediatric Surgery International*, vol. 14, no. 1-2, pp. 102–103, 1998.

[5] J. B. Pillai, A. Vegas, and S. Brister, "Thoracic complications of nasogastric tube: review of safe practice," *Interactive Cardiovascular and Thoracic Surgery*, vol. 4, no. 5, pp. 429–433, 2005.

[6] T. D. Chou, S. T. Ue, C. H. Lee, T. W. Lee, T. M. Chen, and H. J. Wang, "Duodenal perforation as a complication of routine endoscopic nasoenteral feeding tube placement," *Burns*, vol. 25, no. 1, pp. 86–87, 1999.

[7] G. G. Tsiotos, C. J. Mullany, S. Zietlow, and J. A. van Heerden, "Abdominal complications following cardiac surgery," *The American Journal of Surgery*, vol. 167, no. 6, pp. 553–557, 1994.

[8] A. M. Gharib, E. J. Stern, V. L. Sherbin, and C. A. Rohrmann, "Nasogastric and feeding tubes: the importance of proper placement," *Postgraduate Medicine*, vol. 99, no. 5, pp. 165–176, 1996.

[9] M. J. O. E. Bertleff, J. A. Halm, W. A. Bemelman et al., "Randomized clinical trial of laparoscopic versus open repair of the perforated peptic ulcer: the LAMA trial," *World Journal of Surgery*, vol. 33, no. 7, pp. 1368–1373, 2009.

[10] S. Sauerland, F. Agresta, R. Bergamaschi et al., "Laparoscopy for abdominal emergencies: evidence-based guidelines of the European Association for Endoscopic Surgery," *Surgical Endoscopy and Other Interventional Techniques*, vol. 20, no. 1, pp. 14–29, 2006.

[11] S. Gupta, R. Kaushik, R. Sharma, and A. Attri, "The management of large perforations of duodenal ulcers," *BMC Surgery*, vol. 5, pp. 15–19, 2005.

[12] J. Boey, N. W. Lee, J. Koo, P. H. Lam, J. Wong, and G. B. Ong, "Immediate definitive surgery for perforated duodenal ulcers: a prospective controlled trial," *Annals of Surgery*, vol. 196, no. 3, pp. 338–344, 1982.

[13] T. J. Crofts, K. G. Park, R. J. Steele, S. S. Chung, and A. K. Li, "A randomized trial of nonoperative treatment for perforated peptic ulcer," *The New England Journal of Medicine*, vol. 320, no. 15, pp. 970–973, 1989.

12

A Challenging Case of a Large Gastroduodenal Artery Pseudoaneurysm after Surgery of a Peptic Ulcer

Rocio Santos-Rancaño,[1] Esteban Martín Antona,[1] and José Vicente Méndez Montero[2]

[1]*Division of Hepatobiliopancreatic Surgery, Department of General Surgery, San Carlos Clinic Hospital of Madrid, Madrid, Spain*
[2]*Unit of Abdomen Imaging Diagnosis and Interventional Radiology, Department of Radiology and Imaging, San Carlos Clinic Hospital of Madrid, Madrid, Spain*

Correspondence should be addressed to Rocio Santos-Rancaño; rociosantosr@hotmail.com

Academic Editor: Muthukumaran Rangarajan

We report a 48-year-old man in whom a chronic postbulbar duodenal ulcer destroyed much of the back wall of the duodenum and gastroduodenal artery causing pseudoaneurysm. The lesion was found and evaluated by contrast-enhanced computed tomography (that revealed a large pseudoaneurysm of 83 mm × 75 mm in diameter) and by angiography and then treated with transcatheter embolization leading to a complete resolution of the lesion. The case is rare and important for several reasons. First, we demonstrate that pseudoaneurysm of the gastroduodenal artery caused by a duodenal ulcer can occur and present a diagnostic challenge (as far as we know, only three cases have been reported previously in the literature). Second, this case report focuses on the importance of ligation of the gastroduodenal artery when bleeding of peptic ulcers occurs. Additionally, we present an overview of the relevant literature.

1. Introduction

Pseudoaneurysms of the gastroduodenal artery are very rare (less than 50 cases reported; 0.01%–0.2% of the autopsies) with the splenic artery being the most common vessel. In addition, their incidence is probably underreported in the literature [1]. They occur as critical complications following pancreatitis and much rarer after gastric or pancreatic surgery or trauma [2]. They are serious because they may be difficult to diagnose and because they may become a life threatening condition if they get ruptured. Therefore, early diagnosis and adequate therapeutic interventions are imperative. At present, the selective embolization of pseudoaneurysms provides a noninvasive tool to manage a disorder that used to be managed by surgery, with a significant reduction of morbi-mortality.

Herewith we present a challenging case of a 48-year-old man in whom a chronic postbulbar duodenal ulcer eroded gastroduodenal artery causing a giant pseudoaneurysm that was treated with transcatheter embolization leading to a complete resolution of the lesion.

2. Case Report

A 48-year-old male patient was admitted to the hospital for hematemesis and melena. His past medical history included chronic alcohol abuse, intense smoking habit, chronic antral gastritis due to *Helicobacter pylori* that had not been eradicated, and longstanding epigastric pain treated with proton pump inhibitors.

The patient was lucid, but anemic, with a fine radial pulse of 120 beats per minute and a blood pressure of 60/40 mm Hg. The abdominal examination showed no elements suggesting peritoneal irritation.

On initial presentation, his hemoglobin level was 7.0 g/dL so the patient management began with the transfusion of two packed red cells and intravenous fluids and posteriorly a gastroscopy was performed revealing a posterior bulbar ulcer of 15 mm, with blood oozing. Hemostasis was achieved using 1/10,000 adrenaline. But the ulcer continued bleeding and, after assuring it was not safe to repeat the sclerosis, we decided to perform an urgent duodenotomy, suture of the penetrated ulcer in the posterior wall and Graham patch.

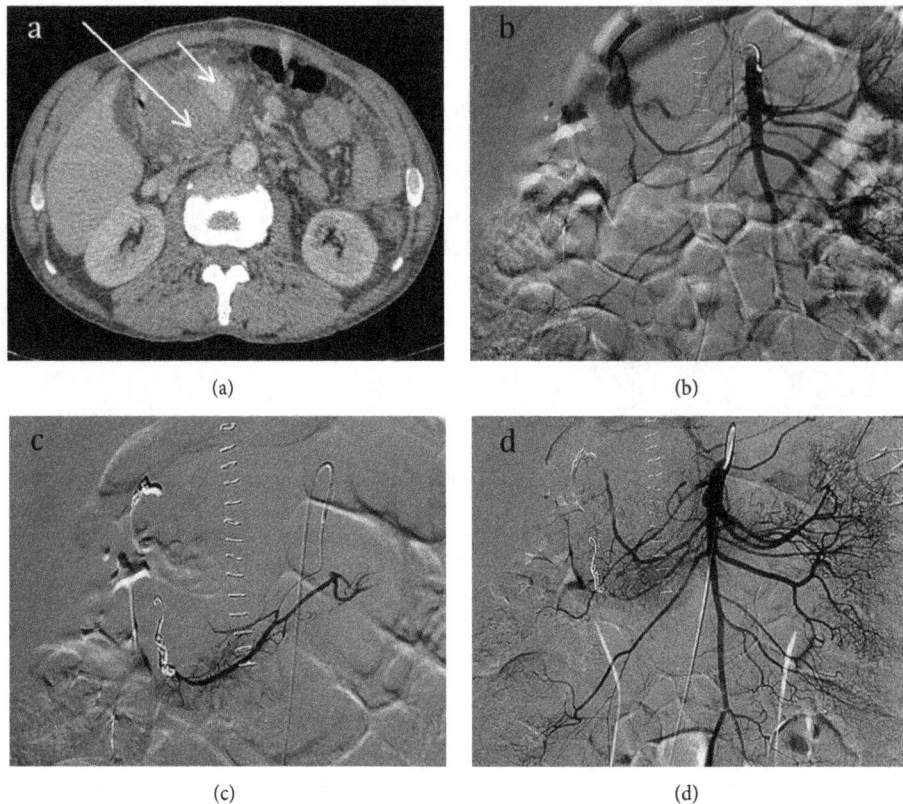

(a)

(b)

(c)

(d)

FIGURE 1: (a) Contrast-enhanced axial CT image shows a giant pseudoaneurysm of 8.3 × 7.5 cm in size originating from the gastroduodenal artery (long arrow). The intravenous contrast showed filling of the mass, certifying its vascular origin (short arrow). (b) Aortography shows the blood circulation of the aneurysm in continuity with the gastroduodenal artery. (c) Angiogram after selective coil-embolization of the gastroduodenal artery through the celiac trunk and the inferior pancreaticoduodenal artery, through the superior mesenteric artery. (d) Angiographic control confirmed the complete exclusion of the pseudoaneurysm.

Due to placement of the ulcer and the inflammation of the tissues around, the gastroduodenal artery was not ligated. The patient developed well and was discharged 6 days after. But he presented again to our hospital two days after with a history of persistent epigastric pain associated. He was afebrile and hemodynamically stable; moreover, physical examination revealed a palpable beating mass in the epigastrium.

The contrast-enhanced CT scan documented the presence of a large (8.3 × 7.5 cm) pseudoaneurysm of the gastroduodenal artery supplied by the superior mesenteric artery.

Selective arterial embolization through a femoral approach was successfully performed to treat the pseudoaneurysm. We decided to occlude the gastroduodenal artery first to stop the backflow into the pseudoaneurysm and it was embolized with two 3 mm × 4 cm coils. Subsequently, the inferior pancreaticoduodenal artery was embolized with two 3 mm × 5 cm coils through the superior mesenteric artery. An angiographic control uncovered a marginal filling of the pseudoaneurysm and an additional embolization using the liquid embolic agent lipiodol/ethibloc mixture was performed. Angiographic control confirmed the complete exclusion of the pseudoaneurysm (Figure 1).

The patient's hospital stay was uneventful and he could be discharged after 4 days without any signs of bleeding or

intestinal ischemia. A contrast-enhanced follow-up CT scan (4 weeks after embolization) showed the pseudoaneurysm excluded completely and no changes in its size, which was still thrombosed by the coils.

3. Discussion

Pseudoaneurysms represent contained ruptures after injury to one or more layers of a vascular wall. Most of them are a consequence of pancreatitis, much rarer after operative trauma or Whipple procedure, where an enzymatic leak from the pancreaticojejunostomy reconstruction may occasionally lead to breakdown of the ligature on the GDA stump, leading to catastrophic hemorrhage.

In our case a chronic postbulbar duodenal ulcer destroyed much of the back wall of the duodenum, which eroded gastroduodenal artery causing a giant pseudoaneurysm of 8.3 mm × 7.5 mm in diameter. To the best of our knowledge, only three cases have been reported previously in the literature.

The potential for rapid growth and high mortality rates associated with a false aneurysm rupture (up to 100%) emphasizes the importance of early diagnosis and treatment, as in our case [3]. The risk of rupture is not dependent on the size of the aneurysm. Hence, it is advocated that all gastroduodenal artery aneurysms, regardless of size, be treated actively at the time of the diagnosis.

CT is an excellent modality and demonstrates the features of pseudoaneurysm in the majority of cases in the initial differential diagnosis. Angiography also plays a critical role and is considered the gold standard for diagnosis of aneurysms in the peripancreatic vessels [4].

Conservative management of pseudoaneurysms is burdened by a death rate of more than 90%. Endovascular therapies are often favored over surgery, given their less invasive approach, its efficacy rate ranges from 70 to 100% and they have a lower rate of morbimortality. Embolization is done with coils or using percutaneous or endoscopic ultrasound guided thrombin injection [5], as in the present case where the occlusion of the pseudoaneurysm was achieved by filling it with numerous coils and finally with a mixture of ethibloc/lipiodol.

We highlight the importance of this case in several aspects. First, we demonstrate that pseudoaneurysm of the gastroduodenal artery caused by a duodenal ulcer is a possibility with a challenging diagnosis. We also focus on the importance of ligation of the gastroduodenal artery when bleeding of peptic ulcers occurs. Furthermore, our patient did not suffer a serious gastrointestinal bleeding. Additionally, we present an overview of the relevant literature.

Authors' Contribution

All the authors have read and approved the final paper.

References

[1] S. B. Pasha, P. Gloviczki, A. W. Stanson, and P. S. Kamath, "Splanchnic artery aneurysms," *Mayo Clinic Proceedings*, vol. 82, no. 4, pp. 472–479, 2007.

[2] M. A. Volpi, E. Voliovici, F. Pinato et al., "Pseudoaneurysm of the gastroduodenal artery secondary to chronic pancreatitis," *Annals of Vascular Surgery*, vol. 24, no. 8, pp. 1136.e7–1136.e11, 2010.

[3] K. Harris, M. Chalhoub, and A. Koirala, "Gastroduodenal artery aneurysm rupture in hospitalized patients: an overlooked diagnosis," *World Journal of Gastrointestinal Surgery*, vol. 2, no. 9, pp. 291–294, 2010.

[4] G. T. Fankhauser, W. M. Stone, S. G. Naidu et al., "The minimally invasive management of visceral artery aneurysms and pseudoaneurysms," *Journal of Vascular Surgery*, vol. 53, no. 4, pp. 966–970, 2011.

[5] N. Habib, S. Hassan, R. Abdou et al., "Gastroduodenal artery aneurysm, diagnosis, clinical presentation and management: a concise review," *Annals of Surgical Innovation and Research*, vol. 7, no. 1, article 4, 2013.

13

Management of a Gastrobronchial Fistula Connected to the Skin in a Giant Extragastric Stromal Tumor

Emilio Muñoz, Fernando Pardo-Aranda, Noelia Puértolas, Itziar Larrañaga, Judith Camps, and Enrique Veloso

Hospital Universitari Mutua Terrassa, 08221 Barcelona, Spain

Correspondence should be addressed to Fernando Pardo-Aranda; fparanda@gmail.com

Academic Editor: Shin-Ichi Kosugi

Introduction. Gastrointestinal stromal tumors first treatment should be surgical resection, but when metastases are diagnosed or the tumor is unresectable, imatinib must be the first option. This treatment could induce some serious complications difficult to resolve. *Case Report.* We present a 47-year-old black man with a giant unresectable gastric stromal tumor under imatinib therapy who presented serious complications such as massive gastrointestinal bleeding and a gastrobronchial fistula connected with the skin, successfully treated by surgery and gastroscopy. *Discussion.* Complications due to imatinib therapy can result in life threatening. They represent a challenge for surgeons and digestologists; creative strategies are needed in order to resolve them.

1. Introduction

Gastrointestinal stromal tumors (GIST) are originated in the interstitial cell of Cajal [1] and have initial intramural growth. They can be intraluminal or extraluminal reaching a progressive bulky size and becoming giant tumors, especially in the stomach, which represents around 60% of all GIST [2].

In these giant gastric tumors necrotic intratumor cavities communicated to gastric lumen are quite common and can be infected, cause bowel obstruction, suffer a spontaneous rupture, or even bleed [3–6].

Some tumors can be unresectable because of their large size that affects nearby organs or metastatic disease at the time of clinical presentation. Imatinib plays an important role in these situations but may not always give the expected response. Besides acquired resistances [7, 8], it could induce serious complications because of massive necrosis. Although rare, these complications represent a therapeutic challenge for surgeons, like the case we present.

2. Case Report

The patient is a 47-year-old black male, with no medical history reported, diagnosed with a giant, cavitated, and unresectable gastric stromal tumor (GIST) (Figures 1(a) and 1(b)) with high mitotic index and *c-kit gene* exon 11 mutations, fistulized to the stomach lumen (Figures 2(a) and 2(b)), and liver metastases. The patient was started to be treated in March 2013 with imatinib 400 mg daily for a month. In May 2013, he was admitted to the Emergency Department due to melena. At the time of his admission the hemoglobin was 5 g/dL, blood pressure was 80/40 mmHg, and heart rate was 90 lpm.

Once hemodynamically stable, a gastroscopy was performed, with findings of a stomach full of blood clots and heavy bleeding coming from the tumor cavity, which was also full of clotted blood and its irregular walls were oozing blood that was not controllable with argon beam; therefore, an urgent laparotomy was carried out to achieve hemostasis. Intraoperatively, a huge intra-abdominal mass was found blocking nearly three-quarters of the abdominal cavity with strong fibrotic adhesions to the diaphragm, abdominal viscera, and abdominal wall, which made it inadvisable to resect. A gastrotomy was performed through anterior gastric wall to remove all blood clots and the intragastric fistula hole was closed with interrupted absorbable suture. The tumor cavity was opened through the softer tumor area and complete hemostasis was achieved using diathermia and homeostatic

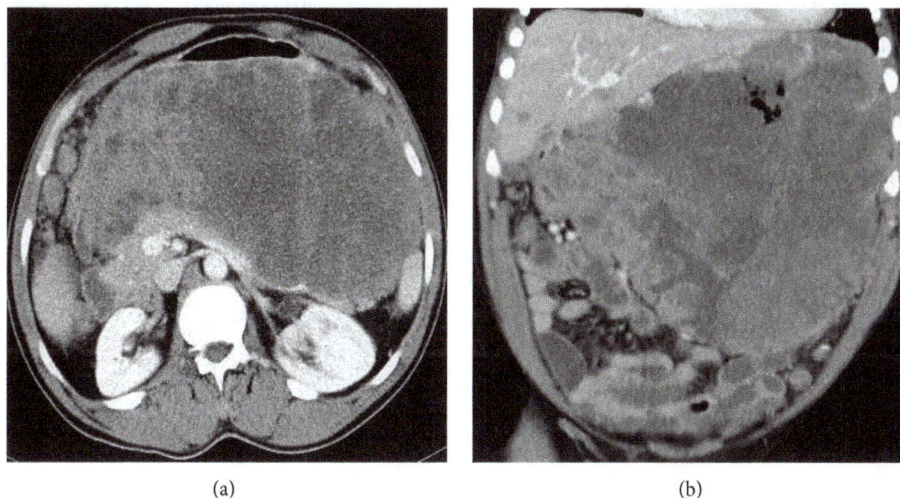

(a)   (b)

FIGURE 1: (a) Coronal section: giant GIST with aerial bubbles inside. (b) Axial section: giant gastric GIST.

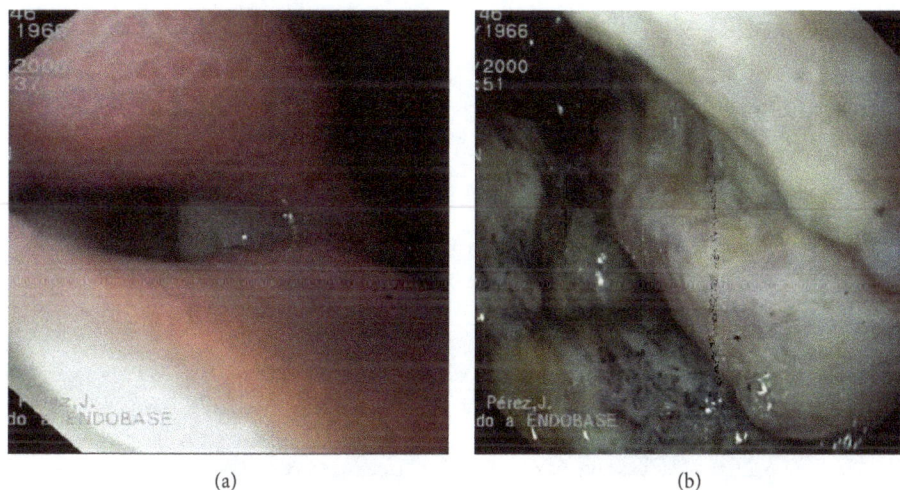

(a)   (b)

FIGURE 2: (a) Gastric fistula hole. (b) Necrotic intratumoral cavity.

biological sheets (Tachosil, Surgicel). A closed drainage was left in the tumor cavity. Patient recovered uneventfully and was discharged on postop day 14, in order to continue his treatment in the outpatient clinics. In August 2013, he started suffering from vomiting and imatinib was reduced to a dose of 300 mg daily, being well tolerated.

The patient was readmitted to the Emergency Department four months later, with fever (37.8°C), weight loss, persistent cough, pus leaking through the old drainage scar, and left pleural effusion. A sample of sputum was obtained. CT imaging showed persistence of liver metastases without relevant changes, but the primary tumor had experienced a very impressive shrinkage. The CT scan also showed a left pleural effusion with atelectasis and a left subphrenic abscess that was not suitable for percutaneous drainage; therefore, a surgical debridement and drainage were indicated.

Intraoperatively, a complete blockage of the supramesocolic abdomen was found. Several biopsies were taken (all of which were negative for GIST). Following the old drain tract,

a collection with chronic appearance was debrided and sent for culture. A double closed drainage was left in the abscess cavity and a feeding jejunostomy was placed. Microbiological culture of the sputum and collection samples were positive for MRSA and *Candida*. The patient was treated with appropriate antibiotics and antifungals.

Postoperatively, after an early clinical improvement, we realized that performing flushes through the double drain tube caused intense cough. A left bronchial fistula (Figure 3(a)) and a gastric fistula were confirmed. Both were connected with the abscess cavity and skin through the abscess drainage. The attempt to close twice a small gastric hole using over-the-scope clips (OTSC) not only was unsuccessful but also made the gastric fistula bigger, worsening the bronchial symptoms.

As the performance status was inappropriate for a left thoracotomy and taking into account the complete frozen upper abdomen, it was decided to isolate the bronchial fistula organizing a controlled gastrocutaneous fistula tract.

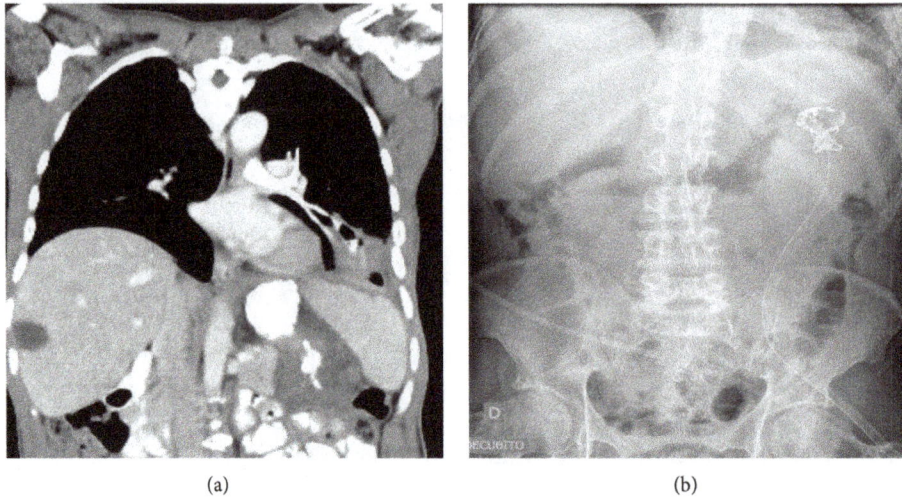

(a)   (b)

FIGURE 3: (a) Left bronchial tree full of contrast from stomach and abscess cavity. (b) PEG tube from stomach to the skin cavity isolating bronchial fistula tract.

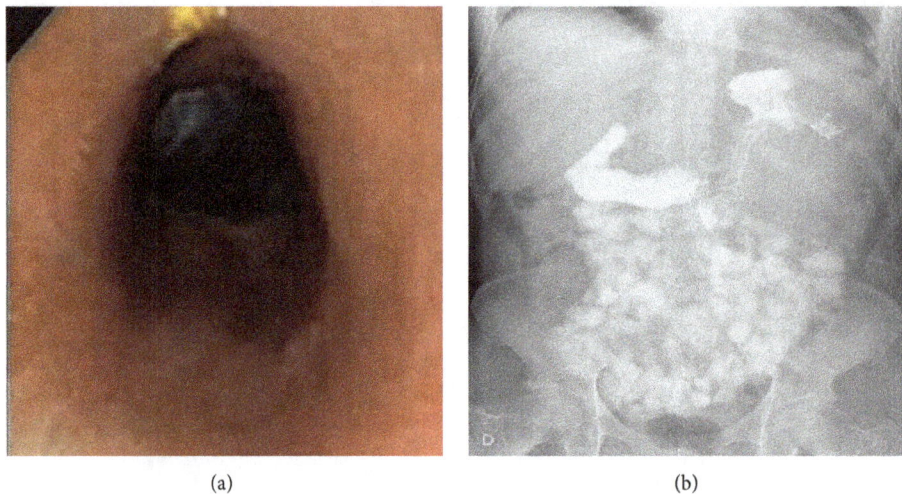

(a)   (b)

FIGURE 4: (a) Uniform duct fistula 18 cm long from stomach to the skin. Obtained with pediatric gastroscope. (b) Gastrografin transit without any leakage. OTSC still remains near the old fistulous opening.

Using a pediatric gastroscope, a transgastric abscess cavity examination was performed. Once in the abscess cavity, the tip of the drain was identified, and as it was being removed, it was followed by the pediatric endoscope until the skin was reached. A nylon guide was introduced and a 20 Fr percutaneous gastrostomy (PEG) tube was placed from stomach to skin (Figure 3(b)).

Progressive hyperproteic enteral feeding was given up to 5,25 kcal/kg/hour. Two weeks later, the cough, pleural effusion, and atelectasis had disappeared. In 2 months, the patient had gained 12 kg (to reach 54 kg), and a regular 18 cm long gastrocutaneous fistulous tract had been achieved (Figure 4(a)). Gastrografin transit showed no leakage (Figure 4(b)) and once the PEG tube was removed, the fistula tract closed completely in 6 days and the patient was discharged with oral intake and imatinib treatment. Although liver metastases are still in regression, the abdominal mass has

not recurred and the patient is having a good quality of life sixteen months later.

3. Discussion

Imatinib therapy is justified for locally advanced GIST and for metastatic, recurrent, and unresectable disease [8]. It should be used indefinitely as long as the tumor does not progress and patient tolerance permits [9, 10].

Complications under imatinib therapy due to tumor necrosis appear when the treatment has its higher effect during the first six months of therapy [11, 12].

We found in the literature some unusual cases of GIST bleeding caused by imatinib therapy [13]. Nevertheless, complications such as gastrobronchial fistula are exceptional, and we have not found any similar case in the literature. Probably, necrosis induced by imatinib must play an important role, but we cannot be sure about the exact pathophysiology of this serious complication. Two explanations may be posited: (a) gastric GIST was invading diaphragm and left lung, and necrosis tumor resulted in the formation of the fistula; (b) GIST are rarely infiltrative tumors, so that we believe that communication between the gastric lumen and tumor necrotic area was set up as a result of gastric wall necrosis progression under imatinib therapy. Consequently, an infection in left subphrenic space occurred and turned out into chronic abscess that drained through the weakest area such as diaphragm adhered to the lung.

Regardless of the pathophysiology, the fact was that we have a complex disease like a gastrobronchial fistula, also connected to the skin through a drainage tube, in a patient with poor general condition.

Taking into account patient's performance status and the abdominal blockade, surgical approach was not the best option. Bad as this situation was, we thought that the most feasible solution should be as simple as possible.

"Over-the-scope clip" (OTSC), which has demonstrated its effectiveness in the treatment of similar gastric holes [14, 15], seemed to be an easier way to fix it but failed, maybe due to gastric wall inflammation. Alternatively, we attempted to convert this complex triple fistula to a simple fistula without any intermediate cavity between the stomach and the skin to isolated bronchial communication and achieve a spontaneous closure.

Once we checked that there was no distal bowel obstruction, a pediatric gastroscope was used to see the fistula tract from the stomach to the skin and a PEG tube properly adjusted to the fistula was placed.

Finally, with appropriate feeding support over four months, expected evolution was achieved.

4. Conclusion

Complications due to imatinib therapy, such as gastrobronchial fistula, can result in life threatening; surgeons and digestologists should be aware of these uncommon complications.

References

[1] L.-G. Kindblom, H. E. Remotti, F. Aldenborg, and J. M. Meis-Kindblom, "Gastrointestinal pacemaker cell tumor (GIPACT): gastrointestinal stromal tumors show phenotypic characteristics of the interstitial cells of Cajal," *American Journal of Pathology*, vol. 152, no. 5, pp. 1259–1269, 1998.

[2] L. Zhou, C. Liu, J.-G. Bai et al., "A rare giant gastrointestinal stromal tumor of the stomach traversing the upper abdomen: a case report and literature review," *World Journal of Surgical Oncology*, vol. 10, article 66, 2012.

[3] K. Kitabayashi, T. Seki, K. Kishimoto et al., "A spontaneously ruptured gastric stromal tumor presenting as generalized peritonitis: report of a case," *Surgery Today*, vol. 31, no. 4, pp. 350–354, 2001.

[4] R. M. Metha, V. O. Sudheer, A. K. John et al., "Spontaneous rupture of gian gastric stromal tumor intro gastric lumen," *Journal of Surgical Oncology*, vol. 3, pp. 11–15, 2005.

[5] T. Osada, A. Nagahara, T. Kodani et al., "Gastrointestinal stromal tumor of the stomach with a giant abscess penetrating the gastric lumen," *World Journal of Gastroenterology*, vol. 13, no. 16, pp. 2385–2387, 2007.

[6] A. Cappellani, G. Piccolo, F. Cardì et al., "Giant gastrointestinal stromal tumor (GIST) of the stomach cause of high bowel obstruction: surgical management," *World Journal of Surgical Oncology*, vol. 11, article 172, 2013.

[7] M. van Glabbeke, J. Verweij, P. G. Casali et al., "Initial and late resistance to Imatinib in advance gastrointestinal tumors are predicted by different prognostic factors: a European Organization for Research and Treatment of cancer-Italian Sarcoma Group-Australasian gastrointestinal trials group study," *Journal of Clinical Oncology*, vol. 23, no. 24, pp. 5795–5804, 2005.

[8] A. T. Van Oosterom, I. Judson, J. Verweij et al., "Safety and efficacy of imatinib (STI571) in metastatic gastrointestinal stromal tumours: a phase I study," *The Lancet*, vol. 358, no. 9291, pp. 1421–1423, 2001.

[9] G. D. Demetri, M. Von Mehren, C. D. Blanke et al., "Efficacy and safety of imatinib mesylate in advanced gastrointestinal stromal tumors," *The New England Journal of Medicine*, vol. 347, no. 7, pp. 472–480, 2002.

[10] M. H. Cohen, A. Farrell, R. Justice, and R. Pazdur, "Approval summary: imatinib mesylate in the treatment of metastatic and/or unresectable malignant gastrointestinal stromal tumors," *Oncologist*, vol. 14, no. 2, pp. 174–180, 2009.

[11] V. Dudeja, L. H. Armstrong, P. Gupta, H. Ansel, S. Askari, and W. B. Al-Refaie, "Emergence of imatinib resistance associated with downregulation of C-Kit expression in recurrent gastrointestinal stromal tumor (GIST): optimal timing of resection," *Journal of Gastrointestinal Surgery*, vol. 14, no. 3, pp. 557–561, 2010.

[12] A. T. van Oosterom, I. R. Judson, J. Verweij et al., "Update of phase I study of imatinib (STI571) in advanced soft tissue sarcomas and gastrointestinal stromal tumors: a report of the EORTC Soft Tissue and Bone Sarcoma Group," *European Journal of Cancer*, vol. 38, pp. S83–S87, 2002.

[13] A. Hecker, B. Hecker, B. Bassaly et al., "Dramatic regression and bleeding of a duodenal GIST during preoperative imatinib therapy: case report and review," *World Journal of Surgical Oncology*, vol. 8, article 47, 2010.

[14] A. Kirschniak, F. Traub, M. A. Kueper, D. Stüker, A. Königsrainer, and T. Kratt, "Endoscopic treatment of gastric perforation caused by acute necrotizing pancreatitis using over-the-scope clips: a case report," *Endoscopy*, vol. 39, no. 12, pp. 1100–1102, 2007.

[15] A. Kirschniak, N. Subotova, D. Zieker, A. Königsrainer, and T. Kratt, "The Over-The-Scope Clip (OTSC) for the treatment of gastrointestinal bleeding, perforations and fistulas," *Surgical Endoscopy*, vol. 25, no. 9, pp. 2901–2905, 2011.

14

Isolated Duodenal Crohn's Disease: A Case Report and a Review of the Surgical Management

Faruk Karateke,[1] Ebru Menekşe,[1] Koray Das,[1] Sefa Ozyazici,[1] and Pelin Demirtürk[2]

[1] Numune Training and Research Hospital, Department of General Surgery, 01170 Adana, Turkey
[2] Numune Training and Research Hospital, Department of Pathology, 01170 Adana, Turkey

Correspondence should be addressed to Faruk Karateke; karatekefaruk@hotmail.com

Academic Editors: G. Lal and M. Rangarajan

Crohn's disease may affect any segment of the gastrointestinal tract; however, isolated duodenal involvement is rather rare. It still remains a complex clinical entity with a controversial management of the disease. Initially, patients with duodenal Crohn's disease (DCD) are managed with a combination of antiacid and immunosuppressive therapy. However, medical treatment fails in the majority of DCD patients, and surgical intervention is required in case of complicated disease. Options for surgical management of complicated DCD include bypass, resection, or stricturoplasty procedures. In this paper, we reported a 33-year-old male patient, who was diagnosed with isolated duodenal Crohn's diseases, and reviewed the surgical options in the literature.

1. Introduction

Duodenal Crohn's disease (DCD) has been reported to occur in 0.5% to 4% of patients with Crohn's disease [1]. The first report of duodenal involvement was described by Gottlieb and Alpert in 1937 [1–3]. Since then, DCD still remains a complex clinical entity with a controversial management of the disease. The most common site of duodenal Crohn's disease is the duodenal bulb, and obstruction is the most frequent presentation [1, 4]. Medical management with anti-inflammatory and antiacid medications is effective in patients without obstruction. However, surgery has been reported to be necessary for as many as 91% of patients with obstruction [1, 5, 6]. Options for surgical management of complicated DCD include bypass, resection, or stricturoplasty. Resection has been abandoned because of associated increased morbidity; therefore, bypass procedures and stricturoplasty have become the accepted surgical options for DCD [5, 7–9]. Although Crohn's disease can involve any segment of the gastrointestinal tract, isolated Crohn's disease of duodenum without extraduodenal involvement is extremely rare. In this report, we described an isolated case of DCD and reviewed the surgical options.

2. Case

A 33-year-old male patient was referred to our clinic with a 6-month history of intermittent, abdominal pain accompanied by progressive nausea, bilious emesis, and weight loss. His defecation habits were normal. On physical examinations, only a slight tenderness and fullness was noted in the epigastric region. Routine blood work revealed a mild normocytic anemia (Hgb: 12,0 g/dL, normal range: 13,5–17,2 g/dL). Biochemical parameters were unremarkable. He subsequently underwent an esophagogastroduodenoscopy (EGD), abdominal computerized tomography (CT), and colonoscopy. EGD revealed a tight stricture with mucosal edema and the longitudinal ulcerations in the duodenal bulb with a near-complete obstruction (Figure 1). The biopsy specimens of the duodenum showed severe inflammation, mixed chronic inflammatory infiltrate in lamina propria, and cryptitis with the evidence of DCD (Figures 2 and 3). CT and colonoscopy were normal. Based on these clinical, radiological, and pathological findings, isolated DCD was diagnosed, and total parenteral nutrition therapy was initiated along with nasogastric decompression. After having the nutritional status of the patient improved, he went on laparoscopic exploration. A stricture was found in the first part of the duodenum

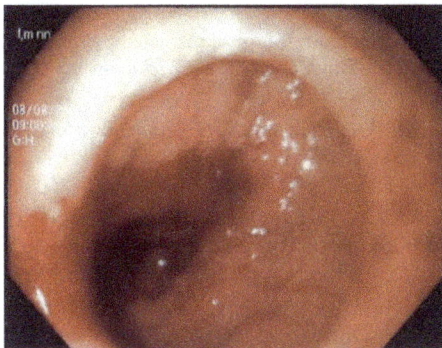

FIGURE 1: Esophagogastroduodenoscopy findings of the patient: a tight stricture with mucosal edema and the longitudinal ulcerations in the duodenal bulb with a near-complete obstruction.

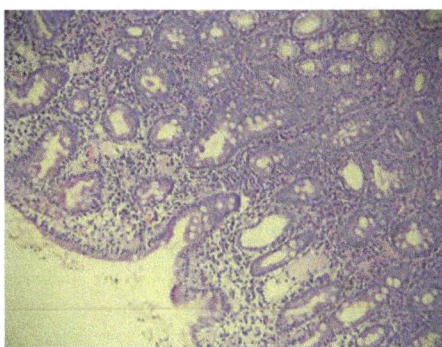

FIGURE 2: Foci of villous blunting, glandular destruction, mixed chronic inflammatory infiltrate in lamina propria, and cryptitis (H&Ex200).

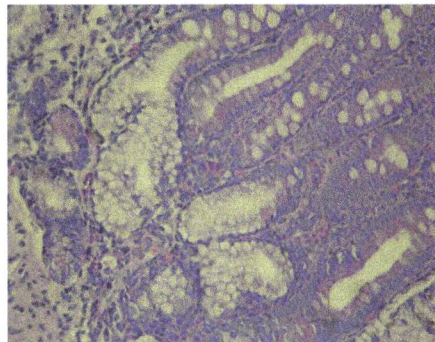

FIGURE 3: Pyloric metaplasia at the base of the crypt (H&Ex400).

with a dilated stomach. A laparoscopic gastrojejunostomy was performed without vagotomy. The patient tolerated the procedure well and was discharged without any adverse event on postoperative 7th day, and thereafter, he was referred to the gastroenterology department for adjuvant therapy. He was noted to be on remission without any complaints during a 9-month followup under proton-pump inhibitors treatment.

3. Discussion

Crohn's disease is a chronic and inflammatory disease characterized by the segmented, transmural involvement of the alimentary tract that can affect any part of the system from the mouth to the anus [10]. Patients with DCD usually present with Crohn's disease affecting other areas of the gastrointestinal tract; however, isolated DCD is a very rare clinical entity [1, 4]. Initially, patients with DCD are managed with a combination of antiacid and immunosuppressive therapy. However, medical treatment fails in the majority of DCD patients, and surgical intervention is required in case of complicated disease. The most common indication for surgical intervention is progressive obstruction, failure of medical management with intractable pain, bleeding, perforation, and fistulous disease [1, 5, 6].

Options for surgical treatment of complicated DCD disease include resection, bypass, or strictureplasty. Resection

procedure that was described by Allen Whipple has been associated with significant morbidity and mortality. Short gut syndrome, diarrhea, chronic malnutrition, electrolyte derangements, vitamin deficiencies, and chronic anemia are the complications of resection [5, 11].

Because of high rates of morbidity and mortality, bypass procedures and strictureplasty have been considered as standard surgical options to preserve the duodenum and prevent related complications of surgical resection.

Strictureplasty was introduced by Lee and Papiaoannu in the 1970s and furthermore popularized by Alexander-Williams [12, 13]. The most common strictureplasty techniques for DCD are the Heineke-Mikulicz procedure for shorter strictures and the Finney strictureplasty for longer segments of disease [11]. In the early 1990s, strictureplasty techniques were preferred constantly over bypass procedures due to reliability, safety, and efficacy with their own pitfalls. However, due to the complexity of the strictureplasty arising from the retroperitoneal location of the duodenum and need for extensive mobilization of the duodenum, bypass procedures have been preferred recently.

Although bypass procedures are more technically feasible and safe compared to strictureplasty, they are associated more frequently with blind-loop syndrome, dumping, bile reflux gastritis, and marginal ulceration [9]. Only a limited number of studies comparing outcomes after strictureplasty and bypass surgery for duodenal disease are available in the recent literature. The results of these studies have been controversial. Worsey et al. performed strictureplasty for 13 patients and bypass procedures for 21 patients. They concluded that duodenal strictureplasty is safe and effective and may in fact have potential anatomic and physiologic advantages over bypass procedures [9].

Yamamoto et al. performed duodenal strictureplasty for 13 patients, 9 of which required further surgical intervention due to early postoperative complications and restricturing at the strictureplasty site ($n = 6$) in a median followup of 143 months. Similarly, 13 patients underwent bypass procedures. In this cases, no patients required reoperation for early postoperative complications; however, 6 patients required further surgical intervention at a later date (median followup 192 months) for stomal ulceration ($n = 2$) and anastomotic obstruction ($n = 4$) [8].

Yamamoto et al. stated that strictureplasty had no patent advantages over bypass and was associated with a higher incidence of early complications and restricturing [8].

One of the largest study published on the surgical management of patients with DCD was conducted by Shapiro et al., which was the first to present the laparoscopic experience in bypass procedures [3]. In this study, thirty patients had surgical intervention for DCD, including 4 patients with isolated disease. The surgical procedures were open bypass for 11 patients, laparoscopic bypass for 13, and strictureplasty for 2 patients. Early complications rate was 8% in laparoscopic procedures and 36% in open bypass procedures, respectively. This lower complication rate was attributed to a decrease in complication rate after laparoscopic surgery. Also Shapiro et al. revealed that there is no role for vagotomy in bypass procedures to prevent marginal ulceration in the era of wide use of proton pump inhibitors (PPI). Adjuvant treatment options after surgery of isolated DCD include PPI, H2 receptor antagonists, sucralfate, or steroids.

The clinical presentation of our patient was progressive obstruction with symptoms of isolated duodenal involvement as his first clinical manifestation of the disease. Based on the previous studies, we performed laparoscopic gastrojejunal bypass for surgical intervention, and he was noted to be on remission after surgery during 9 months under PPI therapy.

4. Conclusion

The optimal management of duodenal Crohn's disease should be individualized on a case-by-case basis. Laparoscopic gastrojejunal bypass can be an alternative in the treatment of DCD.

References

[1] F. W. Nugent and M. A. Roy, "Duodenal Crohn's disease: an analysis of 89 cases," *The American Journal of Gastroenterology*, vol. 84, no. 3, pp. 249–254, 1989.

[2] C. Gottlieb and S. Alpert, "Regional jejunitis," *The American Journal of Roentgenology*, vol. 38, pp. 881–883, 1937.

[3] M. Shapiro, A. J. Greenstein, J. Byrn et al., "Surgical management and outcomes of patients with duodenal Crohn's disease," *Journal of the American College of Surgeons*, vol. 207, no. 1, pp. 36–42, 2008.

[4] T. Yamamoto, R. N. Allan, and M. R. B. Keighley, "An audit of gastroduodenal Crohn disease: clinicopathologic features and management," *Scandinavian Journal of Gastroenterology*, vol. 34, no. 10, pp. 1019–1024, 1999.

[5] J. J. Murray, D. J. Schoetz Jr., F. W. Nugent, J. A. Coller, and M. C. Veidenheimer, "Surgical management of crohn's disease involving the duodenum," *The American Journal of Surgery*, vol. 147, no. 1, pp. 58–65, 1984.

[6] A. Lossing, B. Langer, and K. N. Jeejeebhoy, "Gastroduodenal Crohn's disease: diagnosis and selection of treatment," *Canadian Journal of Surgery*, vol. 26, no. 4, pp. 358–360, 1983.

[7] T. M. Ross, V. W. Fazio, and R. G. Farmer, "Long-term results of surgical treatment for Crohn's disease of the duodenum," *Annals of Surgery*, vol. 197, no. 4, pp. 399–406, 1983.

[8] T. Yamamoto, I. M. Bain, A. B. Connolly, R. N. Allan, and M. R. Keighley, "Outcome of strictureplasty for duodenal Crohn's disease," *British Journal of Surgery*, vol. 86, no. 2, pp. 259–262, 1999.

[9] M. J. Worsey, T. Hull, L. Ryland, and V. Fazio, "Strictureplasty is an effective option in the operative management of duodenal Crohn's disease," *Diseases of the Colon and Rectum*, vol. 42, no. 5, pp. 596–600, 1999.

[10] S. Akbulut, B. Yavuz, T. Köseoğlu, A. Gököz, and U. Saritaş, "Crohn's disease with isolated esophagus and gastric involvement," *Turkish Journal of Gastroenterol*, vol. 15, no. 3, pp. 196–200, 2004.

[11] A. Fichera, R. D. Hurst, and F. Michelassi, "Current methods of bowel-sparing surgery in Crohn's disease," *Journal of Gastroenterology*, vol. 40, pp. 40–50, 2005.

[12] E. C. Lee and N. Papiaoannu, "Minimal surgery for chronic obstruction in patients with extensive or universal Crohn's disease," *Annals of the Royal College of Surgeons of England*, vol. 64, no. 4, pp. 229–233, 1982.

[13] J. Alexander-Williams, "The technique of intestinal strictureplasty," *International Journal of Colorectal Disease*, vol. 1, no. 1, pp. 54–57, 1986.

15

Acute Gastric Dilatation Resulting in Gastric Emphysema Following Postpartum Hemorrhage

Suhail Aslam Khan,[1] Edmond Boko,[1] Haseeb Anwar Khookhar,[1] Sheila Woods,[2] and A. H. Nasr[1]

[1] Department of Surgery, Our Lady of Lourdes Hospital, Drogheda, County Louth, Ireland
[2] Department of Radiology, Our Lady of Lourdes Hospital, Drogheda, County Louth, Ireland

Correspondence should be addressed to Suhail Aslam Khan, tahirkheli73@gmail.com

Academic Editors: C. Foroulis, M. Nikfarjam, and M. Rangarajan

Acute gastric dilatation is a rare entity, with varying aetiologies the majority of which are benign. Delay in diagnosis and treatment could result in sequelae such as gastric emphysema (pneumatosis), emphysematous gastritis, gangrene, and perforation. Gastric emphysema as a result of a benign nongangrenous condition such as gastroparesis, adynamic ileus can be successfully managed conservatively. Here, we present an interesting case of acute gastric dilatation resulting in gastric emphysema following massive postpartum hemorrhage.

1. Introduction

Acute gastric dilatation is a rare entity, with varying aetiologies, the majority of which are benign. Prompt recognition and appropriate management are essential to prevent sequelae such as gastric emphysema (pneumatosis), emphysematous gastritis, gangrene, and perforation [1–4]. Like other sequelae of acute gastric dilatation, the development of gastric emphysema may also reflect other intra-abdominal pathology, and its presence can suggest gangrenous changes of the stomach or colon and, therefore, represents a surgical emergency [1–3]. However, gastric emphysema can also occur as a result of a benign, nongangrenous condition, such as gastroparesis and adynamic illeus and can be successfully managed conservatively [5–7]. Here we are presenting an interesting case of acute gastric dilatation resulting in gastric emphysema following acute management of postpartum hemorrhage.

2. Case Report

A 40-year-old African gravid 3/para 3 woman was admitted to the intensive care unit (ICU) following a caesarian section for placental abruption and fetal distress. She was booked for antenatal care at approximately 34 weeks of pregnancy with antenatal care prior to that done in Africa for this pregnancy. Her initial assessment was satisfactory (Tables 1 and 2), but in the background history, it was noted that she was suffering from constipation and gestational diabetes mellitus in her last pregnancy (Table 2) and was poorly compliant with insulin therapy.

She underwent emergency C-section after she presented with antepartum haemorrhage, and intraoperative findings were a low-lying placenta with large retroplacental clot with abruption. Postoperatively, she continued to bleed per vagina in ICU and received 7 units of red cell concentrate (RCC), 4 units of plasma, 4 pools of platelets, and an oxytocin infusion. Despite treatment, she continued to bleed and was transferred back to theatre, where a uterine tamponade balloon was successfully inserted. Her total blood loss was estimated in excess of 3 litres.

On the same evening, she began to complain of abdominal pain. On examination, her vital signs were within the normal range. Abdominal examination revealed a distended abdomen with tenderness in the epigastrium and left upper quadrant and was tympanic to percussion over the

TABLE 1: Antenatal history.

Date of booking	22/03/2011
LMP, EDD, gestation	28/7/10, 4/5/11, 33 wks, and 6 days
Cycle length	28, regular
Maternal risk category	Low risk
Allergies	Flagyl, Chloroquine
Drugs in pregnancy	Antimalarial tabs and folic acid
Booking BP, pulse	126/76, 74/min
Smoking, alcohol	None
Medical conditions	H/O essential HTN on med for 6 months in 2010, Rec UTIs, gestational diabetes in previous two pregnancies, constipation
Family history	Sickle cell anemia, DM type 1
Surgical history	Appendicectomy
Ultrasound	
EDD by LMP	4/5/11
EDD by USS	4/5/11
BPD	87.8 mm
ABD circumf.	331.3
Placental site	Upper ant
Wt differential	454 gms
Growth centile	>90
Presentation	Cephalic
Fetal cardiac activity	Present
Head circumf.	306.7
Femur length	77 mm
Fetal wt	3113 gms
CTG	Satisfactory

TABLE 2: Record of previous pregnancies.

Year	2001, Nigeria
Gestation	39 wks
Antenatal problems	No record
Mode of delivery	Spontaneous, vertex, hospital
Perineal problems	Infected episiotomy
Outcome	Live birth, 3690 gms male
Year	2003, Ireland
Gestation	40 wks
Antenatal problems	Gestational diabetes
Onset	Spontaneous
Mode of delivery	Spontaneous, vertex, hospital
Outcome	Live birth, 3890 gms female
Year	2006, Ireland
Gestation	40 wks
Antenatal problems	Gestational diabetes, insulin given
Onset	Induced
Mode of delivery	Spontaneous, vertex, hospital
Outcome	Live birth, 3790 gms male
Neonatal problems	Yes; SCBU for BSL monitoring for 3 days

epigastric region. There was no guarding or rigidity noted. An abdominal X-ray showed significant gastric distension with diffusely noted gas pattern consistent with gastric emphysema (Figure 1). CT confirmed air in the stomach wall, with moderate abdominal and pelvic fluid, which was attributed to her earlier C-section (Figure 1). An urgent upper GI endoscopy was arranged which revealed a normal oesophagus, food in the stomach, and, on washing, revealed an oedematous beefy red, friable mucous-coated stomach mucosa extending over greater curvature from midstomach towards the fundus (Figure 2). Following consultation with the upper GI unit in a tertiary referral centre, this patient was managed conservatively with gastric drainage via nasogastric tube, broad-spectrum antibiotic cover, oral sucralfate, and total parenteral nutrition with close monitoring in ICU.

Her further clinical course was uneventful, and she responded very well to conservative management. A repeat CT, one week later, showed absence of gastric wall gas or free air (Figure 3). The large and small bowel loops appeared normal, and she was discharged home.

3. Discussion

Acute gastric dilation was first described by Powell et al. in 2003 [1], and it can be as a result of eating disorders, hemorrhage/trauma resuscitation, volvulus, medications, electrolyte abnormalities, infections, superior mesenteric artery syndrome, diabetes mellitus and slow gut transits causing chronic constipation [1–11]. It can have devastating consequences and has a reported mortality rate of 80% to 100% as a consequence of gastric necrosis and perforation [1–4].

Acute gastric dilatation can result in gastric emphysema, emphysematous gastritis, and ischemic necrosis. Ischemic necrosis, in the case of gastric dilatation, is postulated to be due to venous insufficiency [1, 5, 6]. Pressure in the stomach lumen must be >14 mm Hg to exceed gastric venous pressure and lead to ischemia [1, 3, 4]. Gastric emphysema is also a rare finding with only a few cases reported in the literature. Gastric emphysema resulting from a violation of mucosal integrity followed by forceful entry of air between the gastric layers is called noninfectious gastric emphysema [5, 6]. The other extremely rare condition that was first described by Fraenkel in 1889 as emphysematous gastritis is due to infection [9–11]. The most commonly involved microorganisms are *streptococci, Escherichia coli, Pseudomonas aeruginosa, Clostridium perfringens,* and *Staphylococcus aureus* [10].

Gastric emphysema secondary to mechanical aetiologies is far more common than primary gastric emphysema. Causes include obstruction, trauma, and rupture of pulmonary bullae, enteric tube placement, and upper endoscopic procedures [1–8]. In these cases, the intraluminal gas dissects into the gastric wall through a mucosal tear or defect. The tear usually results from increased intraluminal pressure secondary to an obstruction or as a direct result of trauma. The reported mortality in this group, although lower than the mortality associated with gastric emphysema, is still high at 6% to 41% [3–5]. While other authors

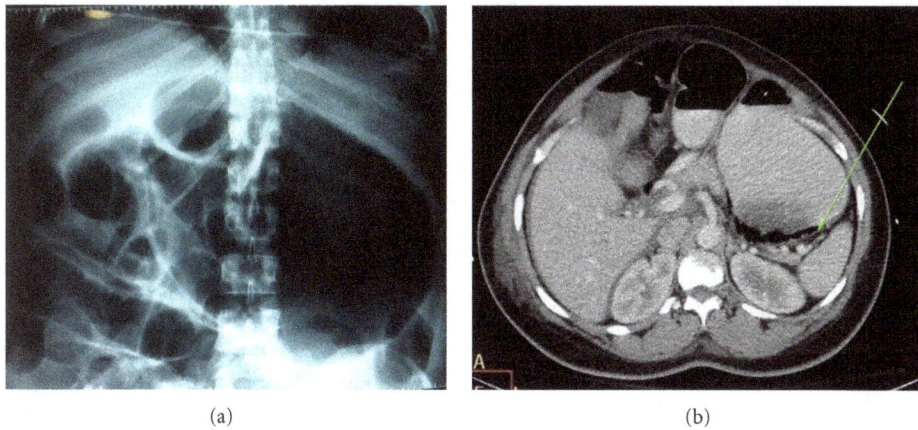

(a)   (b)

FIGURE 1: Plain film of abdomen and CT abdomen showing gastric dilatation of stomach and emphysema (arrow).

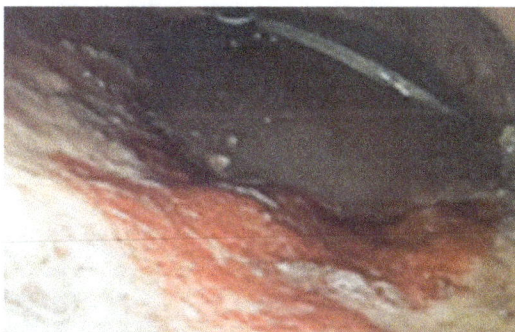

FIGURE 2: Upper GI endoscopy: showing oedamatous beefy red mucosa along the greater curvature of stomach.

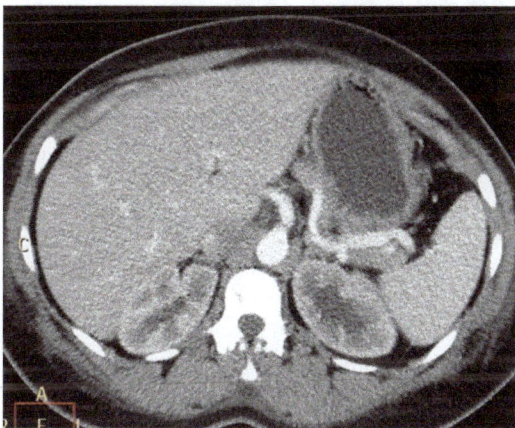

FIGURE 3: Follow-up CT abdomen after a week shows resolution of gastric emphysema.

describe gastric emphysema secondary to bowel or gastric outlet obstruction, Cho et al. highlighted the association of gastric emphysema causing adynamic ileus with postpartum hemorrhage, but gastric emphysema specifically associated with caesarian section and intrapartum hemorrhage has not been reported [7].

Clinically, patients with infectious gastric emphysema appear septic and complain of fever, chills, and abdominal pain [2, 9–11]. These signs and symptoms could be the main differentiating features separating infectious gastritis from symptoms of acute gastric dilation resulting in gastric emphysema, which can be initially vague with progressive abdominal distention and accompanying pain [9–11]. Plain abdominal radiographs or abdominal computed tomography are diagnostic. In the majority of cases, emphysema occurs along the greater curvature of the stomach. The lesser curvature and pyloric regions of the stomach tend to be spared [2, 5, 12, 13]. In a pictorial essay, Johnson et al. presented a series of cases of gastric emphysema. They advocated the use of CT to guide management and to assist in the identification of associated extragastric pathologies [13].

Early endoscopy in the stable patient may be of use, particularly if the CT scan suggests gastric or esophageal involvement. Where diagnosis is emphysematous gastritis, gastroscopy and biopsy are advocated to facilitate a diagnosis, which can show evidence of submucosal abscesses or exudative gastritis [14, 15]. In the above case, where the aetiology is obscure, the endoscopic findings of diffuse inflammation with diffusely friable, oedematous mucosa with mucopurulent exudates and rapid resolution of signs and symptoms may suggest a transient ischemia [5]. Because of transient ischemia, the mucosa may be injured or compromised thus allowing air to penetrate and dissect into the gastric wall. In these patients, nonoperative management and nasogastric decompression resulted in resolution of emphysema in 72 hours [5, 6].

Treatment focuses on early diagnosis, broad-spectrum antibiotic cover, nasogastric decompression of the stomach, and total parenteral nutrition, thus halting the vascular congestion and ensuing ischemia [3–5]. When considering gastric emphysema due to mechanical causes, clinical judgment should be carefully applied when determining which patients require surgical exploration and which can be observed safely. Selective non-operative management has been used successfully in the setting of secondary gastric emphysema, with nongangrenous gastric and esophageal emphysema [5]. Delayed perforation or bleeding is still possible, even following decompression. Surgical exploration is mandated in the presence of instability, perforation or for other indications, such as associated small bowel obstruction or ischemia of the small bowel [1, 4, 7].

In our case, it is reasonable to presume that multiple factors have played a role in the development of acute gastric dilatation and gastric emphysema. This patient's co-morbidities, gestational diabetes with poor diabetic control leading to gastroparesis, and chronic constipation are likely to have been a factor in the development of acute gastric dilatation and subsequently gastric emphysema. It is also likely that other factors can potentially aggravate the condition in this patient such as increase in intra-abdominal pressure because of gastric dilatation and acute massive haemorrhage, leading to transient poor perfusion of the gastrointestinal tract. Also the use of opiates for pain relief can further potentiate depression of gut motility. From the above case report and discussion, it is clear that the diagnosis and treatment of underlying cause of gastric emphysema are most important for a favourable outcome then simple gastric decompression.

References

[1] J. L. Powell, J. Payne, C. L. Meyer, and P. R. Moncla, "Gastric necrosis associated with acute gastric dilatation and small bowel obstruction," *Gynecologic Oncology*, vol. 90, no. 1, pp. 200–203, 2003.

[2] P. A. McKelvie and M. A. Fink, "A fatal case of emphysematous gastritis and esophagitis," *Pathology*, vol. 26, no. 4, pp. 490–492, 1994.

[3] S. Luncă, A. Rikkers, and A. Stănescu, "Acute massive gastric dilatation: severe ischemia and gastric necrosis without perforation," *Romanian Journal of Gastroenterology*, vol. 14, no. 3, pp. 279–283, 2005.

[4] S. Lewis, A. Holbrook, and P. Hersch, "An unusual case of massive gastric distension with catastrophic sequelae," *Acta Anaesthesiologica Scandinavica*, vol. 49, no. 1, pp. 95–97, 2005.

[5] S. A. Mclaughlin and J. H. Nguyen, "Conservative management of nongangrenous esophageal and gastric pneumatosis," *The American Surgeon*, vol. 73, no. 9, pp. 862–864, 2007.

[6] T. Nagai, M. Yokoo, T. Tomizawa, and M. Mori, "Acute gastric dilatation accompanied by diabetes mellitus," *Internal Medicine*, vol. 40, no. 4, pp. 320–323, 2001.

[7] F-N. Cho, C.-B. Liu, J.-Y. Li, S.-N. Chen, and K. J. Yu, "Adynamic ileus and acute colonic pseudo-obstruction occurring after cesarean section in patients with massive peripartum hemorrhage," *Journal of the Chinese Medical Association*, vol. 72, no. 12, pp. 657–662, 2009.

[8] P. Y. Lin, M. S. Tsai, J. H. Chang, W. J. Chen, and C. H. Huang, "Gastric distension: a risk factor of pneumoperitoneum during cardiopulmonary resuscitation," *The American Journal of Emergency Medicine*, vol. 24, no. 7, pp. 878–879, 2006.

[9] E. Fraenkel, "Ueber einen Fall von Gastritis acuta emphysematosa wahrscheinlich mykotischen Ursprungs," *Archiv für Pathologische Anatomie und Physiologie und für Klinische Medicin*, vol. 118, no. 3, pp. 526–535, 1889.

[10] C. E. Yale and E. Balish, "The natural course of Clostridium perfringens—induced pneumatosis cystoides intestinalis," *Journal of Medicine*, vol. 23, no. 3-4, pp. 279–288, 1992.

[11] A. Ocepek, P. Skok, M. Virag, B. Kamenik, and M. Horvat, "Emphysematous gastritis—case report and review of the literature," *Zeitschrift fur Gastroenterologie*, vol. 42, no. 8, pp. 735–738, 2004.

[12] P. T. Johnson, K. M. Horton, B. H. Edil, E. K. Fishman, and W. W. Scott, "Gastric pneumatosis: the role of CT in diagnosis and patient management," *Emergency Radiology*, vol. 18, no. 1, pp. 65–73, 2011.

[13] F. Lassandro, M. L. M. Di Santo Stefano, A. Maria Porto, R. Grassi, M. Scaglione, and A. Rotondo, "Intestinal pneumatosis in adults: diagnostic and prognostic value," *Emergency Radiology*, vol. 17, no. 5, pp. 361–365, 2010.

[14] M. S. Soon, H. H. Yen, A. Soon, and O. S. Lin, "Endoscopic ultrasonographic appearance of gastric emphysema," *World Journal of Gastroenterology*, vol. 11, no. 11, pp. 1719–1721, 2005.

[15] N. R. Cordum, A. Dixon, and D. R. Campbell, "Gastroduodenal pneumatosis: endoscopic and histological findings," *The American Journal of Gastroenterology*, vol. 92, no. 4, pp. 692–695, 1997.

16

Five-Year Survival after Surgery for Invasive Micropapillary Carcinoma of the Stomach

**Shigeo Ninomiya, Kazuya Sonoda, Hidefumi Shiroshita,
Toshio Bandoh, and Tsuyoshi Arita**

Department of Surgery, Arita Gastrointestinal Hospital, 1-2-6 Maki, Oita 870-0294, Japan

Correspondence should be addressed to Shigeo Ninomiya; sninomiy@med.oita-u.ac.jp

Academic Editors: N. A. Chowdri, M. Rangarajan, and F. Turégano

Invasive micropapillary carcinoma (IMPC) of the breast, urinary bladder, ovary, and colon has been reported. However, few reports have described IMPC of the stomach. In addition, IMPC has been described as a histological indicator for lymphatic invasion and nodal metastasis, resulting in poor prognosis. We report a case of 5-year survival after surgery for IPMC of the stomach. A 69-year-old woman was admitted to our hospital with symptoms of upper abdominal pain. Upper gastrointestinal endoscopy revealed a tumor at the antrum of the stomach. Histological examination of the biopsy specimen indicated poorly differentiated adenocarcinoma. The patient underwent distal gastrectomy with lymph node dissection. Microscopic examination of the specimen revealed that the tumor consisted of an invasive micropapillary component. Carcinoma cell clusters were floating in the clear spaces. The patient recovered uneventfully and remains alive without recurrence 5 years after surgery.

1. Introduction

Invasive micropapillary carcinoma (IMPC) was first reported as a rare subtype of invasive ductal carcinoma of the breast, defined as a carcinoma composed of small clusters of tumor cells lying within clear spaces simulating vascular channels [1]. IMPC has been described as a histological indicator for lymphatic invasion and nodal metastasis, resulting in poor prognosis [2]. After initially being reported as a histological variant of breast cancer [1], IPMC of the urinary bladder [3], ovary [4], colon [5], and ampulla of Vater [6] was also reported. However, reports of IPMC of the stomach have been limited. Herein, we report a case of 5-year survival after surgery for IMPC of the stomach and discuss the clinical findings of this disease according to the previous literature.

2. Case Report

A 69-year-old woman was admitted to our hospital with the complaint of upper abdominal pain. On admission, her abdomen was flat and soft, and no superficial lymph nodes were palpated. Routine laboratory findings were unremarkable, with the exception of an elevated carbohydrate antigen 19-9 level of 544 U/mL. Upper gastrointestinal endoscopy revealed a circumferential tumor located at the antrum of the stomach (Figure 1). Histopathological examination indicated poorly differentiated adenocarcinoma. Computed tomography (CT) also showed a tumor located at the antrum of the stomach, with no invasion of the primary tumor to the adjacent structures and no distant metastasis (Figure 2). Based on all of the preoperative clinical examinations, the tumor was diagnosed to be T3N1M0 stage IIIA according to UICC staging. With a provisional diagnosis of gastric adenocarcinoma, we performed distal gastrectomy with lymph node dissection. Macroscopically, the tumor was 36 × 30 mm in size. Microscopic examination of the specimen revealed that the tumor consisted of an invasive micropapillary component. Carcinoma cell clusters were floating in the clear spaces (Figures 3(a) and 3(b)). Carcinoma cells had invaded the subserous tissue, and two regional lymph node metastases were seen. In addition, there was marked lymphatic invasion, but no obvious venous invasion. The sections were examined immunohistochemically with primary antibodies using the

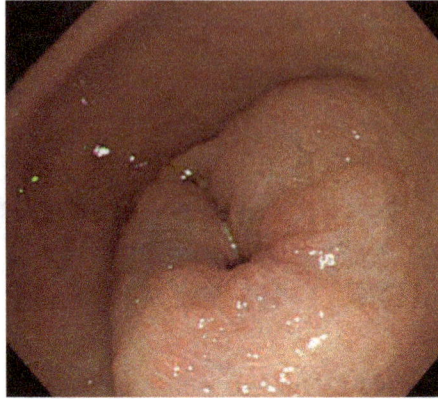

FIGURE 1: Upper gastrointestinal endoscopy revealed a circumferential tumor located at the antrum of the stomach.

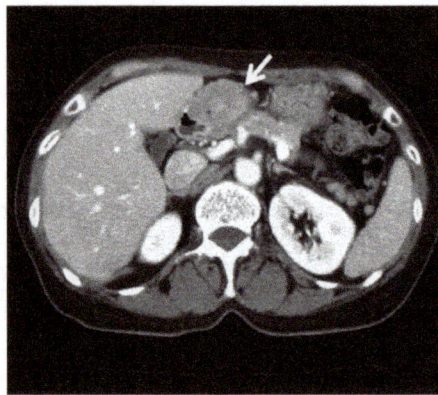

FIGURE 2: Computed tomography showed a tumor located at the antrum of the stomach (arrow), with no invasion of the primary tumor to adjacent structures and no distant metastasis.

streptavidin peroxidase complex method, which revealed carcinoma cells positive for epithelial membrane antigen (EMA) and MUC-1. Also, carcinoma cell membranes at the periphery of the cell clusters were characteristically positive for EMA, indicating an "inside-out" pattern [7] of reactivity (Figures 4(a) and 4(b)).

We administered postoperative adjuvant chemotherapy with S-1 according to the pathological results. Presently, the patient is alive and without recurrence and is doing well 5 years after surgery.

3. Discussion

IMPC was initially described as a histological variant of breast cancer, characterized as a carcinoma composed of small clusters of tumor cells lying within clear spaces simulating vascular channels. IPMC of the breast has a high propensity to invade the lymphatic system with extensive metastasis to the axillary lymph nodes [1]. Although IPMC of the stomach is extremely rare, and this entity has not been fully described, the pathological features of IPMC of the stomach have been reported recently. Ushiku et al. [7] identified an incidence of nodal metastasis in 82% of cases, and lymphovascular invasion was present in all 17 cases. Fujita et al. [8] also reported an incidence of nodal metastasis of 100% and

lymphatic invasion of 78.5% in their 14-case series. Therefore, the clinicopathological features of IPMC of the stomach could be similar to those of IPMC of the breast, with a high incidence of nodal metastasis and lymphatic invasion.

The prognosis for patients with IPMC of the stomach has not been clarified. Some reports have shown survival rates no poorer than those of patients with IPMC of the breast. Fujita et al. [8] noted that significant differences were observed in the 3-year disease-free survival rate of patients with IPMC of the stomach compared with that for the stage-matched controls. Eom et al. [9] reported that overall 5-year survival rates for patients with IPMC of the stomach were significantly worse than those for patients with stage I and II non-IPMC. However, Roh et al. [10] found no significant differences in overall survival rates between patients with IPMC of the stomach and non-IPMC. These previous reports have some limitations in that the numbers of patients with IMPC of the stomach were very small. Our case is a rare report of 5-year survival from IPMC of the stomach successfully treated by surgery and adjuvant chemotherapy. Further examination is necessary to clarify the prognosis for patients with IPMC of the stomach.

Optimal treatment strategy for IPMC of the stomach has not been established. This rare histological type frequently shows aggressive tumor behavior with marked lymphatic

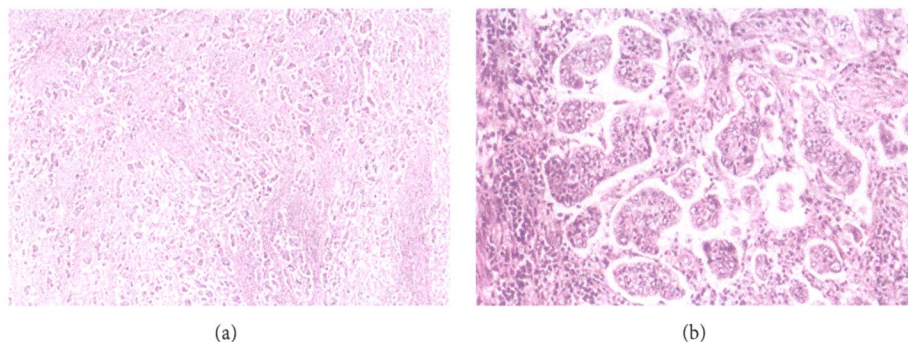

(a)   (b)

FIGURE 3: Histological examination of the specimen revealed that the tumor consisted of an invasive micropapillary component. Carcinoma cell clusters were floating in the clear spaces. (a) Hematoxylin-eosin stain, original magnification, ×40. (b) Hematoxylin-eosin stain, ×200.

MUC-1   EMA

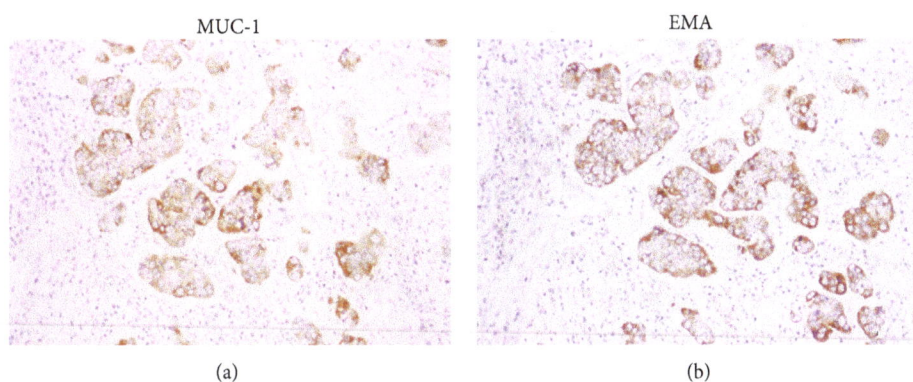

(a)   (b)

FIGURE 4: Immunohistochemical staining showed the carcinoma cells to be positive for epithelial membrane antigen (EMA) and MUC-1. Carcinoma cell membranes at the periphery of the cell clusters were characteristically positive for EMA and MUC-1, indicating an "inside-out" pattern of reactivity.

invasion and nodal metastasis in various organs. With recent chemotherapeutic advances, it is expected that adjuvant chemotherapy would result in a survival benefit after surgery for stages II and III gastric cancer [11]. Eom et al. [9] reported that IPMC of the stomach was predictive of worse patient survival rate especially in patients with stages I and II cancer. Adjuvant chemotherapy should be administered for the patients with IPMC of the stomach at high risk for recurrence. Additionally, a few reported cases of early-stage IPMC of the stomach exist in the literature [7, 10]. With the technical advance of endoscopic submucosal dissection (ESD), most early-stage gastric cancer could be treated without surgery. However, it is important not to hesitate to carry out surgery when pathological examination of the specimen after ESD reveals early-stage gastric cancer with an invasive micropapillary component.

4. Conclusion

We reported a case of 5-year survival after surgery for IPMC of the stomach. To clarify the features of IPMC of the stomach, including responses to chemotherapy, further investigations with a large number of cases are required.

References

[1] S. Siriaunkgul and F. A. Tavassoli, "Invasive micropapillary carcinoma of the breast," *Modern Pathology*, vol. 6, no. 6, pp. 660–662, 1993.

[2] M. Paterakos, W. G. Watkin, S. M. Edgerton, D. H. Moore, and A. D. Thor, "Invasive micropapillary carcinoma of the breast: a prognostic study," *Human Pathology*, vol. 30, no. 12, pp. 1459–1463, 1999.

[3] H. Samaratunga and K. Khoo, "Micropapillary variant of urothelial carcinoma of the urinary bladder; a clinicopathological and immunohistochemical study," *Histopathology*, vol. 45, no. 1, pp. 55–64, 2004.

[4] S. Moritani, S. Ichihara, M. Hasegawa et al., "Serous papillary adenocarcinoma of the female genital organs and invasive micropapillary carcinoma of the breast. Are WT1, CA125, and GCDFP-15 useful in differential diagnosis?" *Human Pathology*, vol. 39, no. 5, pp. 666–671, 2008.

[5] K. Sakamoto, M. Watanabe, C. De La Cruz, H. Honda, H. Ise, and K. Mitsuki, "Primary invasive micropapillary carcinoma of the colon," *Histopathology*, vol. 47, pp. 479–484, 2005.

[6] T. Fujita, M. Konishi, N. Gotohda et al., "Invasive micropapillary carcinoma of the ampulla of Vater with extensive lymph node metastasis: report of a case," *Surgery Today*, vol. 40, no. 12, pp. 1197–1200, 2010.

[7] T. Ushiku, K. Matsusaka, Y. Iwasaki, Y. Tateishi, N. Funata, and Y. Seto, "Gastric carcinoma with invasive micropapillary pattern and its association with lymph node metastasis," *Histopathology*, vol. 59, pp. 1081–1089, 2011.

[8] T. Fujita, N. Gotohda, Y. Kato, T. Kinoshita, S. Takahashi, and M. Konishi M, "Clinicopathological features of stomach cancer with invasive micropapillary component," *Gastric Cancer*, vol. 15, pp. 179–187, 2012.

[9] D. W. Eom, G. H. Kang, S. H. Han et al., "Gastric micropapillary carcinoma: a distinct subtype with a significantly worse prognosis in TNM stages I and II," *American Journal of Surgical Pathology*, vol. 35, no. 1, pp. 84–91, 2011.

[10] J. H. Roh, A. Srivastava, G. Y. Lauwers et al., "Micropapillary carcinoma of stomach: a clinicopathologic and immunohistochemical study of 11 cases," *American Journal of Surgical Pathology*, vol. 34, no. 8, pp. 1139–1146, 2010.

[11] S. Sakuramoto, M. Sasako, T. Yamaguchi et al., "Adjuvant chemotherapy for gastric cancer with S-1, an oral fluoropyrimidine," *New England Journal of Medicine*, vol. 357, no. 18, pp. 1810–1820, 2007.

17

Reexpansion Pulmonary Edema following Laparoscopy-Assisted Distal Gastrectomy for a Patient with Early Gastric Cancer: A Case Report

Kazuhito Yajima,[1] Tatsuo Kanda,[1] Ryo Tanaka,[1] Yu Sato,[1] Takashi Ishikawa,[1] Shin-ichi Kosugi,[1] Tadayuki Honda,[2] and Katsuyoshi Hatakeyama[1]

[1] *Division of Digestive and General Surgery, Niigata University Graduate School of Medical and Dental Sciences, 1-757 Asahimachi-dori, Niigata 951-8510, Japan*
[2] *Advanced Disaster Medical and Emergency Critical Care Center, Niigata University Medical and Dental Hospital, 1-754 Asahimachi-dori, Niigata 951-8520, Japan*

Correspondence should be addressed to Kazuhito Yajima, yajikazu@nifty.com

Academic Editors: G. Rallis, M. Rangarajan, and C. Schmitz

We report here a case of reexpansion pulmonary edema following laparoscopy-assisted distal gastrectomy (LADG) for early gastric cancer. A 57-year-old Japanese woman with no preoperative comorbidity was diagnosed with early gastric cancer. The patient underwent LADG using the pneumoperitoneum method. During surgery, the patient was unintentionally subjected to single-lung ventilation for approximately 247 minutes due to intratracheal tube dislocation. One hour after surgery, she developed severe dyspnea and produced a large amount of pink frothy sputum. Chest radiography results showed diffuse ground-glass attenuation and alveolar consolidation in both lungs without cardiomegaly. A diagnosis of pulmonary edema was made, and the patient was immediately intubated and received ventilatory support with high positive end-expiratory pressure. The patient gradually recovered and was weaned from the ventilatory support on the third postoperative day. This case shows that single-lung ventilation may be a risk factor for reexpansion pulmonary edema during laparoscopic surgery with pneumoperitoneum.

1. Introduction

Due to advances in instruments and surgical techniques, laparoscopic surgery has been widely used in recent years for the treatment of early gastric cancer [1]. The many advantages of laparoscopic gastrectomy, including reduced surgical invasiveness, less postoperative pain, better cosmetic outcomes, and faster recovery after surgery, are well documented [2, 3]. Although surgical stress and tissue damage are minimized by laparoscopic techniques, laparoscopic surgery is associated with the risk of serious adverse events that are laparoscopic specific. These complications are mainly a result of prolonged pneumoperitoneum with concomitant high intraabdominal pressure. Reexpansion pulmonary edema (RPE) is a potentially life-threatening complication. Morbidity is caused by the rapid reexpansion of collapsed lungs, a process associated with the treatment of pleural effusion, pneumothorax, and single-lung ventilation. We herein report a case of reexpansion pulmonary edema following laparoscopy-assisted distal gastrectomy (LADG) associated with unintended single-lung ventilation.

2. Case Report

A 57-year-old Japanese woman (body height: 146 cm; body weight: 54.3 kg; body mass index: 25.3 kg/m^2) was diagnosed with early adenocarcinoma of the middle third of the stomach. She had no history of smoking, lung disease, or heart disease. Preoperative laboratory data were normal. Respiratory function tests showed that her vital capacity was 2160 mL, and forced expiratory volume in one second was 1640 mL. Chest radiography did not reveal any notable findings. Blood gas analysis (BGA) was not performed preoperatively.

Upper gastrointestinal endoscopy revealed a depressed-type tumor in the greater curvature of the middle third of the stomach. The tumor was classified as a moderately to poorly differentiated adenocarcinoma by biopsy. Endoscopically, the tumor invasion was evaluated as not reaching the submucosa, but the tumor had a concomitant peptic ulcer scar (Figure 1). Accordingly, distal gastrectomy using a laparoscopic approach was recommended for this early gastric cancer (cT1N0M0, stage IA).

The LADG procedure in the present case was carried out as follows: the patient was positioned in the supine position with the legs apart and head-up tilt. A pneumoperitoneum was created using carbon dioxide via a Veress needle, and the maximum pneumoperitoneum pressure was set at 10 mmHg. Distal gastrectomy was completed with laparoscopic manipulations through five trocars, and a D1 lymphadenectomy with dissection of stations 8a, 9, and 11p [4] was also performed. The resected stomach was removed from a 5 cm minilaparotomy placed in the upper middle abdomen, and a gastrojejunostomy was made extracorporeally using the Roux-en-Y procedure. Intraoperative findings are shown in Figure 2. The total operative time and the duration of pneumoperitoneum were 309 minutes and 214 minutes, respectively. The blood loss was less than 10 mL.

General anesthesia was induced using propofol (1% Diprivan injection, AstraZeneca Co., Osaka, Japan) and rocuronium bromide (Eslax Intravenous, MSD K.K., Tokyo, Japan). Remifentanil hydrochloride (Ultiva, Janssen Pharmaceutical K.K., Tokyo, Japan) was also administered. An epidural anesthesia using ropivacaine hydrochloride hydrate (Anapeine injection, AstraZeneca Co., Osaka, Japan) was also administered. The intratracheal tube (7.0 mm ID) was inserted transorally and placed 21 cm from the incisors and inflated with 4 mL of cuff air. Upon noticing a decrease in the monitored SpO_2 levels, the intratracheal tube was pulled back 1 cm under bronchofiberscopic observation 247 minutes after the start of anesthesia. The results of BGA during anesthesia and the postoperative course are shown in Table 1.

The total time under anesthesia was 409 minutes. The total administered fluid intake was 2560 mL, and urine output during surgery was 330 mL. Blood pressure and heart rate remained stable throughout the surgery. Figure 3(a) shows the chest radiograph that was taken in the operating room just after surgery was completed.

The patient was extubated in the operating room and returned to the surgical ward as her respiratory condition was regarded as acceptable. One hour after surgery, the patient complained of dyspnea and rapidly developed respiratory failure: pulse oximetry revealed that the blood oxygen saturation decreased to 85% despite the use of an oxygen mask (10 L/min). Arterial BGA indicated the following results: pH 7.237, pO_2 56.2 mmHg, and pCO_2 63.9 mmHg. A large amount of pink frothy sputum was discharged from the airway and nasogastric tube. A chest radiograph demonstrated progression of diffuse ground glass

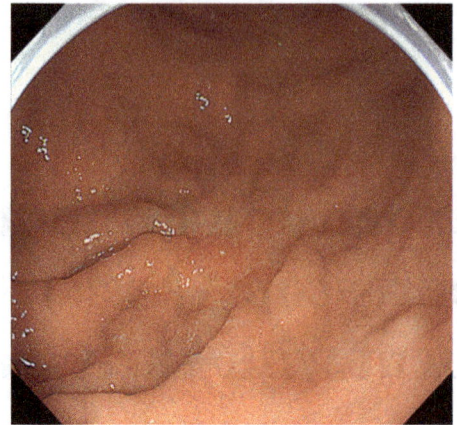

FIGURE 1: Gastrointestinal endoscopy revealed a depressed-type tumor in the greater curvature of the middle third of the stomach. Biopsy specimens showed a moderately to poorly differentiated adenocarcinoma of the stomach.

attenuation and the appearance of alveolar consolidation (Figure 3(b)). On the basis of these findings, a diagnosis of pulmonary edema was made.

The patient was immediately intubated and received ventilatory support using the Puritan Bennett 840 Ventilator System (Covidien, Tokyo, Japan), set on the synchronized intermittent mandatory ventilation plus pressure support (PS) mode, with a tidal volume of 450 mL, frequency of 20 breaths/minutes, positive end-expiratory pressure (PEEP) of 10 mmHg, PS of 8 mmHg, and FiO_2 of 100%, in the intensive care unit. A dose of 500 mg of methylprednisolone sodium succinate (Solu-Medrol, Pfizer Japan, Tokyo, Japan) was administered by intravenous bolus, and sivelestat sodium hydrate (Elaspol, Ono Pharmaceutical Co., Ltd, Osaka, Japan), a selective inhibitor of neutrophil elastase, was also administered (0.23 mg/kg/hr) for three days. Fiber optic bronchoscopy revealed that the frothy secretions originated from both lungs.

The patient's respiratory condition improved gradually, and she was extubated on the third postoperative day (POD) (Figure 3(c)). Thereafter, the patient recovered uneventfully. She started a diet on the fifth POD and was discharged on the 15th POD.

3. Discussion

We have described a 57-year-old woman who developed severe bilateral pulmonary edema following LADG for early gastric cancer. To characterize this rare but life-threatening disease, we searched the PUBMED and Japana Centra Revuo Medicina (Vor.5) databases using the keywords "laparoscopy" and "pulmonary edema." As of October 2011, there were only nine case reports including reference lists describing pulmonary edema following laparoscopic surgery. The nine published cases and the current case are summarized in Table 2 [5–12]. Four cases were from Japan [5, 6, 9, 10], three from South Korea [7, 11, 12], and the remaining two from the United States [8].

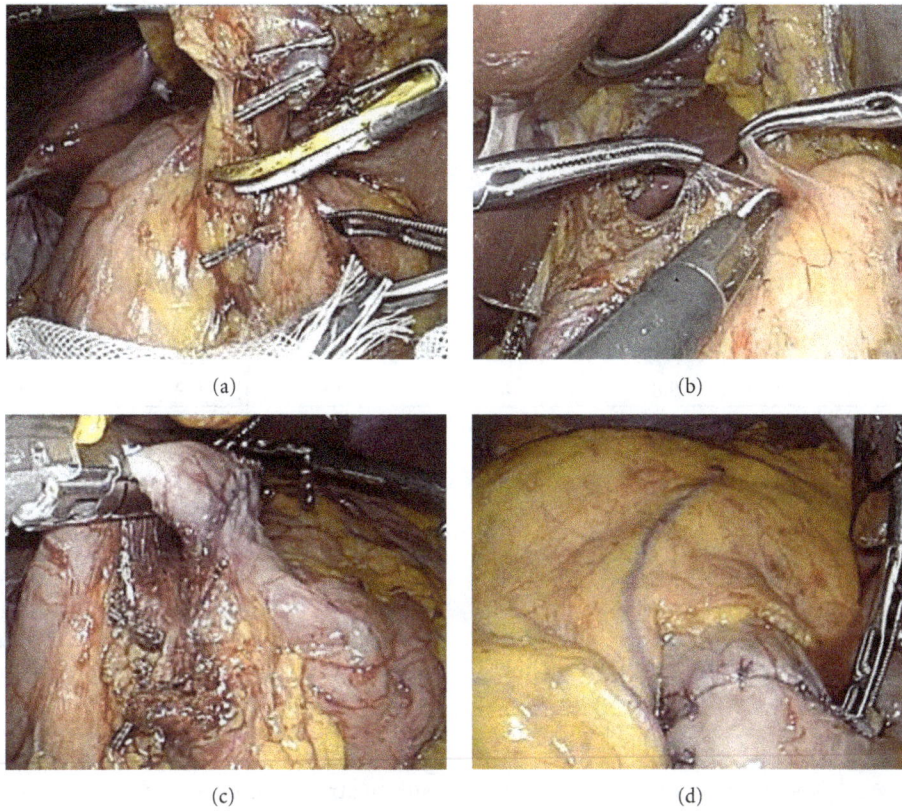

FIGURE 2: Intraabdominal findings from the laparoscopy-assisted distal gastrectomy with lymphadenectomy. (a) Dissection of the infrapyloric lymph nodes (station 6) from the pancreatic head: the right gastroepiploic vessels were exposed and divided. (b) Dissection of lymph node stations 7, 8a, 9, and 11p: suprapancreatic lymph nodes and lymph nodes around the celiac axis were dissected along the common hepatic artery and the splenic artery. (c) Transection of the duodenum: the duodenum was cut 1 cm distal to the pylorus using an endoscopic stapling device (Endo GIA, Duet TRS, Covidien, Tokyo, Japan). (d) Anastomosis: a Roux-en Y gastrojejunostomy was made. The jejunal limb was pulled up through the retrocolic route.

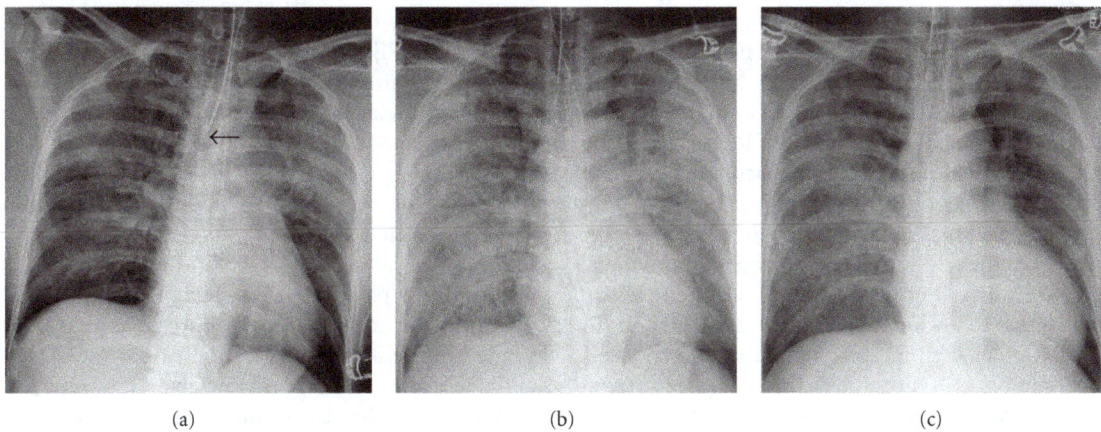

FIGURE 3: (a) A postoperative chest radiograph taken in the operating room showed bilateral diffuse ground glass attenuation. The central shadow was not widened: the cardiopulmonary rate was 48%. The tip of the intratracheal tube was located near the tracheal bifurcation (black arrow). (b) A chest radiograph demonstrated progression of the diffuse ground glass attenuation and appearance of alveolar consolidation. The photograph was taken in the intensive care unit 2 hours after surgery. (c) A chest radiograph revealed significant resolution of pulmonary abnormalities 3 days after the operation.

TABLE 1: Perioperative ventilatory support information and arterial blood gas analysis results.

	Start of anesthesia	During surgery*	Bedroom	Reintubation	1 POD	3 POD	7 POD
Respirator mode	SIMV	SIMV		[†]SIMV (VC) + PS	[†]SIMV (VC) + PS	[†]Spont/PEEP + PS	
Tidal volume	400 mL	400 mL		450 mL	450 mL	450 mL	
Frequency	20 times	20 times	None	20 times	20 times	20 times	None
PS	0 mmHg	0 mmHg		10 mmHg	12 mmHg	10 mmHg	
PEEP	0 mmHg	0 mmHg		10 mmHg	10 mmHg	5 mmHg	
BGA							
FiO_2	0.4	0.5	10 L mask	1.0	0.65	0.4	Room air
pH	7.414	7.384	7.237	7.328	7.338	7.397	7.420
pO_2 (mmHg)	178.5	86.2	56.2	158.6	137.6	74.4	88.2
pCO_2 (mmHg)	41.6	41.4	63.9	39.4	48.5	53.4	42.3
B.E. (mmol/L)	1.3	0.8	−2.4	−2.0	−0.9	6.4	1.0

SIMV: synchronized intermittent mandatory ventilation; VC: volume control; PS: pressure support; Spont: spontaneous respiration; PEEP: positive end-expiratory pressure; BE: base excess; POD: postoperative day; BGA: blood gas analysis; *During surgery: 229 minutes after the initiation of surgery. [†]Puritan Bennett 840 Ventilator System.

Of the 10 cases with pulmonary edema following laparoscopic surgery (Table 2), five patients were men and five were women with a median age of 44.5 years (range: 23–73 years). Three patients had preoperative comorbidity: however, only one patient had preoperative cardiopulmonary comorbidities (Case 7). Three patients had a malignant disease, which included cecal cancer, prostate cancer, and gastric cancer. In three patients, pulmonary edema was associated with accidental single-lung ventilation during surgery. The median operative time was 166 minutes (range: 50–330 minutes), and median infusion during the surgery was 2225 mL (range: 1750–8000 mL). The pulmonary edema was unilateral in five patients and bilateral in five patients.

Common causes of pulmonary edema include heart failure with left ventricular dysfunction, fluid overload, and renal failure. Morrisroe et al. [8] reported two cases of pulmonary edema following laparoscopic living-donor nephrectomy. The infusion volumes during surgery for these two nephrectomy cases were 7700 mL in 5 hours and 8000 mL in 5.5 hours, respectively. The authors presumed that the infusion overload may have been the main cause of the postoperative pulmonary edema. Patient position during an operation is also an important issue to consider when determining the association between volume overload and perioperative pulmonary edema. Several reports suggested that a steep Trendelenburg position could be one of the risks for perioperative pulmonary edema [5, 11–13]. Stoelting [13] reported a case of severe pulmonary edema following total pelvic exenteration in a 30-year-old woman with alveolar rhabdomyosarcoma of the pelvis. Stoelting [13] presumed that the steep Trendelenburg position was a possible cause: the steep position led to further elevation of the high central venous pressure thereby provoking the development of pulmonary edema.

In the present case, the chest radiograph taken at the end of the operation did not show cardiomegaly, and the infused volume for this patient (2560 mL lactated Ringer's solution

in 5 hours) did not appear to be an overload. Moreover, the patient was positioned with a head-up tilt during the laparoscopic surgery. Cardiac failure or fluid overload was unlikely to account for perioperative pulmonary edema in the present case.

RPE is a particular form of pulmonary edema. In general, RPE is well known as a complication associated with treatment for pleural effusion and pneumothorax [14]. The reported incidence rate of RPE following spontaneous pneumothorax ranges from 0.9% to 14% [15, 16]. The clinical presentations of RPE are rapid onset of dyspnea and/or tachypnea. Pink frothy sputum is one of the important signs used to make a clinical diagnosis. Mahfood et al. [17] reviewed 47 cases of RPE reported between 1958 and 1987. Based on their study, 64% of the patients developed RPE within one hour of lung reexpansion, and the remainder developed it within 24 hours. Interestingly, RPE could occur not only in the collapsed lung but also in the contralateral lung or in both lungs. It is noteworthy that the study indicated that middle-aged women were more likely to be affected by RPE: the cohort was composed of 9 men and 38 women with an average age of 42 years.

RPE associated with surgery can occur after single-lung ventilation, although the exact pathophysiology is still unknown. Many cases of RPE following single-lung ventilation occurred in patients undergoing thoracoscopic surgery, which requires intentional single-lung ventilation [18–21]. Hong et al. [7] reported a case of RPE that occurred in a patient with a body mass index of 38.6 kg/m^2 who underwent laparoscopic gastric banding. In that case, single-lung ventilation accidentally occurred during surgery and continued for approximately 50 minutes. Cephalad movement of the carina during laparoscopic surgery was confirmed to cause this and may have been associated with high insufflation pressure [22]. In the present case, the results of BGA worsened with time during surgery after initiation of pneumoperitoneum. Moreover, a chest radiograph indicated that the top of the intubation tube was positioned just above the tracheal bifurcation even though the tube

TABLE 2: Reported cases of pulmonary edema following laparoscopic surgery.

Case	Year [Ref.]	Age	Sex	Comorbidity	Disease	Laparoscopic procedure	Position	Single-lung ventilation	Operation time	Infusion	Urinary output	Pulmonary edema
1	1995 [5]*	32 y	F	None	Sterility	Diagnostic laparotomy	Trendelenburg	Present	80 min	2000 mL	ND	Unilateral
2	2000 [6]	31 y	F	Obesity, pregnancy	Cushing's synd.	Adrenalectomy	Lateral	None	150 min	2150 mL	1100 mL	Unilateral
3	2005 [7]	23 y	F	Obesity	Obesity	Bariatric surgery	ND	Present	140 min	2400 mL	120 mL	Unilateral
4	2007 [8]	32 y	M	None	Donor	Nephrectomy	Lateral	None	300 min	7700 mL	1550 mL	Unilateral
5	2007 [8]	44 y	M	None	Donor	Nephrectomy	Lateral	None	330 min	8000 mL	2750 mL	Unilateral
6	2010 [9]*	45 y	M	None	Cecal cancer	Ileocecal resection	ND	None	182 min	3460 mL	1330 mL	Bilateral
7	2010 [10]*	73 y	M	HT, DM, angina	Cholecystitis	Cholecystectomy	ND	None	128 min	2150 mL	290 mL	Bilateral
8	2010 [11]	25 y	F	None	Ectopic pregnancy	ND	Trendelenburg	None	50 min	1750 mL	ND	Bilateral
9	2010 [12]	63 y	M	None	Prostate cancer	Prostatectomy	Trendelenburg	None	256 min	2500 mL	800 mL	Bilateral
10	2011†	57 y	F	None	Gastric cancer	Distal gastrectomy	Head-up tilt	Present	309 min	2150 mL	290 mL	Bilateral

* Reported in Japanese with English abstract; † our case; Ref.: reference number; ND: not described; HT: hypertension; DM: diabetes mellitus; Synd.: syndrome.

was relocated during surgery. These findings suggested that unintended single-lung ventilation, which might be caused by upward-migration of the diaphragm associated with pneumoperitoneum, triggered RPE in the present case.

Carbon dioxide (CO_2) is generally used for pneumoperitoneum because it is quickly absorbed from the peritoneal cavity into the circulation. However, the absorbed CO_2 might induce hemodynamic, pulmonary, renal, splanchnic, and endocrine pathophysiological changes [23]. Pulmonary complications of laparoscopic surgery with CO_2 pneumoperitoneum are represented by hypercapnia, hypoxemia, acidosis, barotrauma, pulmonary edema, atelectasis, gas embolism, and pneumothorax. Karapolat et al. [24] demonstrated histologically that CO_2 pneumoperitoneum caused oxidative stress injury to lung tissue including intra-alveolar hemorrhage, congestion, and leukocyte infiltration in a rodent model. However, at present there is no clinical evidence indicating that CO_2 pneumoperitoneum is a risk for pulmonary edema. The clinical significance of hypercapnia associated with pneumoperitoneum is more important, because an increasing number of cancer surgeries are being performed using a laparoscopic approach, a process that requires prolonged pneumoperitoneum and has an increased risk for hypercapnia.

The treatment for pulmonary edema is supplementary oxygen and ventilatory support with a high PEEP. The use of steroids, diuretics, and bronchodilators is also beneficial. As rapid reexpansion of a collapsed lung or a sudden increase in the negative intrapleural pressure can lead to fluid transudation across the capillaries and alveolar membranes, inhibitors of neutrophil elastase may serve as a rational treatment for patients with RPE. Trachiotis et al. [25] recommended that the lateral decubitus position was beneficial because it facilitated the recovery of insulted lungs from reduced perfusion and interstitial edema. Differential lung ventilation was recently advocated as a useful treatment for RPE [26]. Tung et al. [27] reported a case of severe RPE that developed bilaterally, in which they successfully cured the patient using extracorporeal membrane oxygenation. The reported mortality rate for RPE is very high. Mahfood et al. [17] reported that 11 of 47 patients with RPE died: the mortality rate is estimated as higher than 20%. It is likely that the early introduction of ventilatory support with high PEEP and the timely use of steroids and a neutrophil elastase inhibitor were beneficial for the complete recovery of the patient in the present case.

In conclusion, we have described a case of RPE following an uneventful LADG for early gastric cancer. Single-lung ventilation may be a risk factor for RPE during laparoscopic surgery with pneumoperitoneum. Surgeons and anesthesiologists involved in laparoscopic surgery should be aware of the risk for this life-threatening disease.

References

[1] S. Nomura and M. Kaminishi, "Surgical treatment of early gastric cancer," *Digestive Surgery*, vol. 24, no. 2, pp. 96–100, 2007.

[2] K. Shehzad, K. Mohiuddin, S. Nizami et al., "Current status of minimal access surgery for gastric cancer," *Surgical Oncology*, vol. 16, no. 2, pp. 85–98, 2007.

[3] S. Kitano, N. Shiraishi, I. Uyama et al., "A multicenter study on oncologic outcome of laparoscopic gastrectomy for early cancer in Japan," *Annals of Surgery*, vol. 245, no. 1, pp. 68–72, 2007.

[4] Japanese Gastric Cancer Association, "Japanese classification of gastric carcinoma—2nd English Edition," *Gastric Cancer*, vol. 1, pp. 10–24, 1998.

[5] K. Koshiba, F. Suzuki, F. Asato, and F. Goto, "Unilateral pulmonary edema following accidental endobronchial intubation," *Journal of Clinical Anesthesia*, vol. 19, pp. 1201–1202, 1995.

[6] Y. M. Nakashima, Y. Itonaga, H. Inoue, and S. Takahashi, "Pulmonary edema after laparoscopic adrenalectomy in a pregnant patient with Cushing's syndrome," *Journal of Anesthesia*, vol. 14, no. 3, pp. 157–159, 2000.

[7] S. J. Hong, J. Y. Lee, J. H. Choi, H. J. Lee, and C. H. Choi, "Pulmonary edema following laparoscopic bariatric surgery," *Obesity Surgery*, vol. 15, no. 8, pp. 1202–1206, 2005.

[8] S. N. Morrisroe, R. T. Wall, and A. D. Lu, "Unilateral pulmonary edema after laparoscopic donor nephrectomy: report of two cases," *Journal of Endourology*, vol. 21, no. 7, pp. 760–762, 2007.

[9] T. Yamada, K. Kito, M. Kawamura, H. Ohata, and S. Ota, "Acute pulmonary edema after extubation," *Journal of Clinical Anesthesia*, vol. 34, pp. 603–604, 2010.

[10] R. Takabayashi, O. Tajiri, H. Ito, and Y. Yago, "A case of pulmonary edema due to excessive hypertension following extubation," *Japanese Journal of Anesthesiology*, vol. 59, no. 12, pp. 1487–1489, 2010.

[11] J. H. Shim, W. J. Shin, and S. H. Lee, "Bilateral upper lobe pulmonary edema during gynecologic laparoscopic surgery in the Trendelenberg position," *Korean Journal of Anesthesiology*, vol. 59, pp. S163–S166, 2010.

[12] J. Y. Hong, Y. J. Oh, K. H. Rha, W. S. Park, Y. S. Kim, and H. K. Kil, "Pulmonary edema after da Vinci-assisted laparoscopic radical prostatectomy: a case report," *Journal of Clinical Anesthesia*, vol. 22, no. 5, pp. 370–372, 2010.

[13] R. K. Stoelting, "Acute pulmonary edema during anesthesia and operation in a healthy young patient," *Anesthesiology*, vol. 33, no. 3, pp. 366–369, 1970.

[14] S. M. Neustein, "Reexpansion pulmonary edema," *Journal of Cardiothoracic and Vascular Anesthesia*, vol. 21, no. 6, pp. 887–891, 2007.

[15] J. Rozenman, A. Yellin, D. A. Simansky, and R. J. Shiner, "Re-expansion pulmonary oedema following spontaneous pneumothorax," *Respiratory Medicine*, vol. 90, no. 4, pp. 235–238, 1996.

[16] Y. Matsuura, T. Nomimura, H. Murakami, T. Matsushima, M. Kakehashi, and H. Kajihara, "Clinical analysis of reexpansion pulmonary edema," *Chest*, vol. 100, no. 6, pp. 1562–1566, 1991.

[17] S. Mahfood, W. R. Hix, B. L. Aaron, P. Blaes, and D. C. Watson, "Reexpansion pulmonary edema," *Annals of Thoracic Surgery*, vol. 45, no. 3, pp. 340–345, 1988.

[18] A. P. C. Yim and H. P. Liu, "Complications and failures of video-assisted thoracic surgery: experience from two centers

in Asia," *Annals of Thoracic Surgery*, vol. 61, no. 2, pp. 538–541, 1996.

[19] W. R. Smythe, N. D. Bridges, J. W. Gaynor, S. Nicolson, B. J. Clark, and T. L. Spray, "Reexpansion pulmonary edema after VATS successfully treated with continuous positive airway pressure," *Annals of Thoracic Surgery*, vol. 70, no. 2, pp. 669–671, 2000.

[20] N. Barbetakis, G. Samanidis, D. Paliouras, and C. Tsilikas, "Re-expansion pulmonary edema following video-assisted thoracic surgery for recurrent malignant pleural effusion," *Interactive Cardiovascular and Thoracic Surgery*, vol. 7, no. 3, pp. 532–534, 2008.

[21] C. Y. Chang, M. H. Hung, H. C. Chang et al., "Delayed onset of contralateral pulmonary edema following reexpansion pulmonary edema of a collapsed lung after video-assisted thoracoscopic surgery," *Acta Anaesthesiologica Taiwanica*, vol. 47, no. 2, pp. 87–91, 2009.

[22] N. Morimura, K. Inoue, and T. Miwa, "Chest roentgenogram demonstrates cephalad movement of the carina during laparoscopic cholecystectomy," *Anesthesiology*, vol. 81, no. 5, pp. 1301–1302, 1994.

[23] C. N. Gutt, T. Oniu, A. Mehrabi et al., "Circulatory and respiratory complications of carbon dioxide insufflation," *Digestive Surgery*, vol. 21, no. 2, pp. 95–105, 2004.

[24] S. Karapolat, S. Gezer, U. Yildirim et al., "Prevention of pulmonary complications of pneumoperitoneum in rats," *Journal of Cardiothoracic Surgery*, vol. 6, no. 1, article 4, 2011.

[25] G. D. Trachiotis, L. A. Vricella, B. L. Aaron, and W. R. Hix, "Reexpansion pulmonary edema: updated in 1997," *Annals of Thoracic Surgery*, vol. 63, no. 4, pp. 1206–1207, 1997.

[26] S. R. Cho, S. L. Jeong, and S. K. Mun, "New treatment method for reexpansion pulmonary edema: differential lung ventilation," *Annals of Thoracic Surgery*, vol. 80, no. 5, pp. 1933–1934, 2005.

[27] Y. W. Tung, F. Lin, M. S. Yang, C. W. Wu, and K. S. Cheung, "Bilateral developing reexpansion pulmonary edema treated with extracorporeal membrane oxygenation," *Annals of Thoracic Surgery*, vol. 89, no. 4, pp. 1268–1271, 2010.

18

Jejunojejunal Intussusception as the Initial Presentation of Non-Hodgkin's B-Cell Lymphoma in an Adult Patient

V. Stohlner, N. A. Chatzizacharias, M. Parthasarathy, and T. Groot-Wassink

Department of Surgery, Ipswich Hospital, Ipswich, Suffolk IP4 5PD, UK

Correspondence should be addressed to N. A. Chatzizacharias; nickchatzizachariasmd@yahoo.com

Academic Editors: K. Honma, H. Kawai, and M. L. Quek

Introduction. Intussusception is a rare cause of bowel obstruction in adults and is usually associated with an underlying pathology, benign, or malignant. This is a report of a case of jejunojejunal intussusception secondary to non-Hodgkin's B-cell lymphoma in an adult patient. *Case Presentation.* A 74-year-old male with no previous significant medical history presented with symptoms of acute intestinal obstruction. A CT scan of the abdomen and pelvis revealed 2 areas of jejunojejunal intussusception, which were surgically managed successfully. Histopathological examination of the specimen revealed the presence of high grade diffuse large B-cell-type non-Hodgkin's lymphoma, and the patient was referred to the oncology team for further management. *Discussion.* B-cell lymphoma is a rare but well-documented cause of intussusception in adults, with most cases being at the ileocolic region. We present a rare case of jejunojejunal intussusception as the initial presentation of non-Hodgkin's B-cell lymphoma in an adult patient.

1. Introduction

Intussusception of the bowel, first reported in 1674, can be described as the telescoping of a proximal segment of the intestine within the lumen of the adjacent segment [1]. It is considered a rare cause of bowel obstruction in adults with approximately 95% of the total number of cases of intussusception seen in children. A small number of cases seen in adults are idiopathic, with no lead point lesion identified. However, the majority of cases are secondary to pathology, such as carcinoma, polyps, diverticulum, or other lesions [1].

Lymphoma is a very rare cause of adult intussusception, with only 36 cases reported in the literature between 2000 and 2011 [2]. Of these 11 were due to the non-Hodgkin's B-cell type.

We report a rare case of non-Hodgkin's B-cell lymphoma presenting with 2 areas of jejunojejunal intussusception. A similar presentation, with one area of jejunojejunal intussusception, has been reported only once previously [3].

2. Case Presentation

The patient was a 74-year-old male who presented to the emergency department of our hospital complaining of severe abdominal pain associated with vomiting and failure to defecate for three days. A detailed history revealed that his symptomatology included a 2 month history of significant weight loss (12 Kg over 2-months) and poor appetite. He also complained of a recent change in bowel habit, alternating between constipation and loose motions, and an intermittent colicky abdominal pain, which was relieved by passing flatus and defecation.

Clinical examination revealed a distended, soft abdomen, with generalised tenderness, but no peritonism, organomegaly, or masses. Bowel sounds were reduced and rectal examination was unremarkable. All other aspects of the examination were normal. Initial blood investigations showed raised inflammatory markers (CRP 231 mg/L, white blood cells 17.1×10^9/L) and anaemia (haemoglobin 9.5 g/dL, MCV 71 fL). An abdominal X-ray showed distended loops of small bowel.

An initial diagnosis of bowel obstruction was made and the patient was admitted for conservative management. Further investigations with a computer tomography (CT) scan of the abdomen and pelvis with contrast showed a 9 cm circumferential wall thickening of the small bowel inferior to the transverse colon, associated with two areas of intussusception and further abnormal loops of bowel (Figure 1). A decision for an emergency laparotomy was reached. Intraoperative findings confirmed two separate areas of jejunojejunal intussusception. The involved parts of the bowel were resected and an end-to-end anastomosis was performed. Furthermore, during inspection of the bowel numerous thick stalked polyps were identified within the jejunum. The seven largest of these were resected by separate enterotomies.

Postoperatively the patient was managed on the Intensive Care Unit and was discharged to the ward on day 6. His course was complicated with an upper gastrointestinal bleed on day 7 due to a Mallory-Weis tear, which was managed with an emergency esophagogastroscopy. The remaining of the recovery period was uncomplicated and the patient was discharged after a total of 26 days of hospital stay.

The histopathological examination of the specimens revealed features of high grade non-Hodgkin's B-cell lymphoma of the diffuse large B-cell type (Figure 2). Therefore the patient was referred to the oncology team for appropriate further management.

3. Discussion

Primary lymphoma of the gastrointestinal tract accounts for 30–40% of lymphomas arising extranodally and comprises 10–15% of all non-Hodgkin lymphomas [4]. Symptomatology varies and can include any combination of the following: dyspepsia, epigastric pain, abdominal pain, nausea, vomiting, diarrhoea, weight loss, malabsorption, obstruction, anaemia, and to a lesser extent ulceration, perforation, and intussusceptions [5–7]. In the Western population, 60% to 80% of intestinal lymphomas are B-cell lymphomas, mostly of the diffuse type. Most commonly they are derived from the B cells in the lymphoid tissue of the lamina propria and submucosa of the ileum, where the greatest concentration of gut-associated lymphoid tissue is located [6, 7].

Intussusception is rarely considered clinically in the differential diagnosis of adult patients with vague abdominal complaints. Therefore diagnosis is usually made on CT or during exploratory laparoscopy/laparotomy [8]. The clinical importance of intussusception in adults is that it is usually due to an underlying pathology. Therefore, surgical resection, with adequate margins in case of suspected malignancy, is considered as the definitive management in this population [2, 3, 9]. Although rare, intussusception is a recognised presenting feature of lymphoma [2, 5–7, 9]. The most common recognised site is the ileocolic region [2, 5–9]. We report a case of non-Hodgkin's B-cell lymphoma presenting with 2 areas of jejunojejunal intussusception. This is the first case with more than one area of small intestinal intussusception due to lymphoma in the published literature, with

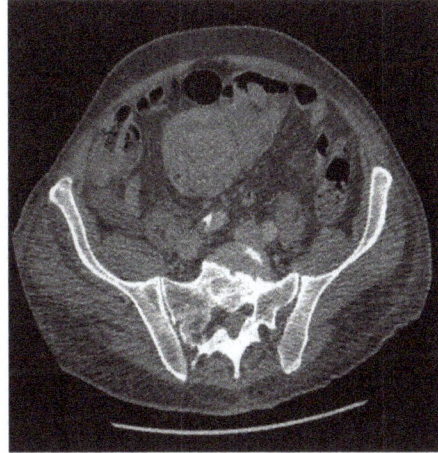

FIGURE 1: CT scan illustrating the area of intussusception.

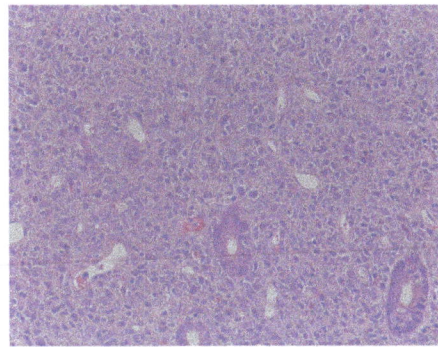

FIGURE 2: Hematoxylin and eosin stain showing intestinal glands surrounded by large pleomorphic lymphoid cells (magnification ×200).

one case of a single intussusception been also described [3]. These two cases demonstrate that lymphoma polyps in any part of the small bowel can cause intussusception. Excision of such polyps with critical size at the time of surgery appears advisable. Urgent chemotherapy is required to prevent enlargement of other smaller lesions.

In conclusion, intussusception in the adult population is usually associated with an underlying cause, including lymphoma. This report illustrates a rare case of a jejunojejunal intussusception secondary to a high grade diffuse large B-cell-type non-Hodgkin's lymphoma.

References

[1] A. Marinis, A. Yiallourou, L. Samanides et al., "Intussusception of the bowel in adults: a review," World Journal of Gastroenterology, vol. 15, no. 4, pp. 407–411, 2009.

[2] S. Akbulut, "Unusual cause of adult intussusception: diffuse large B-cell non-Hodgkin's lymphoma: a case report and review," European Review for Medical and Pharmacological Sciences, vol. 16, pp. 1938–1946, 2012.

[3] N. S. Salemis, E. Tsiambas, C. Liatsos, A. Karameris, and E. Tsohataridis, "Small bowel intussusception due to a primary non-hodgkin's lymphoma. An unusual presentation and clinical

course," *Journal of Gastrointestinal Cancer*, vol. 41, no. 4, pp. 233–237, 2010.

[4] M. A. Bautista-Quach, C. D. Ake, M. Chen, and J. Wang, "Gastrointestinal lymphomas: morphology, immunophenotype and molecular features," *Journal of Gastrointestinal Oncology*, vol. 3, pp. 209–225, 2012.

[5] E. G. Ford, "Gastrointestinal tumors," in *Pediatric Surgical Oncology*, R. J. Andrassy, Ed., pp. 289–304, WB Saunders, Philadelphia, Pa, USA, 1st edition, 1998.

[6] M. P. LaQuaglia, C. J. H. Stolar, M. Krailo et al., "The role of surgery in abdominal non-Hodgkin's lymphoma: experience from the childrens cancer study group," *Journal of Pediatric Surgery*, vol. 27, no. 2, pp. 230–235, 1992.

[7] P. Domizio, R. A. Owen, N. A. Shepherd, I. C. Talbot, and A. J. Norton, "Primary lymphoma of the small intestine: a clinicopathological study of 119 cases," *American Journal of Surgical Pathology*, vol. 17, no. 5, pp. 429–442, 1993.

[8] G. Gayer, R. Zissin, S. Apter, M. Papa, and M. Hertz, "Adult intussusception—a CT diagnosis," *British Journal of Radiology*, vol. 75, no. 890, pp. 185–190, 2002.

[9] L. Yin, C. Q. Chen, C. H. Peng et al., "Primary small-bowel non-Hodgkin's lymphoma: a study of clinical features, pathology, management and prognosis," *Journal of International Medical Research*, vol. 35, no. 3, pp. 406–415, 2007.

19

Unusual Case of Metastatic Gastrointestinal Adenocarcinoma to the Cervical Spine without a Detectable Primary Source in a Patient with Acquired Immunodeficiency Syndrome: A Case Report

Paul E. Kaloostian,[1] Marc Barry,[2] and James Fred Harrington[1]

[1] *Department of Neurosurgery, The University of New Mexico, MSC 10 5615, Albuquerque, NM 87131-0001, USA*
[2] *Department of Pathology, The University of New Mexico, MSC 10 5615, Albuquerque, NM 87131-0001, USA*

Correspondence should be addressed to Paul E. Kaloostian, paulkaloostian@hotmail.com

Academic Editors: K. Honma, E. Ishikawa, S. H. Jeon, and Y. Rino

The authors report a case of metastatic gastrointestinal adenocarcinoma to the cervical spine in a patient with acquired immunodeficiency syndrome (AIDS) being treated with antiretroviral therapy. The source of this tumor could not be identified despite a thorough evaluation. A 49-year-old male being treated for AIDS presents with worsening neck pain and left distal arm weakness. MRI demonstrated an erosive mass within the cervical four vertebral body extending through the pedicle on the left side. Patient underwent needle biopsy followed by combined anterior and posterior fusion procedures. Pathology demonstrated metastatic gastrointestinal adenocarcinoma without known primary origin. He is currently undergoing palliative radiotherapy. This is an unusual case of metastatic gastrointestinal adenocarcinoma to the cervical spine. This should be included on the differential diagnosis of spinal lesions in this patient population and may represent a unique tumor in patients with HIV/AIDS who are on immunosuppressive therapy.

1. Introduction

The authors report an unusual case of symptomatic metastatic gastrointestinal adenocarcinoma without known primary tumor to the cervical spine in a patient with AIDS on chronic antiretroviral therapy.

2. Case Presentation

We report the case of a 49-year-old homosexual male being treated for AIDS who presented with worsening neck pain and left distal arm and hand weakness. MRI demonstrated an erosive mass within the C4 vertebral body extending through the pedicle on the left side and causing severe spinal stenosis (Figures 1 and 2). Additionally, multiple cervical spine vertebral bodies were involved in this pathological process with the fourth cervical body being the most remarkable.

PET scan, CT scan of chest/abdomen/pelvis, prior recent colonoscopy, and upper endoscopy were all performed demonstrating no obvious source. No other lesions were noted elsewhere.

Patient underwent needle biopsy followed by anterior cervical corpectomy and fusion and finally posterior lateral mass instrumentation and fusion (Figure 3). Pathological examination demonstrated metastatic adenocarcinoma composed of infiltrating glands and focal sheets of moderately differentiated tumor (Figure 4). Immunohistochemical staining with appropriate controls shows that the tumor cells are positive for cytokeratin 7, cytokeratin 20, and CDX-2 and are negative for TTF-1 and napsin. The morphologic and immunohistochemical findings are most consistent with tumor origin from a gastrointestinal primary tumor, in particular from an upper gastrointestinal or pancreaticobiliary primary tumor.

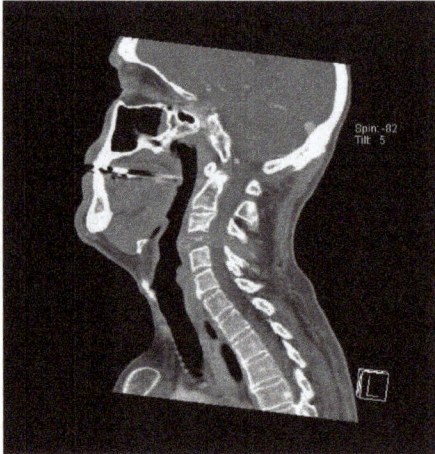

FIGURE 1: CT of the neck demonstrating erosive metastatic tumor of the C4 vertebral body.

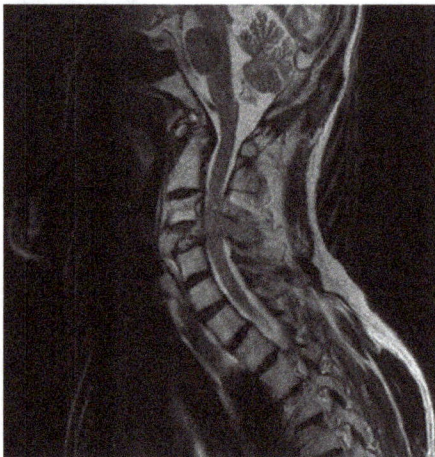

FIGURE 2: MRI of the cervical spine demonstrating erosive metastatic tumor of the C4 vertebral body.

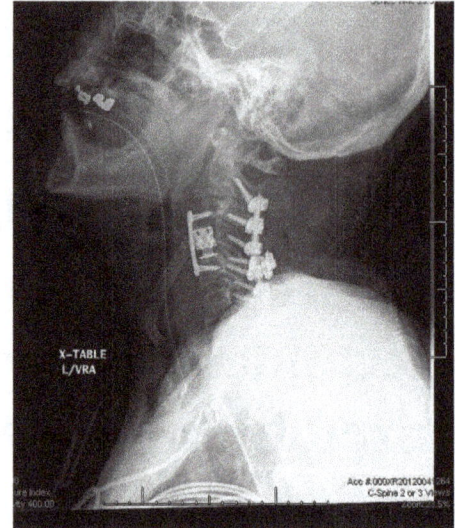

FIGURE 3: Postoperative cervical spine X rays demonstrating cervical corpectomy with placement of cage and posterior lateral mass instrumentation.

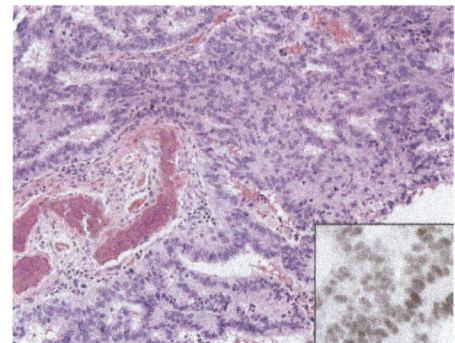

FIGURE 4: Metastatic adenocarcinoma involving trabecular bone (H&E, 200x), with (inset) immunoperoxidase staining of tumor for CDX-2 (400x).

The patient was successfully treated for post-operative cerebrospinal fluid collection in the neck with a lumbar drain. His neurological examination returned to its baseline. His CD4 counts remained stable preoperatively and postoperatively. He is currently undergoing palliative radiotherapy with 37.5 Gy over 15 fractions to his cervical spine.

3. Discussion

AIDS-defining cancers, such as Kaposi's sarcoma, non-Hodgkin's lymphoma, and cervical cancer, are quite common in patients with end-stage AIDS [1–3]. Over the last few decades with the advent of antiretroviral therapy, the incidence of these cancers has increased significantly [1, 3]. Additionally, the incidence of non-AIDS-defining cancers has increased in this patient population due to the increased longevity of patients on such medications [3–5]. These include such malignancies as anal cancer, lung cancer, hepatocellular cancer, and head and neck cancers [3–5]. Over the last few decades, a mortality in mortality in this patient

population has in fact been associated with these non-AIDS-defining malignancies [3]. It is hypothesized that the long-term immunosuppression, increased longevity with AIDS, and exposure to various carcinogens such as tobacco and drugs contribute to this increased incidence [3–5].

Some authors have argued that there is an association between chronic AIDS and human immunodeficiency syndrome (HIV) infection and the occurrence of colonic malignancy [4]. Studies have suggested that young age and advanced stage at time of diagnosis carry the greatest weight in classifying a poorer prognosis [3, 4]. It is well known that recipients of organ transplants are similarly known to have an increased incidence of cancer, believed to be related to the length of immunosuppressive drugs use to prevent rejection [3, 4].

About 10% of all cancer patients develop metastases to the spine [4, 5]. Among immunocompetent adult patients with cancer, 60% of these spinal metastases are either from the breast, lung, or prostate [4, 5]. Renal and gastrointestinal cancers each account for 5% of spinal metastases [4, 5].

In patients with AIDS, this differential diagnosis is quite different. Pathology may include non-Hodgkin's lymphoma, Kaposi's sarcoma, metastasis, and infection. To add to this complexity, unknown primary tumors in patients with clearly biopsy-proven metastatic disease are quite rare [1, 2, 6]. This incidence is in the range of 0.5%–38% [7, 8]. In these patients in whom a primary source could not be identified, antemortem studies have demonstrated definitive pathological diagnosis in 31% of cases, with a range being 7% to 88% in studies looking at patients with spinal metastatic disease [8]. In one study, lung cancer turned out to be the most common cancer found in these patients with initially an unknown primary site 56% of the time [9]. Interestingly, this study also demonstrated a significant increase in survival in patients with noncervical spinal disease as compared to those with isolated cervical metastatic disease [9]. Patients with extraspinal disease at presentation also had poorer survival compared with those who did not, hypothesized to be due to increased tumor burden [9].

Ravalli et al. noted in their seminal report three patients with HIV in less than one year who developed gastrointestinal carcinoma and suggested an increased frequency in this population [5]. Gastrointestinal metastasis to the spine is unusually rare. Reports of esophageal cancer, carcinoid tumor in a patient with multiple endocrine neoplasia, rectal cancer, and colonic adenocarcinoma have been reported [5, 10]. Other than Ravalli et al., a review of the literature noted no reports of patients with AIDS/HIV and associated gastrointestinal adenocarcinoma of unknown primary tumor despite full workup.

This case stimulates interest in a possible association between AIDS/HIV, long-term antiretroviral therapy, and metastatic gastrointestinal adenocarcinoma without a clear primary site. We wonder if this particular metastatic gastrointestinal tumor is a unique tumor of the gastrointestinal system that is associated with chronic HIV/AIDS or chronic immunotherapy. In conclusion, this pathology must be kept on the differential diagnosis list in this patient population and further cases must be documented to clearly confirm this association.

References

[1] H. F. P. Hillen, "Unknown primary tumours," *Postgraduate Medical Journal*, vol. 76, no. 901, pp. 690–693, 2000.

[2] M. Nottebaert, G. U. Exner, A. R. Von Hochstetter, and A. Schreiber, "Metastatic bone disease from occult carcinoma: a profile," *International Orthopaedics*, vol. 13, no. 2, pp. 119–123, 1989.

[3] A. M. Levine, "AIDS-related malignancies: the emerging epidemic," *Journal of the National Cancer Institute*, vol. 85, no. 17, pp. 1382–1397, 1993.

[4] J. F. Yegüez, S. A. Martinez, D. R. Sands, L. R. Sands, and M. D. Hellinger, "Colorectal malignancies in HIV-positive patients," *American Surgeon*, vol. 69, no. 11, pp. 981–987, 2003.

[5] S. Ravalli, A. B. Chabon, and A. A. Khan, "Gastrointestinal neoplasia in young HIV antibody-positive patients," *American Journal of Clinical Pathology*, vol. 91, no. 4, pp. 458–461, 1989.

[6] G. R. Varadhachary, J. L. Abbruzzese, and R. Lenzi, "Diagnostic strategies for unknown primary cancer," *Cancer*, vol. 100, no. 9, pp. 1776–1785, 2004.

[7] J. L. Abbruzzese, M. C. Abbruzzese, R. Lenzi, K. R. Hess, and M. N. Raber, "Analysis of a diagnostic strategy for patients with suspected tumors of unknown origin," *Journal of Clinical Oncology*, vol. 13, no. 8, pp. 2094–2103, 1995.

[8] J. L. Abbruzzese, M. C. Abbruzzese, K. R. Hess, M. N. Raber, R. Lenzi, and P. Frost, "Unknown primary carcinoma: natural history and prognostic factors in 657 consecutive patients," *Journal of Clinical Oncology*, vol. 12, no. 6, pp. 1272–1280, 1994.

[9] M. R. Aizenberg, B. D. Fox, D. Suki, I. E. Mccutcheon, G. Rao, and L. D. Rhines, "Surgical management of unknown primary tumors metastatic to the spine: clinical article," *Journal of Neurosurgery: Spine*, vol. 16, no. 1, pp. 86–92, 2012.

[10] M. Ohnuma, T. Uchiyama, T. Abe et al., "A case of advanced colon cancer with metastases to both para-aortic lymph nodes and cervical vertebrae effectively treated by TS-1 therapy," *Gan to Kagaku Ryoho*, vol. 33, no. 4, pp. 521–524, 2006.

20

Unusual Appearance of a Pendulated Gastric Tumor: Always Think of GIST

Kristel De Vogelaere,[1] Vanessa Meert,[2] Frederik Vandenbroucke,[3]
Georges Delvaux,[1] and Anne Hoorens[4]

[1] Department of Abdominal Surgery, UZ Brussel, Laarbeeklaan 101, 1090 Brussels, Belgium
[2] Department of Pathology, OLV Aalst, Moorselbaan 163, 9300 Aalst, Belgium
[3] Department of Radiology, UZ Brussel, Laarbeeklaan 101, 1090 Brussels, Belgium
[4] Department of Pathology, UZ Brussel, Laarbeeklaan 101, 1090 Brussels, Belgium

Correspondence should be addressed to Kristel De Vogelaere, kristel.devogelaere@uzbrussel.be

Academic Editors: M. Nikfarjam, M. Rangarajan, and M. Shimoda

Objective. To investigate the clinicopathological characteristics of gastrointestinal stromal tumor (GIST) with significant cystic changes and to assess the molecular genetic characteristics. *Methods.* In a 68-year-old man, a large abdominal tumoral mass was discovered incidentally. Computed tomography (CT) and magnetic resonance imaging (MRI) confirmed the presence of a large cystic lesion with multiple contrast-enhancing septae and papillary projections. No clear connection with any of the surrounding organs was identified. Malignancy could not be excluded, and surgery was indicated. During surgery, the large mass was found to be attached by a narrow stalk to the large curvature of the stomach. *Results.* The histological features and immunohistochemical profile of the tumor cells (positivity for CD117 and CD34) were consistent with a gastrointestinal stromal tumor with a high risk of progressive disease according to the Fletcher classification. Diagnosis was confirmed by mutational analysis; this demonstrated mutation in exon 14 of PDGFRA. During the followup of 97 months, the patient had a cancer-free survival. *Conclusions.* This case demonstrates that gastrointestinal stromal tumors (GISTs) with extensive cystic degeneration should be considered in the differential diagnosis of a cystic abdominal mass.

1. Introduction

Gastrointestinal stromal tumors (GISTs) are specific mesenchymal tumors of the gastrointestinal tract. GISTs are rare, accounting for only 0.2% of all gastrointestinal tumors [1]. Morphologically they show similarities to other tumor types and were previously misclassified as leiomyomas, leiomyoblastomas, or leiomyosarcomas, but also as schwannomas or malignant peripheral nerve sheath tumors. Since the discovery of KIT (CD117) in 1998, GISTs were identified as a distinct entity [2]. These tumors are believed to originate from the interstitial cells of Cajal or related stem cells [3–6]. Proper identification of GIST has become very important since the availability of a specific pathogenesis-targeted treatment, namely, imatinib. GISTs usually present as solid tumors. We report an incidental finding of a cystic gastric GIST with exophytic pedunculated growth.

2. Case Report

In a 68-year-old man, a large abdominal tumoral mass was discovered incidentally during checkup for vascular insufficiency of the lower limbs. The patient complained of vascular insufficiency and had no symptoms of abdominal pain. Physical examination revealed a palpable mass in the right upper quadrant of the abdomen. Results of blood samples were all within normal values.

Ultrasonography showed a well-defined large cystic mass with several membranous septa with a diameter of

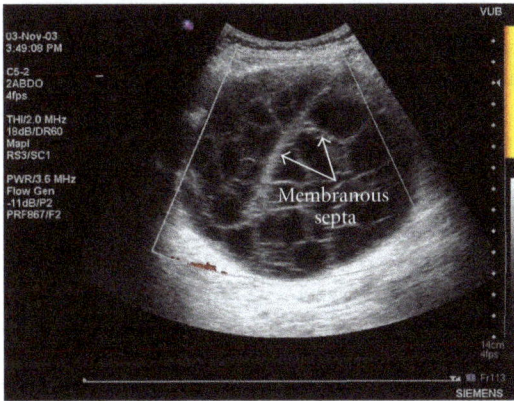

FIGURE 1: Abdominal ultrasonography (US) showing a well-defined large cystic mass in the right hypochondrium with several membranous septa (arrow).

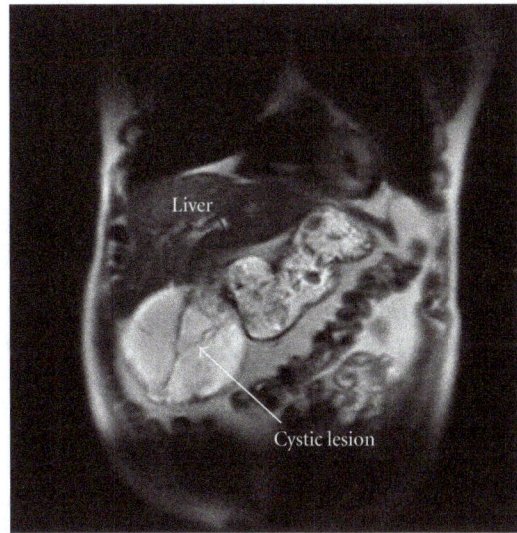

FIGURE 2: Abdominal computed tomography (CT) displaying a large cystic lesion (arrow) adjacent to the right liver lobe, the stomach, and the pancreatic head.

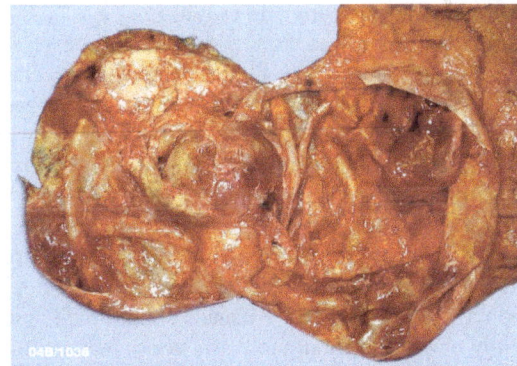

FIGURE 3: On MRI imaging markedly high intensity, compatible with cystic nature (arrow), was revealed in the tumor.

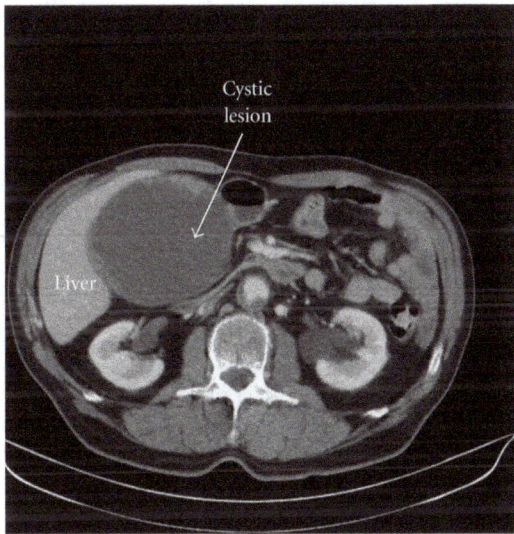

FIGURE 4: Macroscopically, a large unilocular cystic tumor with a smooth outer surface and several membranous septa projecting in the lumen was found.

approximately 12 cm in the right hypochondrium (Figure 1). Subsequent computed tomography (CT) scan demonstrated a large cystic lesion adjacent to the right liver lobe, the stomach, and the pancreatic head (Figure 2). On MRI imaging, markedly high intensity, compatible with cystic nature, was revealed in the tumor. The tumor was lying in contact with the right liver lobe, the stomach, and the pancreatic head (Figure 3).

However, no clear connection with any of these organs was identified. The imaging findings demonstrated no vascularity of the lesion. Malignancy could not be excluded, and surgery was indicated.

At laparotomy a large exophytic mobile mass was found to be attached by a narrow stalk to the larger curvature of the stomach at the level of the antrum. No infiltration into the surrounding tissues was observed.

Surgical resection of the mass along with a wedge resection of the stomach, at the larger curvature, adjoining the stalk and the adherent omentum was performed.

The resected tumor measured almost 12 cm in diameter. Grossly, it was a unilocular cystic tumor filled with serous fluid, with a smooth outer surface and several membranous septa projecting in the lumen (Figure 4). The cyst had a thin wall. The stalk was connecting the cystic tumor with the stomach. The mitotic activity was less than 5 mitoses per 50 HPF. The tumor cells showed positivity for CD117 (KIT) and CD34. The histological features together with the immunohistochemical profile of the tumor cells were consistent with a gastrointestinal stromal tumor (GIST) with a high risk of progressive disease according to the Fletcher classification. Molecular analysis of this tumor showed a mutation in exon 14 of the PDGFRA gene (substitution exon 14, N659 K). Since PDGFRA exon 14 mutant GIST is sensitive to imatinib mesylate (Glivec), this oral treatment was started postoperatively because the high risk of recurrence in this patient (high risk of progressive disease according to the Fletcher classification). Untill now the patient is still free of recurrence.

3. Discussion

Gastrointestinal stromal tumors (GISTs) are rare neoplasms, with an annual incidence of approximately 4 per million [3]. Historically, these tumors were classified as leiomyomas, leiomyoblastomas, and leiomyosarcomas, because of a mistaken belief that they originated from smooth muscle in the wall of the gastrointestinal tract [2].

The cellular origin of GIST recently has been proposed to be the interstitial cell of Cajal, an intestinal pacemaker cell. This postulate is supported by the finding that GISTs display positivity for cell markers similar to those of the normal cell of Cajal [4–6]. The majority (approximately 95%) of GISTs express the CD117 antigen (KIT), a protooncogene product. CD34, a commonly expressed human progenitor cell antigen, is also frequently found positive in GISTs [3]. More than half of the GISTs are located in the stomach followed, by the small intestine, colon and rectum, and esophagus [1, 3, 7].

Complete tumor resection with disease-free resection margins is the treatment of choice for primary nonmetastatic tumors. Lymphadenectomy is not recommended because lymph node involvement is rare. Wedge resection allows full-thickness resection of the stomach wall containing the tumor, with negative resection margins [1, 6].

Grossly, GISTs vary greatly in size and can be more than 30 cm in diameter. These tumors are usually well circumscribed and unencapsulated. GIST can grow in an endophytic or exophytic pattern. They are usually solid. Small cysts are frequently observed, presumably as a consequence of cystic degeneration or necrosis. Larger stromal tumors usually degenerate, and cysts are formed [8–11].

In the present case, the large size of the cyst obscured the origin from the stomach. Imaging showed that the tumor was not originating from the pancreas or any other organ, so the exact origin of the tumor could not be determined preoperatively. Imaging demonstrated no vascularity of the lesion. Since malignancy could not be excluded in our case and the origin of the tumor could not be determined by imaging, surgery was indicated.

Complete tumor resection with disease-free resection margins is the treatment of choice for primary nonmetastatic tumors. Lymphadenectomy is not recommended because lymph node involvement is rare. Wedge resection allows full-thickness resection of the stomach wall containing the tumor, with negative resection margins [1, 6].

Lesions that should be considered in the differential diagnosis of a cystic abdominal mass on radiologic imaging (CT and MRI) include gastric or bowel duplication cysts, cystic mesothelioma, cystic lymphangioma, cystic mucinous retroperitoneal tumors, cystic pancreatic tumors, pseudocysts of the pancreas or peritoneum, cystic teratoma, and GIST [12–14].

In this case, tumor cells showed diffuse and strong positivity for CD117 (KIT) and CD34, which was consistent with a diagnosis of GIST. This was confirmed by molecular biology that showed a mutation in exon 14 of the PDGFRA gene (exon 14 substitution, N659 K).

Wang et al. recently published a series of 7 patients with cystic GISTs and analysis of c-kit and PDGFRA gene. Gene mutation of exon 11 of c-kit was identified in 3 cases [15]. PDGFRA mutant GISTs arise almost exclusively in the stomach, whereas KIT mutant tumors occur at a variety of sites along the gastrointestinal tract. PDGFRA exon 14 mutations may be associated with a reduced risk of recurrence. Limited clinical data are published, but PDGFRA exon 14 mutant GISTs appear; sensitive to imatinib, the sensitivity is similar to KIT exon 11 mutants [16–18].

In summary, GISTs with cystic appearance clearly should be considered in the differential diagnosis of cystic abdominal tumors. Most GISTs (95%) express Kit (CD117) and CD34 (70%). In case of doubt genmutation analysis is necessary. KIT and PDGFRA genotyping is important for GIST diagnosis and assessment of sensitivity to tyrosine kinase inhibitors.

References

[1] R. P. DeMatteo, J. J. Lewis, D. Leung, S. S. Mudan, J. M. Woodruff, and M. F. Brennan, "Two hundred gastrointestinal stromal tumors: recurrence patterns and prognostic factors for survival," *Annals of Surgery*, vol. 231, no. 1, pp. 51–58, 2000.

[2] S. Hirota, K. Isozaki, Y. Moriyama et al., "Gain-of-function mutations of c-kit in human gastrointestinal stromal tumors," *Science*, vol. 279, no. 5350, pp. 577–580, 1998.

[3] M. Miettinen and J. Lasota, "Gastrointestinal stromal tumors—definition, clinical, histological, immunohistochemical, and molecular genetic features and differential diagnosis," *Virchows Archiv*, vol. 438, no. 1, pp. 1–12, 2001.

[4] L. G. Kindblom, H. E. Remotti, F. Aldenborg, and J. M. Meis-Kindblom, "Gastrointestinal pacemaker cell tumor (GIPACT): gastrointestinal stromal tumors show phenotypic characteristics of the interstitial cells of Cajal," *American Journal of Pathology*, vol. 152, no. 5, pp. 1259–1269, 1998.

[5] M. Miettinen, M. Virolainen, and R. Maarit-Sarlomo, "Gastrointestinal stromal tumors—value of CD34 antigen in their identification and separation from true leiomyomas and schwannomas," *American Journal of Surgical Pathology*, vol. 19, no. 2, pp. 207–216, 1995.

[6] M. Koelz, N. Wick, T. Winkler, F. Längle, and F. Wrba, "The impact of c-kit mutations on histomorphological risk assessment of gastrointestinal stromal tumors," *European Surgery*, vol. 39, no. 1, pp. 45–53, 2007.

[7] T. S. Emory, L. H. Sobin, L. Lukes, D. H. Lee, and T. J. O'Leary, "Prognosis of gastrointestinal smooth-muscle (stromal) tumors: dependence on anatomic site," *American Journal of Surgical Pathology*, vol. 23, no. 1, pp. 82–87, 1999.

[8] M. Miettinen and J. Lasota, "Gastrointestinal stromal tumors: review on morphology, molecular pathology, prognosis, and

differential diagnosis," *Archives of Pathology and Laboratory Medicine*, vol. 130, no. 10, pp. 1466–1478, 2006.

[9] I. Naitoh, Y. Okayama, M. Hirai et al., "Exophytic pedunculated gastrointestinal stromal tumor with remarkable cystic change," *Journal of Gastroenterology*, vol. 38, no. 12, pp. 1181–1184, 2003.

[10] I. Pidhorecky, R. T. Cheney, W. G. Kraybill, and J. F. Gibbs, "Gastrointestinal stromal tumors: current diagnosis, biologic behavior, and management," *Annals of Surgical Oncology*, vol. 7, no. 9, pp. 705–712, 2000.

[11] A. D. Levy, H. E. Remotti, W. M. Thompson, L. H. Sobin, and M. Miettinen, "Gastrointestinal stromal tumors: radiologic features with pathologic correlation," *Radiographics*, vol. 23, no. 2, pp. 283–304, 2003.

[12] S. E. Rha, K. M. Sohn, S. Y. Lee, H. S. Jung, S. M. Park, and K. M. Kim, "Pedunculated exogastric leiomyoblastoma presenting as a wandering abdominal mass," *Abdominal Imaging*, vol. 25, no. 5, pp. 545–547, 2000.

[13] J. H. Stanley, D. Ravenel, T. H. Parker, and I. Vujic, "Exogastric leiomyoblastoma: a rare gastric neoplasm mimicking left hepatic mass on computed tomography," *CT: Journal of Computed Tomography*, vol. 10, no. 2, pp. 187–190, 1986.

[14] S. Tabrez, V. Muralidharen, and I. M. Roberts, "Gastrointestinal stromal, (GIST) leiomyosarcoma arising from the stomach mimicking as pseudocyst of the pancreas: a challenging presentation," *The American Journal of Gastroenterology*, vol. 96, no. 9, supplement 1, pp. S249–S250, 2001.

[15] C. Z. Wang, Y. Y. Hou, K. T. Shen et al., "Clinicopathological features and prognosis of cystic gastrointestinal stromal tumor," *Zhonghua Wei Chang Wai Ke Za Zhi*, vol. 14, no. 8, pp. 599–602, 2011.

[16] J. Lasota, A. Dansonka-Mieszkowska, L. H. Sobin, and M. Miettinen, "A great majority of GISTs with PDGFRA mutations represent gastric tumors of low or no malignant potential," *Laboratory Investigation*, vol. 84, no. 7, pp. 874–883, 2004.

[17] F. Medeiros, C. L. Corless, A. Duensing et al., "KIT-negative gastrointestinal stromal tumors: proof of concept and therapeutic implications," *American Journal of Surgical Pathology*, vol. 28, no. 7, pp. 889–894, 2004.

[18] E. Wardelmann, A. Hrychyk, S. Merkelbach-Bruse et al., "Association of platelet-derived growth factor receptor α mutations with gastric primary site and epithelioid or mixed cell morphology in gastrointestinal stromal tumors," *Journal of Molecular Diagnostics*, vol. 6, no. 3, pp. 197–204, 2004.

21

Management of Locally Advanced Renal Cell Carcinoma with Invasion of the Duodenum

Andrew T. Schlussel,[1] Aaron B. Fowler,[2] Herbert K. Chinn,[3] and Linda L. Wong[4]

[1] Department of General Surgery, Tripler Army Medical Center, 1 Jarrett White Road, Honolulu, HI 96859, USA
[2] University of Utah, School of Medicine, 30 North 1900 East, Salt Lake City, UT 84132, USA
[3] Department of Urology, Queens Medical Center, 1329 Lusitana Street, Suite 108, Honolulu, HI 96813, USA
[4] Department of Surgery, University of Hawaii School of Medicine, 550 South Beretania Street, Suite 403, Honolulu, HI 96813, USA

Correspondence should be addressed to Linda L. Wong; hepatoma@aol.com

Academic Editors: J. Griniatsos, M. Nikfarjam, O. Olsha, G. Sandblom, and G. Santori

Renal cell carcinoma (RCC) is rare but aggressive, with greater than 20% of patients presenting with stage III or IV, disease. Surgical resection of the primary tumor regardless of stage is the treatment of choice, and en bloc resection of involved organs provides the only potential chance for cure. This case report describes a patient with metastatic right-sided RCC with invasion of the inferior vena cava and duodenum managed by en block resection and pancreaticoduodenectomy. This report will review the workup and treatment of locally advanced RCC, as well as the role of cytoreductive nephrectomy in the setting of metastatic disease.

1. Introduction

Renal cell carcinoma (RCC) is a relatively rare cancer that comprises approximately 2% of newly diagnosed visceral cancers in the United States. Tobacco and obesity are the most significant risk factors and are present in 20% and 30% of renal cell carcinoma, respectively [1]. RCC most often develops in the sixth and seventh decades of life with a male-to-female ratio of 2 : 1. It is estimated that in 2012 there will be 64,770 new cases of renal cancer and 13,570 deaths from this malignancy [2].

The most common site of invasion for right-sided renal cell carcinoma is the inferior vena cava (IVC) causing thrombus formation. Previous studies have demonstrated that surgical intervention with enbloc removal of the tumor thrombus in these cases improves overall survival [3]. To date, the mainstay of therapy for RCC invading the IVC involves a radical nephrectomy, cavotomy, and thrombus extraction followed by immunotherapy [4]. Haferkamp et al. demonstrated that surgical resection alone increases survival, but when combined with adjuvant immunotherapy these rates were dramatically increased [4].

Although uncommon, metastatic renal cell carcinoma to the duodenum has been described; however, direct invasion from the kidney into the duodenum has not been reported [5]. Furthermore, there have been no reports of renal cell carcinoma invading both the duodenum and IVC. We present a case of a patient with RCC of the right kidney with invasion of the inferior vena cava and duodenum as well as subsequent treatment.

2. Case Report

This is a case of a 53-year-old Filipino male with a past medical history significant for hypertension and diabetes mellitus, who presented with symptoms of melena, fatigue, and lightheadedness. He denied abdominal pain, nausea, vomiting, fevers, chills, anorexia, or weight loss. He otherwise had an excellent performance status and no family history of cancer. His physical exam was normal without any dominant palpable abdominal mass or leg edema to suggest venous congestion or thrombus. The laboratory workup was significant for a hemoglobin of 6.6 gm/dL for which he received a transfusion of six units of packed red blood cells. He underwent an esophagogastroduodenoscopy that showed a bleeding mass involving the second portion of the duodenum. Hemostasis was achieved and a biopsy was performed that was consistent with renal cell carcinoma. Subsequently, a computed tomography (CT) scan was performed and showed a large mass arising off the anterior cortex of the lower pole of the right kidney with brisk arterial and peripheral enhancement consistent with renal cell carcinoma. The dimensions of this mass were estimated to be approximately 10.1 cm by 8.0 cm by 10.0 cm, protruding into the lumen of the duodenum and displacing it medially (Figure 1). Coronal reformatted images obtained of the portal venous phase demonstrated extension of the mass into the lumen of the inferior vena cava (Figure 2). It appeared that the majority of the infrarenal IVC was displaced and compressed medially. Magnetic resonance imaging (MRI) confirmed the findings on CT scan, and a positron emission tomography (PET) scan was also performed, which demonstrated a large hypermetabolic mass involving the right kidney without evidence of regional metastasis. CT-guided imaging of the patient's chest revealed a cluster of pulmonary nodules and irregular opacities in the left upper lobe and right upper lobe that were hypermetabolic on PET scan and consistent with metastatic disease. The patient was evaluated in a multidisciplinary tumor board, and based on the current literature it was the consensus that surgical resection be attempted with the plan for adjuvant immunotherapy postoperatively [6–8].

Exploratory laparotomy revealed a 12 cm by 15 cm tumor in the right kidney with extension into the inferior vena cava as well as a second 3 cm by 4 cm irregular mass partially adherent to the right renal vein and obstructing the vena cava. There was no evidence of intraabdominal metastases outside these areas. There was extension of the tumor into the second portion of the duodenum but not obstructing the bile duct or invading the portal vein (Figures 3 and 4). Therefore, a right radical nephrectomy was performed with en bloc pancreaticoduodenectomy and resection of the inferior vena cava tumor thrombus with the use of a modified venovenous bypass. A 17-French catheter was inserted in the left femoral vein with blood return at a flow rate of 1.5 L/min to three large bore catheters placed in the bilateral internal jugular veins. The IVC was temporarily clamped for approximately 15 minutes in order to remove the intravascular tumor. At the completion of the procedure, the IVC appeared to be slightly narrowed at about 1.8 cm, but this was distal to the insertion of the left renal vein, and the flow appeared to be adequate. Histological evaluation demonstrated a pT4pN0M1 stage IV, grade 3, clear cell renal carcinoma with direct involvement of the duodenum. The patient tolerated the procedure well without any major intraoperative complications. The total operative time was approximately six hours and his blood loss was five liters. He required a transfusion of ten units of packed red blood cells, eight units of fresh frozen plasma, and one unit of platelets. He had an uncomplicated postoperative course. His creatinine initially increased to a maximum of 1.7 mg/dL from a baseline of 0.9 mg/dL, but at the time of discharge the value had decreased and stabilized at 1.1 mg/dL. His diet was advanced slowly and he underwent gastrografin swallowing

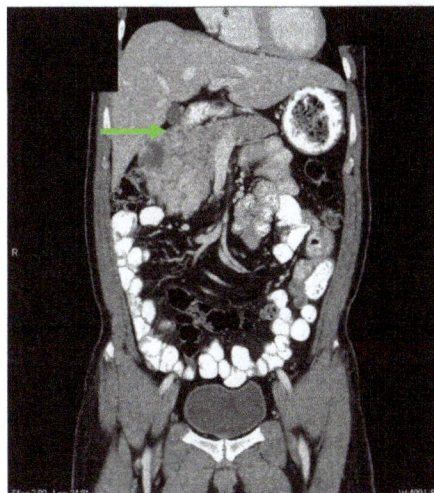

FIGURE 1: Displacement of duodenum by right kidney mass. Arrow indicates duodenum.

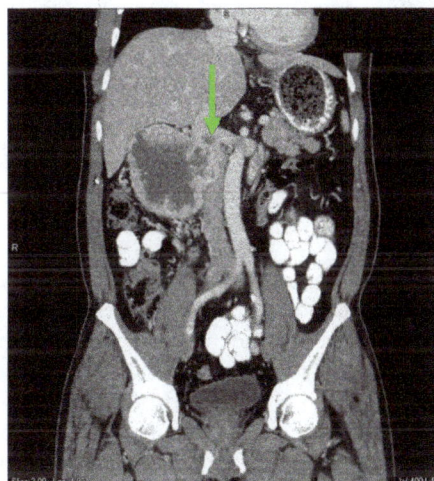

FIGURE 2: Extension of right kidney mass into the lumen of the inferior vena cava. Arrow annotates the inferior vena cava and tumor thrombus.

study on postoperative day seven, which demonstrated no evidence of anastomotic leak, stenosis, or delayed gastric emptying. He was discharged home on postoperative day ten tolerating a soft diet and in stable condition. The patient has recovered and is now three months after surgery without any complications. He is expected to undergo adjuvant therapy with interleukin-2 in the near future.

3. Discussion

Locally advanced RCC occurs in about 2% of the population, and at initial presentation 26.7% are diagnosed with stage II or III disease, with up to 22.7% having metastatic spread [9]. En bloc resection of all involved organs is the only potential curable operation [10]. Typically patients at this stage of the disease will present with pain due to invasion of the posterior abdominal wall, nerve roots, and paraspinous muscles. It is

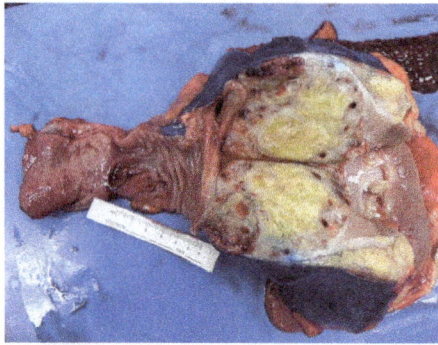

FIGURE 3: Right renal mass invading the duodenum. Ruler demonstrates length of duodenal invasion.

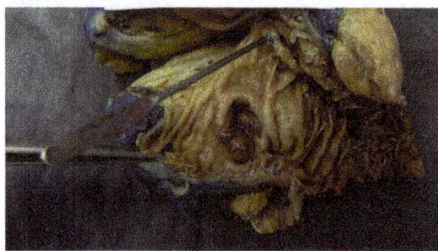

FIGURE 4: Luminal view of duodenum with invasion of the second portion.

uncommon for these tumors to invade adjacent organs to include the liver, duodenum, and pancreas. Unfortunately such extensive disease portends a poor prognosis with reports of a 5% survival rate at 5 years after margin negative resection [10].

Being a technically challenging operation, a combined radical nephrectomy with pancreaticoduodenectomy and IVC resection is rarely performed, and the indications are not well defined [10]. Left-sided RCC with pancreatic invasion has also been described, where en bloc resection with distal pancreatectomy was the treatment of choice [11]. In one study, only 5 out of 180 patients, over 6 years, required a concomitant nephrectomy and pancreaticoduodenectomy. The procedure was performed for three retroperitoneal sarcomas, one locally advanced transitional-cell carcinoma, with only adherence to the duodenal wall not true invasion, and an ampullary cancer with a concurrent right renal cell tumor. All patients did well, with three (60%) reported to have complications related to the pancreaticoduodenal resection, a procedure alone that has a significantly high morbidity rate [12, 13].

Metastatic renal cell carcinoma to the duodenum has been reported and is rare [14]. Pancreatic metastases occur in 1.3–1.9% of patients based on autopsy results. This occurs via the hematogenous route and is classically seen in patients many years after resection of the primary tumor. More common sites for metastatic disease include the lungs, bone, liver, renal fossa, and brain, where the small intestine comprises only 1-2% of all metastases from any tumor. Surgical resection for metastatic RCC is associated with a 5-year survival rate of 29%–35%, and pancreaticoduodenectomy has

been described as a method to clear disease [14]. Attempt at complete resection maintains the best outcome; however, arteriography with embolization of the gastroduodenal artery and duodenal wedge resection has also been described for palliation in the event of a massive gastrointestinal bleed due to duodenal metastasis [5, 14–16].

The workup and management of locally advanced RCC with direct invasion of the duodenum are complex and can only be extrapolated from that of metastatic RCC and the knowledge of other locally invasive cancers requiring pancreaticoduodenectomy [10, 17]. Although these renal tumors demonstrate an aggressive biology, it has been shown in patients with pancreatic metastasis that there is a more favorable prognosis than with resection for a primary pancreatic carcinoma [13]. The patient described here is complicated further by the involvement of the inferior vena cava, which occurs in 4%–10% of patients with renal cell carcinoma. This was once thought to have a very poor prognosis; however, early surgical intervention has been shown to have a 5-year survival rate of 45%–69%, but when confined to the kidney alone [10].

Cytoreductive nephrectomy, an upfront aggressive surgical resection of the renal primary tumor in the face of known metastatic disease, remains the standard treatment of stage IV RCC [6–8]. However, such a radical resection should only be attempted in patients with good performance status, those with minimal comorbidities, an overall low surgical risk, no hepatic, brain or skeletal metastasis, and when 75% if the tumor bulk can be excised [9]. Flanigan and colleagues were able to demonstrate an overall survival benefit of 13.3 months versus 7.8 months with the use of cytoreductive nephrectomy and interferon (IFN) compared to IFN alone in metastatic RCC [7]. Interleukin-2 has also demonstrated some benefit in the adjuvant setting, with complete response rates occurring between 5 and 9% of the time. These therapies, although effective, are associated with significant toxicity [9]. Currently there is no other prospective analysis proving the efficacy of adjuvant therapy. Phase III trials are currently studying the safety of sunitinib in combination with cytoreductive nephrectomy [9]. There is also no conclusive evidence that recommends the use of neoadjuvant therapy for locally advanced RCC [18]. There are some reports that therapy may decrease or downstage the caval tumor thrombus, but partial tumor response is low and complete response is rare. This remains a controversial subject, and prospective studies are ongoing evaluating the potential benefit, timing, and safety of neoadjuvant therapies [8, 9].

In conclusion, this patient was successfully managed based on the current medical literature of locally advanced RCC with IVC involvement. The patient had an extensive preoperative workup with a high-quality CT scan and MRI, which provided appropriate preparation for the surgical team. He received an aggressive and an oncologically sound operation, providing the best potential chance for survival.

References

[1] J. K. McLaughlin, L. Lipworth, and R. E. Tarone, "Epidemiologic aspects of renal cell carcinoma," *Seminars in Oncology*, vol. 33, no. 5, pp. 527–533, 2006.

[2] R. Siegel, D. Naishadham, and A. Jemal, "Cancer statistics, 2012," *CA: A Cancer Journal for Clinicians*, vol. 62, no. 1, pp. 10–29, 2012.

[3] V. F. Marshall, R. G. Middleton, G. R. Holswade, and E. I. Goldsmith, "Surgery for renal cell carcinoma in the vena cava," *Journal of Urology*, vol. 103, no. 4, pp. 414–420, 1970.

[4] A. Haferkamp, P. J. Bastian, H. Jakobi et al., "Renal cell carcinoma with tumor thrombus extension into the vena cava: prospective long-term followup," *Journal of Urology*, vol. 177, no. 5, pp. 1703–1708, 2007.

[5] R. Adamo, P. J. Greaney Jr., A. Witkiewicz, E. P. Kennedy, and C. J. Yeo, "Renal cell carcinoma metastatic to the duodenum: treatment by classic pancreaticoduodenectomy and review of the literature," *Journal of Gastrointestinal Surgery*, vol. 12, no. 8, pp. 1465–1468, 2008.

[6] R. C. Flanigan, S. E. Salmon, B. A. Blumenstein et al., "Nephrectomy followed by interferon alfa-2b compared with interferon alfa-2b alone for metastatic renal-cell cancer," *The New England Journal of Medicine*, vol. 345, no. 23, pp. 1655–1659, 2001.

[7] R. C. Flanigan, G. Mickisch, R. Sylvester, C. Tangen, H. Van Poppel, and E. D. Crawford, "Cytoreductive nephrectomy in patients with metastatic renal cancer: a combined analysis," *Journal of Urology*, vol. 171, no. 3, pp. 1071–1076, 2004.

[8] S. P. Stroup, O. A. Raheem, K. L. Palazzi et al., "Does timing of cytoreductive nephrectomy impact patient survival with metastatic renal cell carcinoma in the tyrosine kinase inhibitor era? A multi-institutional study," *Urology*, 2013.

[9] K. Thillai, S. Allan, T. Powles, S. Rudman, and S. Chowdhury, "Neoadjuvant and adjuvant treatment of renal cell carcinoma," *Expert Review of Anticancer Therapy*, vol. 12, no. 6, pp. 765–776, 2012.

[10] J. Wein, L. Kavoussi, A. Novick, A. Partin, and C. Peters, *Wein: Campbell-Walsh Urology*, Elsevier Saunders, Philadelphia, Pa, USA, 10th edition, 2012.

[11] C. G. Huscher, A. Mingoli, G. Sgarzini, and A. Mereu, "Laparoscopic left nephrectomy with, "en bloc" distal splenopancreatectomy," *Annals of Surgical Oncology*, vol. 19, no. 2, p. 693, 2012.

[12] M. Nikfarjam, N. J. Gusani, E. T. Kimchi, R. P. Mahraj, and K. F. Staveley-O'Carroll, "Combined right nephrectomy and pancreaticoduodenectomy. Indications and outcomes," *Journal of the Pancreas*, vol. 9, no. 4, pp. 449–455, 2008.

[13] C. Bassi, E. Molinari, G. Malleo et al., "Early versus late drain removal after standard pancreatic resections: results of a prospective randomized trial," *Annals of Surgery*, vol. 252, no. 2, pp. 207–214, 2010.

[14] M. Hashimoto, Y. Miura, M. Matsuda, and G. Watanabe, "Concomitant duodenal and pancreatic metastases from renal cell carcinoma: report of a case," *Surgery Today*, vol. 31, no. 2, pp. 180–183, 2001.

[15] H. Zhao, K. Han, J. Li et al., "A case of wedge resection of duodenum for massive gastrointestinal bleeding due to duodenal metastasis by renal cell carcinoma," *World Journal of Surgical Oncology*, vol. 10, article 199, 2012.

[16] J. Yang, Y. B. Zhang, Z. J. Liu, Y. F. Zhu, and L. G. Shen, "Surgical treatment of renal cell carcinoma metastasized to the duodenum," *Chinese Medical Journal*, vol. 125, no. 17, pp. 3198–3200, 2012.

[17] E. T. Kimchi, M. Nikfarjam, N. J. Gusani, D. M. Avella, and K. F. Staveley-O'Carroll, "Combined pancreaticoduodenectomy and extended right hemicolectomy: outcomes and indications," *HPB*, vol. 11, no. 7, pp. 559–564, 2009.

[18] P. A. Kenney and C. G. Wood, "Integration of surgery and systemic therapy for renal cell carcinoma," *Urologic Clinics of North America*, vol. 39, no. 2, pp. 211–231, 2012.

22

Laparoscopic Resection of an Intra-Abdominal Esophageal Duplication Cyst: A Case Report and Literature Review

Ikuo Watanobe,[1] Yuzuru Ito,[1] Eigo Akimoto,[1] Yuuki Sekine,[1] Yurie Haruyama,[1] Kota Amemiya,[1] Fumihiro Kawano,[1] Shohei Fujita,[1] Satoshi Omori,[1] Shozo Miyano,[1] Taijiro Kosaka,[1] Michio Machida,[1] Toshiaki Kitabatake,[1] Kuniaki Kojima,[1] Asumi Sakaguchi,[2] Kanako Ogura,[2] and Toshiharu Matsumoto[2]

[1]*Department of General Surgery, Juntendo University Nerima Hospital, 3-1-10 Takanodai, Nerima, Tokyo 177-8521, Japan*
[2]*Department of Diagnostic Pathology, Juntendo University Nerima Hospital, 3-1-10 Takanodai, Nerima, Tokyo 177-8521, Japan*

Correspondence should be addressed to Ikuo Watanobe; nobei@juntendo.ac.jp

Academic Editor: Boris Kirshtein

Duplication of the alimentary tract is a rare congenital malformation that occurs most often in the abdominal region, whereas esophageal duplication cyst develops typically in the thoracic region but occasionally in the neck and abdominal regions. Esophageal duplication cyst is usually diagnosed in early childhood because of symptoms related to bleeding, infection, and displacement of tissue surrounding the lesion. We recently encountered a rare adult case of esophageal duplication cyst in the abdominal esophagus. A 50-year-old man underwent gastroscopy, endoscopic ultrasonography, computed tomography, and magnetic resonance imaging to investigate epigastric pain and dysphagia that started 3 months earlier. Imaging findings suggested esophageal duplication cyst, and the patient underwent laparoscopic resection followed by intraoperative esophagoscopy to reconstruct the esophagus safely and effectively. Histopathological examination of the resected specimen revealed two layers of smooth muscle in the cystic wall, confirming the diagnosis of esophageal duplication cyst.

1. Introduction

As reported by Ladd and Gross, duplication of the alimentary tract is a rare congenital malformation that develops potentially anywhere in the gastrointestinal tract, from the root of the tongue to the anus [1]. Several theories have been suggested to explain the cause of duplication [2]. Popular theories include persistence of fetal gut diverticula, abnormal recanalization of the solid stage of development of the primitive gut, partial twinning, and a split notochord. We recently encountered a case of asymptomatic esophageal duplication cyst (EDC) that was not discovered until the age of 50 years. EDCs account for 20% of all the gastrointestinal duplication cysts [3]. In this case, the EDC in the lower esophageal region was treated laparoscopically because it was continuous with the mediastinum and abdominal cavity. The postoperative course was excellent. Here, we report this adult case of EDC and review the literature.

2. Case Presentation

A 50-year-old man had a history of an operation for lumbar herniated disc at the age of 37 and hypertension since the age of 42 that was controlled with medication. He visited a nearby clinic because of epigastric pain and dysphagia that started 3 months earlier. He was referred to our hospital because of gastroscopic findings of extrinsic compression.

The initial physical examination revealed normal heart and lung sounds, a flat and soft abdomen, and no tenderness on palpation. No superficial lymph nodes were palpable. Hematological and biochemical findings were normal. Gastroscopy performed at our hospital revealed a submucosal tumor with a smooth surface at the 9 o'clock position in the lower esophagus (Figure 1). Barium esophagogram showed extrinsic compression from the lower esophagus to the gastroesophageal junction (Figure 2). Good expansion and smooth mucosa were noted. Endoscopic ultrasonography

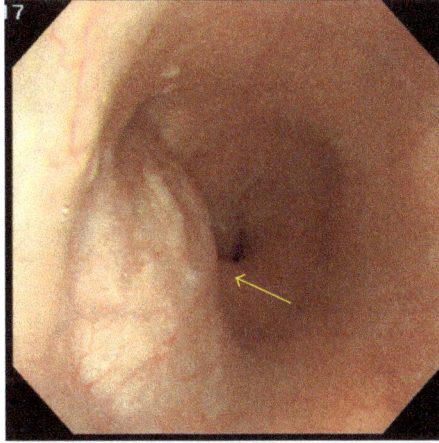

FIGURE 1: Transnasal gastroscopy. A submucosal tumor (arrow) of approximately 2 cm is visible at the 9 o'clock position in the lower esophagus, 41 cm from the tip of the nose. The surface of the tumor is smooth, and all the findings indicate gastrointestinal stromal tumor.

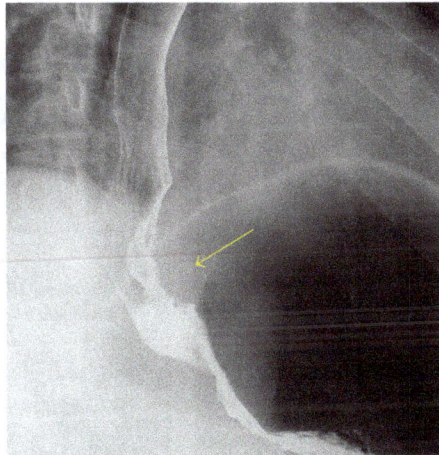

FIGURE 2: Barium esophagography. The image reveals extrinsic compression by a mass with a smooth surface (arrow) in the intra-abdominal esophageal region. Extension of the esophageal wall was good.

showed a cystic mass in the esophageal wall extending from the lower esophagus to the cardiac region of the stomach (Figure 3), with the suspected presence of viscous fluid inside the cyst. Computed tomography (CT) showed an iso-enhanced dumbbell-shaped mass (3.5×3 cm) with a smooth surface and homogeneous content, which extended from the lower thoracic esophagus to the cardiac region of the stomach (Figure 4). Magnetic resonance imaging showed a mass that was hyperintense and moderately hyperintense on T1- and T2-weighted imaging, respectively, with and without fat suppression (Figure 5). Although gastrointestinal stromal tumor and leiomyoma were also suspected, the patient was diagnosed as having EDC based on imaging findings and underwent laparoscopic resection.

Intraoperatively, the mass was soft and elastic and had a smooth surface in the lesser curvature of the stomach near the cardiac region and along the esophagus when approached from the mediastinum by partially dissecting the crus of the diaphragm. The mass was carefully resected along the esophagus in the abdominal cavity toward the mediastinum.

At the resection site, normal mucosa was left in some areas, but in other areas resection extended through all layers. Using a 3-0 synthetic absorbable suture, the surgical site was closed under intraoperative esophagoscopic observation to ensure proper closure and prevent esophageal stricture due to suturing. Cystic fluid in the resected specimen was mucous and reddish brown, with no cellular components (Figure 6). Histopathological findings revealed that the cyst consisted of two layers of smooth muscle and the inside of the cavity was lined with pseudostratified columnar epithelium (Figure 7). These findings, with no evidence of malignancy, led to the definitive diagnosis of EDC. The postoperative course was unremarkable, and the patient resumed a normal diet on postoperative day 4 and was discharged on postoperative day 10.

3. Discussion

Duplication of the alimentary tract is rare malformation observed in 1 of 25,000 deliveries [4]. In 1940, Ladd and

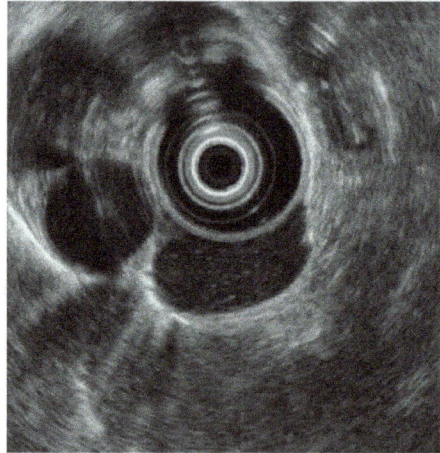

FIGURE 3: Endoscopic ultrasonography. The image shows a cystic mass extending from the lower esophagus to the cardiac region of the stomach and is filled with viscous components. No echoic debris indicative of bleeding or solid components was observed.

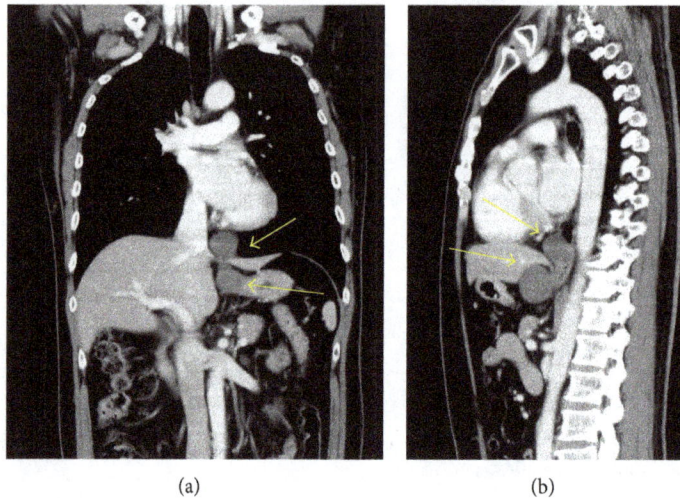

(a)   (b)

FIGURE 4: Computed tomography. The images reveal a dumbbell-shape iso-enhanced mass with a smooth surface, which extends parallel to the esophagus and spreads over and below the esophageal hiatus.

Gross reported that diseases with common features but were named differently as enteric cyst, enterogenous cyst, giant diverticula, ileum duplex, and inclusion cysts were the same disease and should be collectively called duplication of the alimentary tract [1]. Duplications of the alimentary tract are hollow structures that have a muscular coat, usually composed of two layers, and are lined with epithelium similar to that found in the colon or some other portions of the gastrointestinal tract. These lesions are always contiguous to some portion of the alimentary tube, and they were strongly adherent to it in all but 1 reported case. The type of epithelium lining in the duplication cyst does not necessarily correspond to that in the alimentary tract to which it is attached. However, due to their morphological and histological variation, even duplications located away from the gastrointestinal tract and those with no muscular layers are now classified as

alimentary tract duplication. The pathogenic mechanisms of EDC are unknown but are thought to be associated with abnormal esophageal development in the fifth to eighth weeks of gestation, when the posterior primitive foregut coalesces to form a single esophageal lumen. In more than 80% of cases, EDC is diagnosed before the age of 2 years when the patient experiences acute abdominal or bowel obstruction or other associated complications. A minority of cases remain asymptomatic until adulthood [5]. After bronchogenic cyst, EDC is the second most common benign posterior mediastinal lesion in children. EDC is relatively common in children presenting with mediastinal masses and accounts for 30% of all pediatric posterior mediastinal masses [6]. Differentiating between bronchogenic and esophageal cysts is more difficult because both derive from the foregut and contain ciliated epithelium. The difference between bronchogenic cysts and

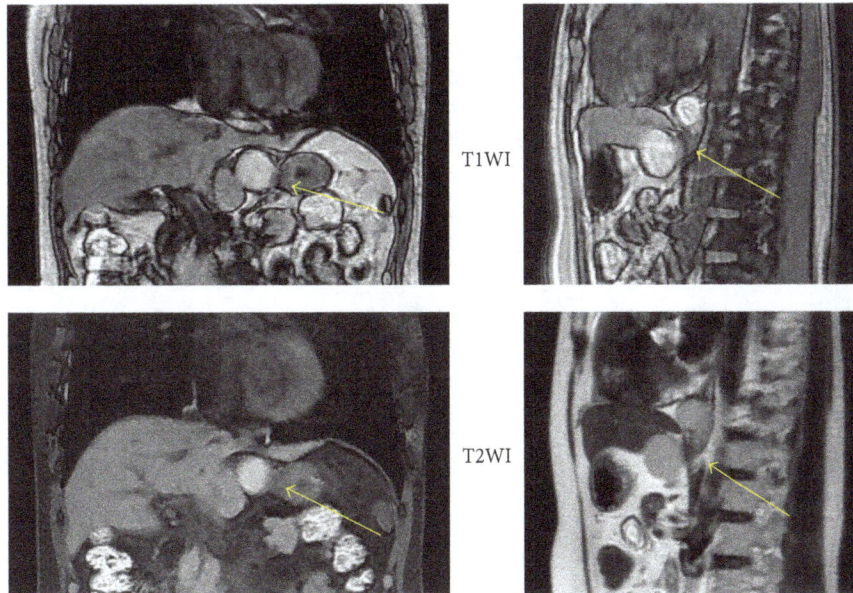

FIGURE 5: Magnetic resonance imaging. The images reveal a cystic mass extending from the lower esophagus to the cardiac region of the stomach. The mass appears to be located in or even outside the muscular layer and may contain mucin, high protein fluid, or blood.

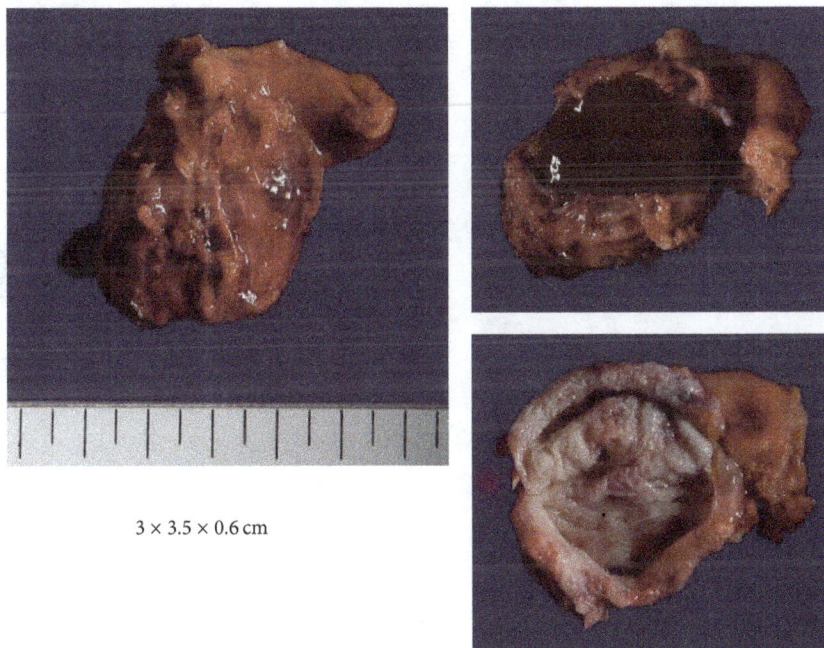

$3 \times 3.5 \times 0.6$ cm

FIGURE 6: Resected specimen. The images show a $3 \times 3.5 \times 0.6$ cm soft mass with no solid components. The content of the mass is a highly mucous, reddish brown fluid with no odor.

EDCs is that duplication cysts of bronchogenic origin do not have two layers of smooth muscle; instead they contain cartilage, bronchogenic glands, or both.

The present case is extremely rare because intra-abdominal EDC was discovered because of the onset of epigastric pain and dysphagia at the age of 50 years. A literature search extracted only 18 published case reports of intra-abdominal EDC [7–23], making the present case the 19th case (Table 1). In 7 of the previous 18 cases, EDC

was incidentally diagnosed on CT scans that were taken as a part of comprehensive examination for other diseases. The most common complaint was pain (12 cases), followed by dysphagia. Interestingly, adults ($n = 15$) accounted for 79% of the patients with intra-abdominal EDC even though many duplication cysts of the alimentary tract are diagnosed before 2 years of age. This may be because no structures in the vicinity of the lower esophagus restrict the growth of tumor. EDC size ranged from 1 to 15 cm and no significant

TABLE 1: Published case reports of intra-abdominal esophageal duplication cyst.

	Reference	Year	Age	Sex	Symptoms	Location	Size (cm)	Treatment
(1)	Ruffin and Hansen [7]	1989	38	F	Epigastric pain, nausea, and vomit	Distal esophagus	4	Resection
(2)	Harvell et al. [8]	1996	57	F	Epigastric pain	Superior border of the body of pancreas	2.2	Laparoscopic resection
(3)	Karahasanoglu et al. [9]	1997	51	M	Dysphagia, weight loss, and epigastric pain	Subdiaphragm	11	Esophagogastrectomy
(4)	Janssen and Fiedler [10]	1998	56	F	Incidental (staging CT for rectal tumor)	Superior to the left kidney	8	Open resection
(5)	Rathaus and Feinberg [11]	2000	5	F	Epigastric pain	Between the left lobe of the liver and the cardia	1	Open resection
(6)	Nelms et al. [12]	2002	44	M	Low back pain	Diaphragmatic crura	7	Laparoscopic resection
(7)	Vijayaraghavan and Belagavi [13]	2002	70	F	Incidental (retching, giddiness, and headache)	Midline between the stomach and liver	7.5	Open resection
(8)	Noguchi et al. [14]	2003	26	F	Incidental (anal bleeding)	Right anterior wall of the distal esophagus	4	Laparoscopic resection with esophageal repair (Nissen)
(9)	Kin et al. [15]	2003	51	F	Incidental (staging CT for breast cancer)	Diaphragmatic crura	4.5	Laparoscopic resection with intraoperative esophagoscopy
(10)	Sakurai et al. [16]	2006	62	M	Dysphagia, upper abdominal pain	Bifurcation of the trachea through the proximal portion of the stomach	15	Resection, thoracotomy followed by laparotomy
(11)	Martin et al. [17]	2007	50	F	Left flank pain	Inferior portion of the pancreatic body/tail and the transverse mesocolon	6.5	Open resection
(12)	Martin et al. [17]	2007	60	M	Epigastric pain, gastric outlet obstruction	Dorsal to the second portion of the duodenum and the pancreatic head	10	Open resection
(13)	Aldrink and Kenney [18]	2011	2	M	Incidental (in laparoscopic fundoplication)	Anterior portion of the gastroesophageal junction	3	Laparoscopic resection with fundoplication
(14)	Gümüş et al. [19]	2011	18	F	Dyspeptic complaints	Lower end of the esophagus adjacent to the liver	4.2	Open resection
(15)	Bhamidipati et al. [20]	2013	69	M	Incidental (CT for diverticulitis)	Gastroesophageal junction	4.4	Laparoscopic resection
(16)	Pujar et al. [21]	2013	13	F	Pain in epigastric region	Gastroesophageal junction below the left lobe of the liver	5	Laparoscopic resection
(17)	Mori et al. [22]	2013	9	M	Incidental (CT for hematuria)	Ventral surface of the abdominal esophagus	2	Laparoscopic resection
(18)	Castelijns et al. [23]	2014	20	M	Nausea, colic pain	Gastroesophageal junction	3.2	Laparoscopic resection
(19)	**Our case**	**2014**	**50**	**M**	**Epigastric pain, dysphagia**	**Intra-abdominal esophagus extending to the distal thoracic esophagus**	**3.5**	**Laparoscopic resection with intraoperative esophagoscopy**

CT, computed tomography.

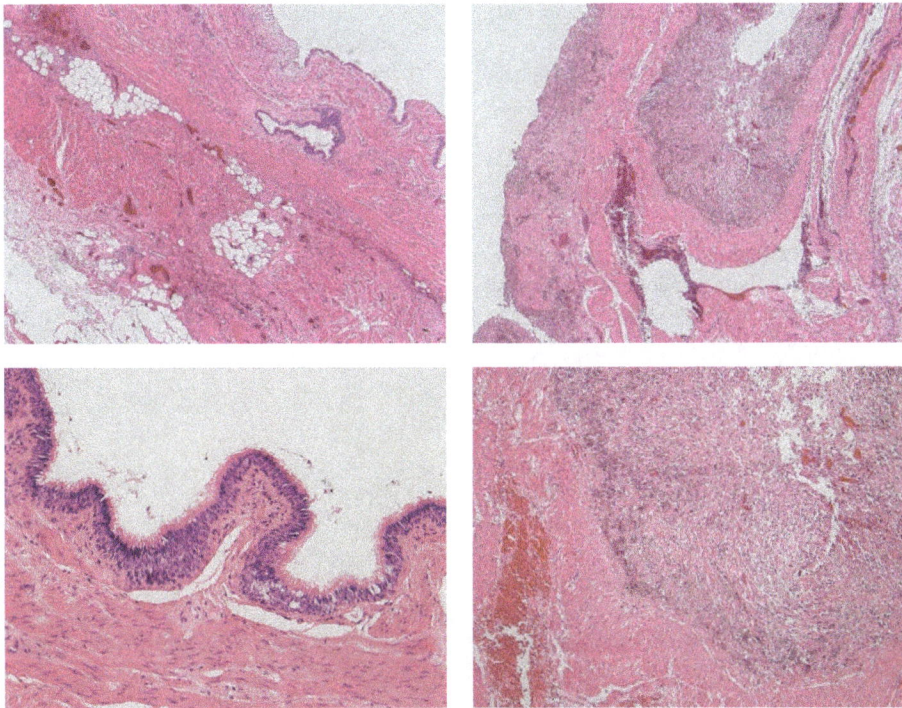

Intra-abdominal esophageal duplication cyst

FIGURE 7: Histopathological examination. The wall of the mass is composed of two layers of smooth muscle fibers, and the cavity is lined with pseudostratified columnar epithelium. Bleeding and hemosiderin deposition are visible in certain areas of the cystic wall.

differences in patient background factors were observed between symptomatic patients and patients whose diagnosis was incidental. In general, the preoperative diagnosis of EDC is made based on CT and endoscopic ultrasonography findings. As in the present study, the definitive diagnosis of EDC is relatively easy for lesions with homogeneous signal intensity and smooth margins. However, it is sometimes difficult to definitively diagnose mediastinal cystic masses because of diverse components, such as hemorrhage, sebum or sebaceous fluid, and proteinaceous fluid. Surgical resection is recommended as the primary treatment for EDC because of reports of malignant transformation of cysts even though the frequency is unknown [24]. Although laparoscopic resection has been widely performed in recent years, it is essential to perform gross total resection because cysts can cause necrosis and fistula formation in nearby structures including the intestines and peritoneum [25] and because recurrence due to incomplete resection has been reported [26]. In our case, intraoperative esophagoscopy was performed after gross total resection of the EDC to ensure the accurate reconstruction of the esophageal wall, and this enabled us to verify the absence of postreconstruction esophageal stricture and to discover fragile areas in the esophagus due to surgical abrasion.

In summary, we reported an extremely rare adult case of intra-abdominal EDC and reviewed the 18 previously published case reports.

References

[1] W. E. Ladd and R. E. Gross, "Surgical treatment of duplication of the alimentary tract," *Surgery, Gynecology & Obstetrics*, vol. 70, pp. 295–307, 1940.

[2] L. E. Stern and B. W. Warner, "Gastrointestinal duplications," *Seminars in Pediatric Surgery*, vol. 9, no. 3, pp. 135–140, 2000.

[3] K. M. Jang, K. S. Lee, S. J. Lee et al., "The spectrum of benign esophageal lesions: imaging findings," *Korean Journal of Radiology*, vol. 3, no. 3, pp. 199–210, 2002.

[4] S. K. Kim, H. K. Lim, S. J. Lee, and C. K. Park, "Completely isolated enteric duplication cyst: case report," *Abdominal Imaging*, vol. 28, no. 1, pp. 12–14, 2003.

[5] H. C. Kuo, H. C. Lee, C. H. Shin, J. C. Sheu, P. Y. Chang, and N. L. Wang, "Clinical spectrum of alimentary tract duplication in children," *Acta Paediatrica Taiwanica*, vol. 45, no. 2, pp. 85–88, 2004.

[6] F. A. M. Herbella, P. Tedesco, R. Muthusamy, and M. G. Patti, "Thoracoscopic resection of esophageal duplication cysts," *Diseases of the Esophagus*, vol. 19, no. 2, pp. 132–134, 2006.

[7] W. K. Ruffin and D. E. Hansen, "An esophageal duplication cyst presenting as an abdominal mass," *The American Journal of Gastroenterology*, vol. 84, no. 5, pp. 571–573, 1989.

[8] J. D. Harvell, J. R. Macho, and H. Z. Klein, "Isolated intra-abdominal esophageal cyst: case report and review of the literature," *The American Journal of Surgical Pathology*, vol. 20, no. 4, pp. 476–479, 1996.

[9] T. Karahasanoglu, A. Ozbal, S. Alcicek, S. Goksel, and M. Altun, "Giant intra-abdominal esophageal duplication cyst," *Endoscopy*, vol. 29, no. 9, pp. S54–S55, 1997.

[10] H. Janssen and P. N. Fiedler, "Isolated intraabdominal esophageal cyst," *The American Journal of Roentgenology*, vol. 170, no. 2, pp. 389–390, 1998.

[11] V. Rathaus and M. S. Feinberg, "Subdiaphragmatic esophageal duplication cyst in a child," *Journal of Clinical Ultrasound*, vol. 28, no. 5, pp. 264–264, 2000.

[12] C. D. Nelms, R. White, B. D. Matthews, W. E. Ballinger Jr., R. F. Sing, and B. T. Heniford, "Thoracoabdominal esophageal duplication cyst," *Journal of the American College of Surgeons*, vol. 194, no. 5, pp. 674–675, 2002.

[13] R. Vijayaraghavan and C. S. Belagavi, "True giant intra-abdominal esophageal cyst," *Indian Journal of Gastroenterology*, vol. 21, no. 5, pp. 198–199, 2002.

[14] T. Noguchi, T. Hashimoto, S. Takeno, S. Wada, K. Tohara, and Y. Uchida, "Laparoscopic resection of esophageal duplication cyst in an adult," *Diseases of the Esophagus*, vol. 16, no. 2, pp. 148–150, 2003.

[15] K. Kin, K. Iwase, J. Higaki et al., "Laparoscopic resection of intra-abdominal esophageal duplication cyst," *Surgical Laparoscopy, Endoscopy & Percutaneous Techniques*, vol. 13, no. 3, pp. 208–211, 2003.

[16] Y. Sakurai, S. Tonomura, K. Inaba et al., "Esophageal duplication cyst continuously extending into the peritoneal cavity on the proximal portion of the stomach," *Esophagus*, vol. 3, no. 3, pp. 113–119, 2006.

[17] N. D. Martin, J. C. Kim, S. K. Verma et al., "Intra-abdominal esophageal duplication cysts: a review," *Journal of Gastrointestinal Surgery*, vol. 11, no. 6, pp. 773–777, 2007.

[18] J. H. Aldrink and B. D. Kenney, "Laparoscopic excision of an esophageal duplication cyst," *Surgical Laparoscopy, Endoscopy & Percutaneous Techniques*, vol. 21, no. 5, pp. e280–e283, 2011.

[19] M. Gümüş, A. Önder, U. Firat, M. Kapan, H. Önder, and S. Gırgın, "Hydatid cyst-like intra-abdominal esophageal duplication cyst in an endemic region," *The Turkish Journal of Gastroenterology*, vol. 22, no. 5, pp. 557–558, 2011.

[20] C. Bhamidipati, M. Smeds, E. Dexter, M. Kowalski, and S. Bazaz, "Laparoscopic excision of gastric mass yields intra-abdominal esophageal duplication cyst," *The Journal of Thoracic and Cardiovascular Surgery*, vol. 61, no. 6, pp. 502–504, 2013.

[21] V. C. Pujar, S. Kurbet, and D. K. Kaltari, "Laparoscopic excision of intra-abdominal oesophageal duplication cyst in a child," *Journal of Minimal Access Surgery*, vol. 9, no. 1, pp. 34–36, 2013.

[22] H. Mori, H. Ishibashi, H. Sato, H. Kuyama, M. Asanoma, and M. Shimada, "Complete laparoscopic surgery for a 9-year-old patient with abdominal esophageal duplication cyst: report of a case," *Shikoku Acta Medica*, vol. 69, no. 5-6, pp. 251–256, 2013.

[23] P. S. S. Castelijns, K. Woensdregt, B. Hoevenaars, and G. A. P. Nieuwenhuijzen, "Intra-abdominal esophageal duplication cyst: a case report and review of the literature," *World Journal of Gastrointestinal Surgery*, vol. 6, no. 6, pp. 112–116, 2014.

[24] R. H. Tapia and V. A. White, "Squamous cell carcinoma arising in a duplication cyst of the esophagus," *The American Journal of Gastroenterology*, vol. 80, no. 5, pp. 325–329, 1985.

[25] M. A. R. Islah and T. Hafizan, "Perforated ileal duplication cyst presenting with right iliac fossa pain mimicking perforated appendicitis," *Medical Journal of Malaysia*, vol. 63, no. 1, pp. 63–64, 2008.

[26] H. Al-Sadoon, N. Wiseman, and V. Chernick, "Recurrent thoracic duplication cyst with associated mediastinal gas," *Canadian Respiratory Journal*, vol. 5, no. 2, pp. 149–151, 1998.

23

A Patient with Advanced Gastric Cancer Presenting with Extremely Large Uterine Fibroid Tumor

Kwang-Kuk Park and Song-I Yang

Department of Surgery, Kosin University College of Medicine, 34 Amnam-dong, Seo-gu, Busan 602-703, Republic of Korea

Correspondence should be addressed to Song-I Yang; tonybin@daum.net

Academic Editors: D. J. Bentrem and M. Zafrakas

Introduction. Uterine fibroid tumors (uterine leiomyomas) are the most common benign uterine tumors. The incidence of uterine fibroid tumors increases in older women and may occur in more than 30% of women aged 40 to 60. Many uterine fibroid tumors are asymptomatic and are diagnosed incidentally. *Case Presentation*. A 44-year-old woman was admitted to our hospital with general weakness, dyspepsia, abdominal distension, and a palpable abdominal mass. An abdominal computed tomography scan showed a huge tumor mass in the abdomen which was compressing the intestine and urinary bladder. Gastroduodenal endoscopic and biopsy results showed a Borrmann type IV gastric adenocarcinoma. The patient was diagnosed with gastric cancer with disseminated peritoneal carcinomatosis. She underwent a hysterectomy with both salphingo-oophorectomy and bypass gastrojejunostomy. Simultaneous uterine fibroid tumor with other malignancies is generally observed without resection. But in this case, a surgical resection was required to resolve an intestinal obstruction and to exclude the possibility of a metastatic tumor. *Conclusion*. When a large pelvic or ovarian mass is detected in gastrointestinal malignancy patients, physicians try to exclude the presence of a Krukenberg tumor. If the tumors cause certain symptoms, surgical resection is recommended to resolve symptoms and to exclude a metastatic tumor.

1. Introduction

Gastric cancer is one of the most commonly diagnosed malignancies in South Korea. Female patients with advanced gastric cancer, in particular premenopausal patients, are also often found to have Krukenberg tumors. Because of this, when a large pelvic or ovarian mass is detected in gastrointestinal malignancy patients, physicians try to exclude the presence of a Krukenberg tumor. The incidence of uterine fibroid tumors increases as women grow older and these tumors may occur from 4 percent in women 20 to 30 years of age to 11 to 18 percent in women 30 to 40 years of age and 33 percent in women 40 to 60 years [1]. Many tumors are asymptomatic and are diagnosed incidentally. Although a causal relationship has not been established, uterine fibroid tumors are associated with menorrhagia, pelvic pain, pelvic or urinary obstructive symptoms, infertility, and pregnancy loss. A patient recently visited our hospital with sudden onset abdominal distension and indigestion. The patient was diagnosed with stomach cancer and suspected metastatic uterine

tumors. We performed a hysterectomy with both a salphingo-oophorectomy and a bypass gastrojejunostomy. A very large uterine mass was histologically revealed to be a uterine fibroid tumor, not a Krukenberg tumor. We report this first case of an extremely large uterine fibroid tumor in a patient with advanced gastric cancer.

2. Case Presentation

A 44-year-old woman was admitted to our hospital with general weakness, dyspepsia, abdominal distension, and a palpable mass that had been present for two weeks. The patient appeared pale and was chronically ill. She stated that she had lost 6 kg over the last two months. On physical examination, she was oriented to time, place, and person. Her vital signs were as follows: blood pressure of 130/75 mmHg, pulse rate of 83 beats/min, and respiration rate of 24 breaths/min. Abdominal examination revealed a mass that was palpable over the entire abdomen. There was no jaundice, cyanosis, or diaphoresis. Neurological and cardiac examinations did not exhibit any pathological findings. Tumor marker levels including carcinoembryonic antigen (CEA), human chorion gonadotropin (HCG), CA19-9, and CA15-3 were all within normal range, but CA125 was high at 171 U/mL. An abdominal computed tomography scan (Figure 1) showed a huge tumor mass in the abdomen which was compressing the intestine and urinary bladder. Gastroduodenal endoscopic and biopsy results showed a Borrmann type IV gastric adenocarcinoma in the prepyloric antrum with gastric outlet obstruction. A F-18 fluorodeoxyglucose (FDG) positron emission tomography/computed tomography (PET-CT) showed a huge pelvic mass and increased FDG uptake from the main pelvic mass and multiple hypermetabolism in the mesentery and peritoneum (Figure 2). An exploratory laparotomy was performed with a long midline incision. After the peritoneal cavity was opened, an enormous circumscribed mass measuring 28.0 × 20.0 × 27.0 cm (Figure 3) was found to be displacing the bowel to the abdominal adhesions periphery. The mass originated from the right corner of the uterus. Multiple peritoneal nodules resembling peritoneal carcinomatosis were observed and a frozen biopsy was carried out. She was diagnosed with peritoneal carcinomatosis of gastric cancer. A total hysterectomy with both salphingo-oophorectomy and bypass gastrojejunostomy was performed. The tumor was sent for histological and cytological assessment, which did not reveal any evidence of malignancy. Due to maladaptation of lung capacity, she complained of difficulty breathing. On the third postoperative day, her breathing was comfortable. The postoperative course was uneventful, and the patient had no further complications. The patient is currently receiving chemotherapy with S-1 plus CDDP (cisplatin), according to the following regimen: S-1 (50 mg/m (2) p.o. b.i.d. from D1 to 14) and cisplatin (70 mg/m (2) on D1), repeated every 3 weeks.

3. Discussion

Female patients with advanced gastric cancer, particularly in the premenopausal state, are subject to Krukenberg tumors [2]. Uterine fibroid tumors are the most common female reproductive tract tumors. They are usually of a unicellular origin, and their growth rate is influenced by estrogen, growth hormone, and progesterone. Although exact process of tumor formation has not been elucidated, uterine fibroid tumors arise during reproductive years and tend to enlarge during pregnancy and regress after menopause.

The use of estrogen agonists is associated with an increased incidence of fibroid tumors [3], and growth hormone appears to act synergistically with estradiol in affecting the growth of uterine fibroid tumors. Some studies have shown increased estrogen receptor mRNA in fibroids compared with normal myometrium [4]. Fibroids overexpress aromatase p450, a synthetase which produces estrogen from androgens, suggesting that local estrogen may play a role in the growth of uterine fibroids [5]. Sex-steroid action is mediated partially via other growth factors such as epidermal

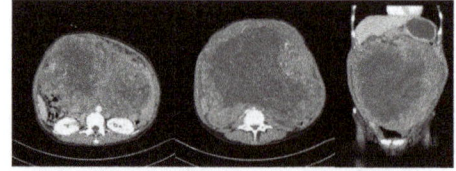

FIGURE 1: Abdominal computed tomography (CT) showing a huge solid mass occupying whole pelvis and abdomen.

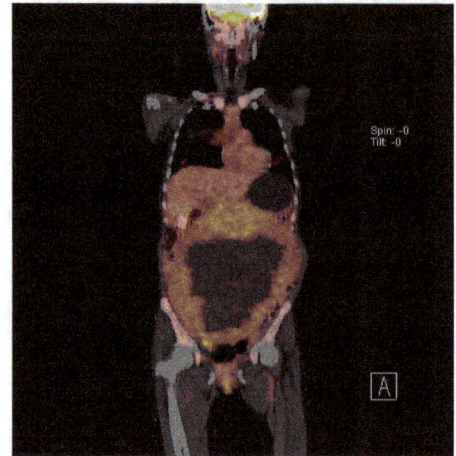

FIGURE 2: F-18 fludeoxyglucose (FDG) positron emission tomography/computed tomography (PET/CT) images.

growth factor and insulin-like growth factor [6]. Estrogen upregulates epidermal growth factors and transforming growth factor-beta1 and transforming growth factor-beta3, all of which play a role in the growth of uterine fibroids [7]. Progesterone is thought to exert a dual action, as it can promote fibroid growth but also may have an inhibitory effect on fibroid growth through downregulating insulin-like growth factor-1 (IGF-1) expression [6]. Several other studies have reported an increased incidence of uterine fibroid tumors in black women [8].

Pelvic pain and pressure are less commonly attributed to uterine fibroid tumors. Individual case reports have described very large tumors that result in pelvic discomfort, respiratory failure, urinary symptoms, and constipation [9–11]. It has been reported that solitary or multiple tumors are possible and may rarely present in a botryose shape [12]. Tumor sizes have been reported to range from microscopic to 3400 g [13]. The fibroid tumor reported here was 7990 g.

The role of uterine fibroid tumors in infertility is controversial. Many studies examining the relationship between these tumors and infertility are retrospective and nonrandomized. Current evidence suggests that submucosal and intramural fibroid tumors that distort the uterine cavity can impair in vitro fertilization attempts [14].

Uterine myomas are classified into subgroups according to their position and relationship to the uterine layers. These tumors become symptomatic based on their position within the uterus and their size. Tumors are usually distinguished by the following characteristics: (a) intramural myomas; (b)

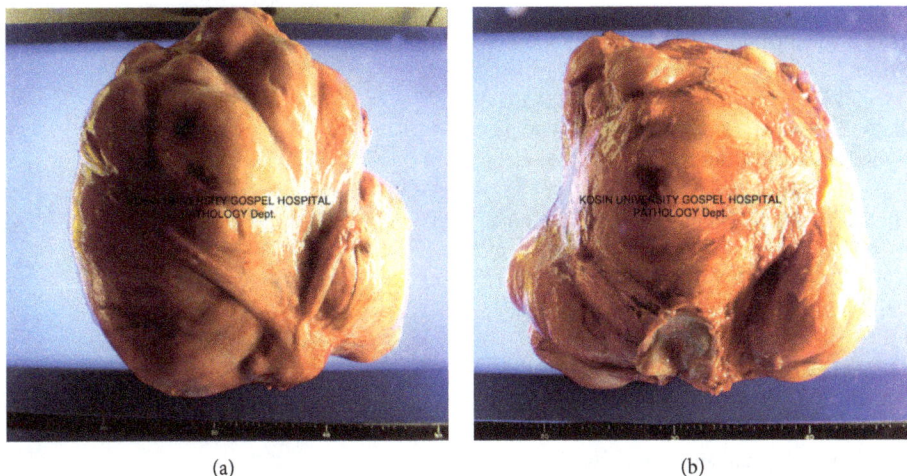

(a)   (b)

FIGURE 3: Macroscopic view of uterine fibroid tumor.

submucosal (endocavitary) myomas, which can be pedunculated or sessile and can extend into the myometrium; (c) subserosal myomas, which can be pedunculated or sessile and are located just beneath the covering peritoneum of the uterine corpus; (d) isthmus or cervical myomas; and (e) extrauterine (intraligamentary or intraovarian) myomas [15].

The treatment for uterine fibroid tumors with no symptoms and a small size is observation at intervals of 6 months. In terms of medical therapy, GnRH agonists, medroxyprogesterone acetate, danazol, and mifepristone (RU 486), which reduces the serum progesterone and estrogen, were reported to reduce the fibroid volume. Surgical treatment can be considered in cases of abnormal bleeding with sustained endometrial hyperplasia or when no improvement is seen with palliative therapy, and uterine artery embolization has been used recently in these cases. A total hysterectomy or myomectomy should be considered based on the patient's age, parity, and future pregnancy plans. Decreases in serum estrogen levels are expected after menopause, which may cause a decrease in the size of the myoma, so surgical removal is therefore not required in most patients who are approaching menopause [13].

4. Conclusion

In this case, a surgical resection was required to resolve an intestinal obstruction and to exclude the possibility of a Krukenberg tumor. We report a surgical resected uterine fibroid tumor in a patient with advanced gastric cancer.

Author's Contribution

The patient was under the care of Kwang-Kuk Park; Song-I Yang operated on the patient. Kwang-Kuk Park and Song-I Yang analyzed and interpreted the data. Kwang-Kuk Park wrote the paper. Song-I Yang added to the paper. Song-I Yang edited the final version of the paper. All authors reviewed and approved the final paper.

References

[1] S. Lurie, I. Piper, I. Woliovitch, and M. Glezerman, "Age-related prevalence of sonographicaly confirmed uterine myomas," *Journal of Obstetrics & Gynaecology*, vol. 25, no. 1, pp. 42–44, 2005.

[2] N. K. Kim, H. K. Kim, B. J. Park et al., "Risk factors for ovarian metastasis following curative resection of gastric adenocarcinoma," *Cancer*, vol. 85, no. 7, pp. 1490–1499, 1999.

[3] E. Chalas, J. P. Costantino, D. L. Wickerham et al., "Benign gynecologic conditions among participants in the Breast Cancer Prevention Trial," *American Journal of Obstetrics & Gynecology*, vol. 192, no. 4, pp. 1230–1239, 2005.

[4] K. A. Kovács, A. Oszter, P. M. Göcze, J. L. Környei, and I. Szabó, "Comparative analysis of cyclin D1 and oestrogen receptor (α and β) levels in human leiomyoma and adjacent myometrium," *Molecular Human Reproduction*, vol. 7, no. 11, pp. 1085–1091, 2001.

[5] M. Shozu, H. Sumitani, T. Segawa et al., "Overexpression of aromatase P450 in leiomyoma tissue is driven primarily through promoter I.4 of the aromatase P450 gene (CYP19)," *The Journal of Clinical Endocrinology & Metabolism*, vol. 87, no. 6, pp. 2540–2548, 2002.

[6] T. Maruo, N. Ohara, J. Wang, and H. Matsuo, "Sex steroidal regulation of uterine leiomyoma growth and apoptosis," *Human Reproduction Update*, vol. 10, no. 3, pp. 207–220, 2004.

[7] A. Barbarisi, O. Petillo, A. Di Lieto et al., "17-beta estradiol elicits an autocrine leiomyoma cell proliferation: evidence for a stimulation of protein kinase-dependent pathway," *Journal Cellular Physiology*, vol. 186, no. 3, pp. 414–424, 2001.

[8] L. A. Wise, J. R. Palmer, E. A. Stewart, and L. Rosenberg, "Age-specific incidence rates for self-reported uterine leiomyomata in the Black Women's Health Study," *Obstetrics & Gynecology*, vol. 105, no. 3, pp. 563–568, 2005.

[9] G. Oelsner, S. E. Elizur, Y. Frenkel, and H. Carp, "Giant uterine tumors: two cases with different clinical presentations," *Obstetrics & Gynecology*, vol. 101, no. 5, part 2, pp. 1088–1091, 2003.

[10] D. Courban, S. Blank, M. A. Harris, J. Bracy, and P. August, "Acute renal failure in the first trimester resulting from uterine leiomyomas," *American Journal of Obstetrics & Gynecology*, vol. 177, no. 2, pp. 472–473, 1997.

[11] R. P. C. Chaparala, A. S. Fawole, N. S. Ambrose, and A. H. Chapman, "Large bowel obstruction due to a benign uterine leiomyoma," *Gut*, vol. 53, no. 3, pp. 386–430, 2004.

[12] A. H. Brand, J. P. Scurry, R. S. Planner, and P. T. Grant, "Grapelike leiomyoma of the uterus," *American Journal of Obstetrics & Gynecology*, vol. 173, pp. 959–961, 1995.

[13] J. S. Berek and E. Novak, *Berek and Novak's Gynecology*, Lippincott Williams & Wilkins, Philadelphia, Pa, USA, 2007.

[14] B. W. Rackow and A. Arici, "Fibroids and in-vitro fertilization: which comes first?" *Current Opinion in Obstetrics & Gynecology*, vol. 17, no. 3, pp. 225–231, 2005.

[15] B. McLucas, "Diagnosis, imaging and anatomical classification of uterine fibroids," *Best Practice and Research*, vol. 22, no. 4, pp. 627–642, 2008.

24

Jejunojejunal Intussusception due to Metastatic Melanoma Seven Years after the Primer

Alexander Giakoustidis,[1] **Thomas Goulopoulos,**[2] **Anastasios Boutis,**[3] **George Kavvadias,**[4] **Aristidis Kainantidis,**[2] **Thomas Zaraboukas,**[5] **and Dimitrios Giakoustidis**[2,6]

[1]Department of HPB Surgery, Royal London Hospital, London, UK
[2]Department of Surgery, European Interbalkan Medical Centre, Thessaloniki, Greece
[3]Department of Oncology, "Theagenion" Anti-Cancer Hospital, Thessaloniki, Greece
[4]Department of Anesthesiology, European Interbalkan Medical Centre, Thessaloniki, Greece
[5]Department of Pathology, European Interbalkan Medical Centre, Thessaloniki, Greece
[6]Division of Transplant Surgery, Department of Surgery, Medical School, Aristotle University of Thessaloniki, Thessaloniki, Greece

Correspondence should be addressed to Dimitrios Giakoustidis; dgiakoustidis@gmail.com

Academic Editor: Boris Kirshtein

Intestinal intussusception in adults is a rare medical condition accounting for less than 5% of all intussusceptions. Herein we present a 45-year-old patient with a history of abdominal pain and loss of weight. CT scan revealed jejunojejunal intussusceptions. The patient was subjected to exploratory operation and small intestine resection due to a mass causing intestinal intussusception. Pathology confirmed suspected diagnosis of metastatic melanoma to small intestine secondary to melanoma, 7 years after the initial manifestation. Postoperative evaluation with 18FDG-PET/CT revealed increased uptake in the thyroid gland. Subsequent total thyroidectomy revealed severe Hashimoto thyroiditis and no signs of metastasis. The patient received adjuvant immunotherapy and is healthy with no signs of recurrence 3 years after the initial diagnosis and treatment.

1. Introduction

Intussusception is a rare condition in the adult population accounting for less than 5% of all intussusceptions [1, 2]. Diagnosis is challenging because it often presents with non-specific symptoms; abdominal pain with obstruction is the common presentation. Intussusception is responsible for 1% of all bowel obstructions [2, 3]. Surgery is the treatment of choice and in most of the cases there is underling malignant pathology involved [1–3]. Even though most small intestine tumors are usually metastatic, with metastatic melanoma being the most common, intussusceptions due to metastasis from melanoma have rarely been described in the literature. We herein present a case of jejunojejunal intussusceptions due to metastatic melanoma in a 45-year-old lady 7 years after the excision of the primer.

2. Case Presentation

A 45-year-old female presented to our clinic with abdominal pain for the last month. In addition the patient presented abdominal fullness, constipation, and loss of weight the last month. On physical examination abdominal discomfort was present. Medical history revealed a prior operation in the left arm for melanoma and axillary lymph node dissection 7 years ago with initial stage unknown and she received adjuvant high-dose interferon (Kirkwood regimen). In May 2014 she developed symptomatic iron-deficiency anemia and diffuse abdominal pain. Imaging exams revealed an obstructing abdominal mass originating from the small bowel and causing intussusception (Figure 1). Laboratory examination revealed no remarkable findings. An exploratory laparotomy was decided and performed. During the operation indeed an

(a)

(b)

(c)

(d)

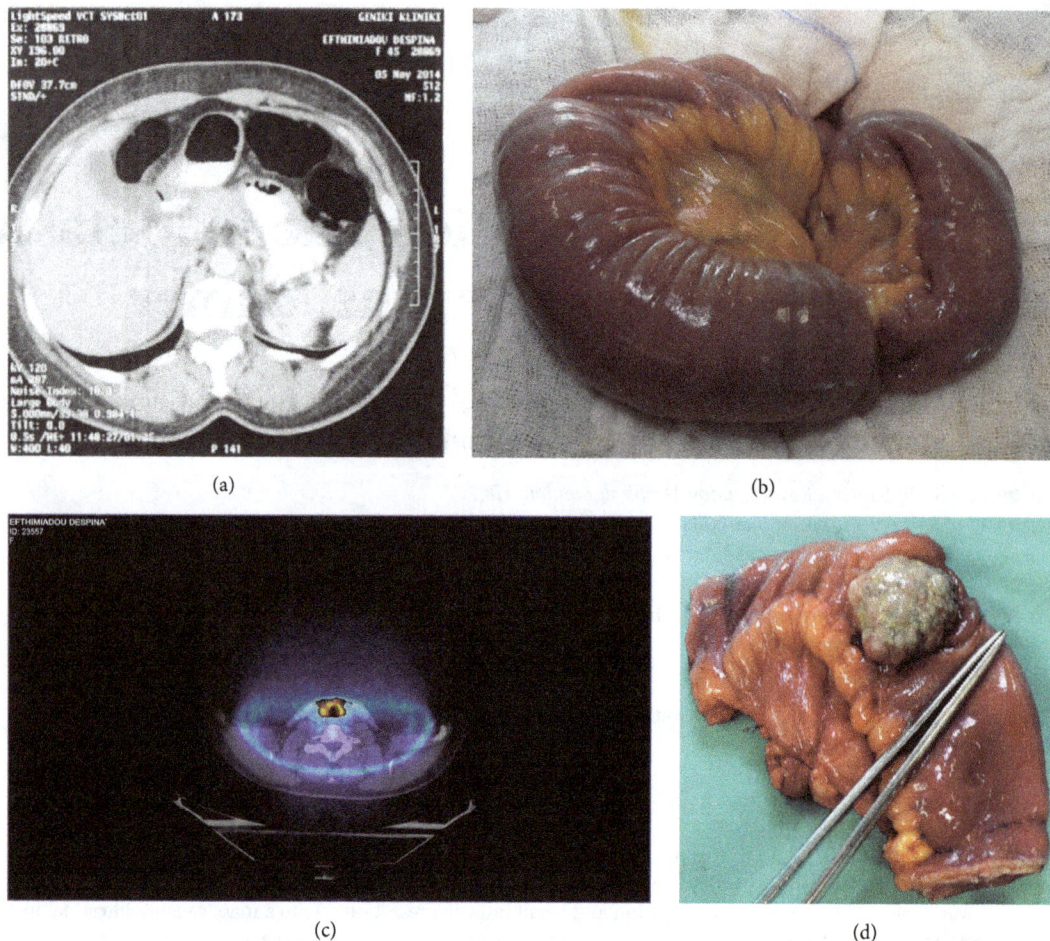

FIGURE 1: (a) CT scan showing an obstructing abdominal mass originating from the small bowel and causing intussusception; (b) intraoperative image of the intussusception; (c) thyroid gland with increased SUV in the 18FDG-PET/CT; (d) intestinal intussusceptions due to what appeared to be a distant melanoma metastasis.

intestinal intussusception was found (Figure 1) due to what appeared to be a distant melanoma metastasis (Figure 1). Intestinal resection was performed with end-to-end hand sewn jejunojejunostomy. After careful checking no other distant metastasis was found in the abdomen. The patient had excellent postoperative course and was discharged at the 4th postoperative day.

Histological examination of the tumor showed a malignant neoplasm consisting of large epithelioid atypical cells in solid arrangement which invades the mucosa, submucosa, and part of the muscularis propria. Immunohistochemistry revealed positivity of the tumor cells for HMB45 and Melan A (Figure 2). One month after the operation the patient was subjected to 18FDG-PET/CT in order to rule out any other distant metastases. 18FDG-PET/CT result was normal except the thyroid gland that showed increased uptake (Figure 1). Consequently it was decided to perform a total thyroidectomy. Two months after the first operation the patient was subjected to a total thyroidectomy. Pathology showed no signs of metastatic melanoma but revealed severe Hashimoto thyroiditis. The patient was referred for adjuvant

immunotherapy. Molecular testing for the b-raf V600E mutation was positive. Between September and November 2014, she received first-line immunotherapy with ipilimumab at standard therapeutic regimen 3 mg/kg q3w for four cycles, which she tolerated without any remarkable toxicity. Subsequent radiologic and clinical controls showed no evidence of disease progression. The patient remains asymptomatic and free of disease 3 years after diagnosis and treatment of metastatic disease. The patient has given his consent for the case reports to be published.

3. Discussion

Intussusception in adults is a rare medical condition appearing in 5% of the total incidents of intussusceptions and represents the cause for 1% of intestinal obstructions [4]. The usual initial clinical signs are those of bowel obstruction while the diagnosis, in contrast with children, is difficult and in the majority of cases it is established intraoperatively [5]. Metastatic melanoma to the GI tract accounts for one-third of all abdominal metastases with small intestine being

(a)

(b)

(c)

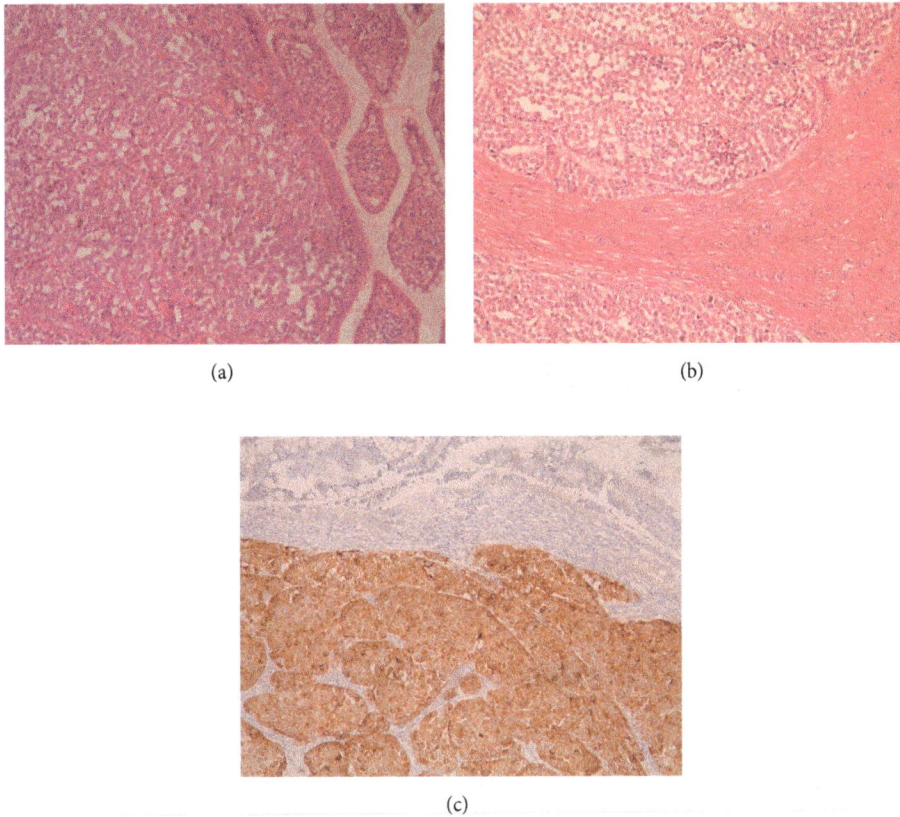

FIGURE 2: (a) Invasion of the mucosa of the small intestine by the melanoma cells (H+EX200). (b) Invasion of the muscularis propria by the melanoma cells (H+EX100). (c) Tumor cells are positive for HMB45 (immunostain ×200).

the most common site [4, 5] and is classified as stage four terminal diseases with an average lifespan of two months to 15 years following diagnosis [6]. Reported incidence of gastrointestinal metastases of melanoma in autopsy series reaches up to 60% [7]. On the contrary patients being clinically diagnosed with malignant melanoma and gastrointestinal metastases are limited to no more than 4% [8, 9]. The risk factors for malignant melanoma spread to the GI tract include superficial spreading melanoma, axial primary tumor, a Clark level III or IV, high degree of histologic regression, ulceration, and high mitotic rate [7, 10, 11]. Herein, we report an uncommon clinical presentation in adults, intussusception, with an underlying pathology, metastatic melanoma to the GI tract, that is rarely diagnosed premortem. This diagnosis should be considered in any patient who presents with gastrointestinal symptoms and a history of malignant melanoma. In our case a 45-year-old female presented with atypical symptoms of abdominal pain, constipation, and loss of weight. Previous history of melanoma in the left arm combined with the intestinal intussusceptions from the CT scan prompts us to operate on the patient with the increased suspicion of metastatic melanoma to the small intestine. Diagnosis was confirmed surgically and subsequently by pathology. The patient was restaged with 18FDG-PET/CT postoperatively showing increased uptake in the thyroid gland. This was

proven false positive sign as we have already described, and this raises a concern over the evaluation of PET/CT. The patient completed the adjuvant immunotherapy and she is in an excellent condition 3 years after the initial diagnosis.

References

[1] S. M. Cera, "Intestinal intussusception," *Clinics in Colon and Rectal Surgery*, vol. 21, no. 2, pp. 106–113, 2008.

[2] T. Azar and D. L. Berger, "Adult intussusception," *Annals of Surgery*, vol. 226, no. 2, pp. 134–138, 1997.

[3] M. Barussaud, N. Regenet, X. Briennon et al., "Clinical spectrum and surgical approach of adult intussusceptions: a multicentric study," *International Journal of Colorectal Disease*, vol. 21, no. 8, pp. 834–839, 2006.

[4] R. H. Stewardson, C. T. Bombeck, and L. M. Nyhus, "Critical operative management of small bowel obstruction," *Annals of Surgery*, vol. 187, no. 2, pp. 189–193, 1978.

[5] H. L. Laws and J. S. Aldrete, "Small-bowel obstruction: a review of 465 cases," *Southern Medical Journal*, vol. 69, no. 6, pp. 733-734, 1976.

[6] Y.-J. Huang, M.-H. Wu, and M.-T. Lin, "Multiple small-bowel intussusceptions caused by metastatic malignant melanoma," *American Journal of Surgery*, vol. 196, no. 3, pp. e1–e2, 2008.

[7] L. M. Schuchter, R. Green, and D. Fraker, "Primary and metastatic diseases in malignant melanoma of the gastrointestinal tract," *Current Opinion in Oncology*, vol. 12, no. 2, pp. 181–185, 2000.

[8] K. Washington and D. McDonagh, "Secondary tumors of the gastrointestinal tract: surgical pathologic findings and comparison with autopsy survey," *Modern Pathology*, vol. 8, no. 4, pp. 427–433, 1995.

[9] D. Blecker, S. Abraham, E. E. Furth, and M. L. Kochman, "Melanoma in the gastrointestinal tract," *The American Journal of Gastroenterology*, vol. 94, no. 12, pp. 3427–3433, 1999.

[10] T. Mucci, W. Long, A. Witkiewicz, M. J. Mastrangelo, E. L. Rosato, and A. C. Berger, "Metastatic melanoma causing jejunal intussusception," *Journal of Gastrointestinal Surgery*, vol. 11, no. 12, pp. 1755–1757, 2007.

[11] K. V. Liang, S. O. Sanderson, G. S. Nowakowski, and A. S. Arora, "Metastatic malignant melanoma of the gastrointestinal tract," *Mayo Clinic Proceedings*, vol. 81, no. 4, pp. 511–516, 2006.

25

Pneumoperitoneum with Subcutaneous Emphysema after Percutaneous Endoscopic Gastrostomy

Yalin Iscan,[1] Bora Karip,[1] Yetkin Ozcabi,[1] Birol Ağca,[1] Yesim Alahdab,[2] and Kemal Memisoglu[1]

[1] *General Surgery, Fatih Sultan Mehmet Eğitim ve Araştırma Hastanesi, İçerenköy, 34752 İstanbul, Turkey*
[2] *Gastroenterology, Fatih Sultan Mehmet Eğitim ve Araştırma Hastanesi, İçerenköy, 34752 İstanbul, Turkey*

Correspondence should be addressed to Yalin Iscan; yaliniscan@gmail.com

Academic Editor: Giovanni Mariscalco

Percutaneous endoscopic gastrostomy is a safe way for enteral nutrition in selected patients. Generally, complications of this procedure are very rare but due to patients general health condition, delayed diagnosis and treatment of complications can be life threatening. In this study, we present a PEG-related massive pneumoperitoneum and subcutaneous emphysema in a patient with neuro-Behçet.

1. Introduction

Percutaneous endoscopic gastrostomy (PEG) has become the most preferred procedure for long-term enteral feeding since its description in the early 1980s [1]. It was reported as the second leading indication for upper gastrointestinal tract endoscopy in the USA [2]. PEG is proven to be safe, cost effective, and feasible. Most of the complications after PEG procedure are clinically minor and the frequency of serious complications is very low. A meta-analysis reported PEG-related morbidity of 9.4% and mortality of 0.53% [3]. With a neuromuscular disease or in a sedated patient, the diagnosis of complications may be delayed.

High clinical suspicion and early screening methods are essential for diagnosis, appropriate treatment, and favourable outcome [4]. In this study, we present a PEG-related massive pneumoperitoneum and subcutaneus emphysema in a patient with neuro-Behçet.

2. Case Presentation

A 45-year-old woman, who was diagnosed as having Neuro-Behçet's disease (NBD), was admitted to our hospital with fever and cough. A PEG was performed 15 days ago due to the swallow dysfunction and standard enteral nutrition

was applied after the procedure without any complaint. Her physical examination revealed a subcutaneous emphysema but there was no sign of peritoneal inflammation and symptoms of acute abdomen due to her neuromuscular disease. Also there was no wound infection around the PEG-tube. Her fever was 38,3 C. The hemoglobin concentration was 9.5 g/dL (12–16 gr/dL), leukocyte count was 9.8 K/uL (4–10 K/uL), platelet count was 215 K/uL (150–450 K/uL), and C-reactive protein level was 6.4 mg/dL (0-1 mg/dL). Liver and renal function tests were normal. Thoracoabdominal computerized tomography (CT) showed the presence of pneumoperitoneum with subcutaneous emphysema over the abdomen wall extending to the cervical and lomber region. The PEG tube was in the stomach in CT but the gastric wall was not attached to the abdominal wall (Figure 1).

After pulling up the PEG-tube and fixing the gastric wall to the abdominal wall, we checked the tube's position by a plain abdominal graph with contrast given through PEG catheter and there was no extra luminal contrast leakage (Figure 2).

Enteral feeding was stopped and intravenous hyperalimentation was given after repositioning of the tube. Because of the fever and high levels of CRP, blood, urine, and deep tracheal aspiration (DTA) cultures were obtained. The culture results of DTA were positive for Klebsiella pneumonia so

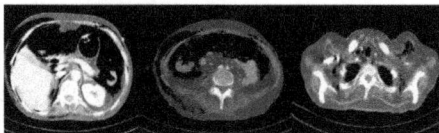

FIGURE 1: Thoracoabdominal CT, showing detached gastric wall from catheter insertion site and massive subcutaneous emphysema through cervical, thoracic, and abdominal region.

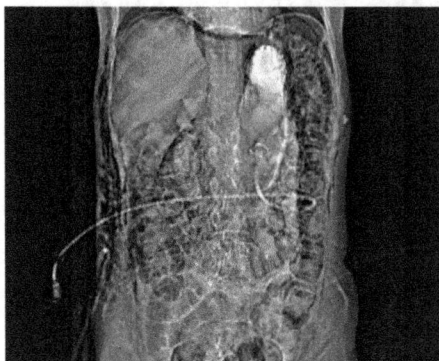

FIGURE 2: Abdominal X ray with contrast given from the PEG catheter. There was no intra-abdominal leakage.

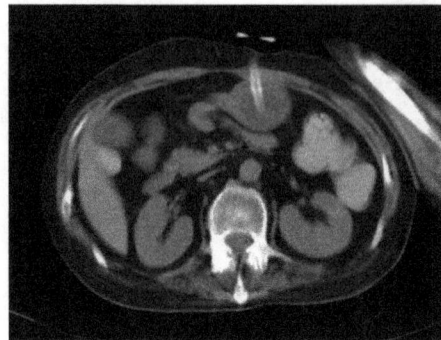

FIGURE 3: Replaced PEG catheter in the stomach and resolved pneumoperitoneum.

Ertapenem therapy was ordered according to the antibiogram results. The subcutaneous emphysema resolved within 7 days. We started enteral nutrition again seven days after admission, but there was a leakage back to the skin around the PEG tube. We replaced the PEG-tube with a 20-F foley catheter and fixed it to the skin with sutures. After this replacement, tube feeding was resumed successfully for seven days. On the fourteenth day of her admission, a new PEG catheter was inserted from another part of the stomach and the transient foley catheter was removed. No recurrence of leakage, pneumoperitoneum, and emphysema developed (Figure 3). She was discharged seventeen days after her admission.

3. Discussion

PEG is the second leading indication for upper gastrointestinal endoscopy in the US [2–5]. The number of patients with PEG tubes has increased significantly and will continue to increase. It is clear that these high volumes will bring higher numbers of complications. Morbidity rates of the procedure range from 9% to 17% but major complications are under 5% and mortality is lower than 1% [6, 7]. Papakonstantinou et al. divided the complications into three subgroups [8] (Table 1).

Pneumoperitoneum is common after PEG procedure, with an incidence of over 50% [9–11]. Probably the etiology of pneumoperitoneum or leakage occurs by insufficient fixation of the PEG, causing leakage of air through the gastric wall which enters the free peritoneal space. It is also explainable that air escapes through the small opening from the stomach during the interval between the initial needle puncture and the PEG tube passage through the abdominal wall. In the absence of symptoms with patients

who have undergone a recent PEG, conservative management in pneumoperitoneum is suggested. Pneumoperitoneum is usually subclinical and self-limiting and should be clinically concerned only when intra-abdominal air is worsening or when it is found in the presence of signs of peritonitis, portal and/or mesenteric venous gas, systemic inflammatory response, and/or sepsis [11].

Subcutaneous emphysema is a very rare complication of PEG [12]. Emphysema was also described after percutaneous gastrostomy in which the catheter was placed under ultrasonography guidance with the asistance of fluoroscopy. It was reported that the evidence of subcutaneous emphysema occured after the fourth day of the procedure [11]. For our patient it was more than two weeks from the PEG insertion to diagnosis of emphysema. And also the patient's complaint was cough and fever which were not specific to emphysema.

Subcutaneous emphysema with gastrointestinal origin is very rare. Peptic ulcer perforation, trauma, carcinoma, diverticulitis, appendicitis, jejunal perforation, colonoscopy, dental surgery, and some acetebular orthopedic surgeries should be kept in mind [13, 14]. For our patients, it was due to the detachment of the gastric wall from abdominal wall.

There is no gold standard for treatment leakage and pneumoperitoneum after PEG. PEG leakage is reported by 58%–78% of patients with long-term PEG tube placement [15]. Leakage from the stoma occurs because of the dilatation of the stoma [16]. Removing the tube for a few days reduces the diameter of the stoma and permits a resized tube replacement [17].

The PEG tract closes in 24–48 hours when the patient is treated with bowel rest with or without nasogastric suction. Subsequent placement of a PEG tube in a new site is often successful. Repositioning or gastric wall fixation by another tube will not always stop the leakage in the same site because all stomas diameters do not reduce always by different manuplations.

Sometimes only repositioning of the catheter is enough. With our patient, although we checked the catheter with X-ray by infusing contrast from the catheter and confirmed it was placed correctly, we faced a leakage problem. An alternative way to solve leakage is the replacement of the PEG tube with a balon catheter or foley catheter. Foley catheters should only be used as temporary replacements to maintain

TABLE 1: Complications of PEG procedure.

Due to the endoscopy procedure	Due to the PEG and the gastrostomy tube	Due to the mode of feeding

(i) Laryngospasm, airway obstruction
(ii) Aspiration and pneumonia
(iii) Respiratory depression or apnea
(iv) Desaturation or respiratory distress and acute respiratory failure
(v) Hypertension
(vi) Fracture of the alveolar ridge while attempting to open the mouth
	(i) Perforation/laceration of the oesophagus or the stomach
	(ii) Transhepatic insertion of the tube
	(iii) Pneumoperitoneum
	(iv) Colonic perforation
	(v) Subcutaneous emphysema
	(vi) Retroperitoneal hemorrhage
	(vii) Aortic perforation
	(viii) Erosion of the gastric mucosa and bleeding
	(ix) Hematoma or infection of the abdominal wall
	(x) Gastrocolic fistula
	(xi) Colocutaneous fistula
	(xii) Hypertrophic granulation tissue at the gastrostomy exit
	(xiii) Buried bumper syndrome
	(xiv) Malpositioning of the tube or leakage
	  (a) To the subcutaneous tissues → cellulitis, myositis, necrotizing fasciitis, subcutaneous abscess
	  (b) To the peritoneal cavity → peritonitis, intraabdominal abscess, sepsis
	(xv) Migration of the tip of the gastrostomy tube
	  (a) To oesophagus (oesophagitis)
	  (b) To pylorus (obstruction or perforation of the duodenum)
	(xvi) Migration of the whole PEG tube up to the terminal ileum
	(xvii) Peristomal hernia or stomal prolapse
	(xviii) Accidental pulling out or cutting off the tube close to the skin during home care
	(xix) Erosion of the tube through the gastric wall
	(xx) Obstruction of the tube lumen
	(xxi) Hub detachment or damage
	(xxii) Later symptomatic gastroesophageal reflux
	(xxiii) Ileus
		(i) Diarrhoea
		(ii) Nausea
		(iii) Vomiting
		(iv) Dumping syndrome
		(v) Ogilvie's syndrome
		(vi) Aspiration pneumonia
		(vii) Constipation and meteorism

the integrity of the fistula. In addition, the catheters should be marked in some way to determine the depth of insertion prior to inflation. Clinicians must pay attention to fix these kinds of catheters to the skin because of the catheter migration risk. By the propulsive force of gastric peristaltism, the head of tube may lead to a mechanical obstruction through duodenum and this may also cause pancreatitis [18]. If there is any doubt as to the location of any replacement tube, the position of the tube should be confirmed radiographically before inflation and the resumption of tube feedings.

In summary, the number of patients with PEG tubes has increased significantly and will continue to increase. An increased awareness of these rare but potentially life threatening complications is important. In this critically ill, comatose patient group, missing possible but rare complications may be lethal.

References

[1] W. L. Gauderer, J. L. Ponsky, and R. J. Izant Jr., "Gastrostomy without laparotomy: a percutaneous endoscopic technique," *Journal of Pediatric Surgery*, vol. 15, no. 6, pp. 872–875, 1980.

[2] M. W. Gauderer, "Twenty years of percutaneous endoscopic gastrostomy: origin and evolution of a concept and its expanded applications," *Gastrointestinal Endoscopy*, vol. 50, no. 6, pp. 879–883, 1999.

[3] B. Wollman, H. B. D'Agostino, J. R. Walus-Wigle, D. W. Easter, and A. Beale, "Radiologic, endoscopic, and surgical gastrostomy: an institutional evaluation and meta-analysis of the literature," *Radiology*, vol. 197, no. 3, pp. 699–704, 1995.

[4] M. R. Taheri, H. Singh, and D. R. Duerksen, "Peritonitis after gastrostomy tube replacement: a case series and review of literature," *Journal of Parenteral and Enteral Nutrition*, vol. 35, no. 1, pp. 56–60, 2011.

[5] J. Z. Potack and S. Chokhavatia, "Complications of and controversies associated with percutaneous endoscopic gastrostomy: report of a case and literature review," *Medscape General Medicine*, vol. 10, no. 6, article 142, 2008.

[6] J. A. DiSario, "Endoscopic approaches to enteral nutritional support," *Best Practice and Research: Clinical Gastroenterology*, vol. 20, no. 3, pp. 605–630, 2006.

[7] H. S. Lin, H. Z. Ibrahim, J. W. Kheng, W. E. Fee, and D. J. Terris, "Percutaneous endoscopic gastrostomy: strategies for prevention and management of complications," *Laryngoscope*, vol. 111, no. 10, pp. 1847–1852, 2001.

[8] K. Papakonstantinou, A. Karagiannis, M. Tsirantonaki et al., "Mediastinitis complicating a percutaneous endoscopic gastrostomy: a case report," *BMC Gastroenterology*, vol. 3, article 11, 2003.

 [9] K. M. Hillman, "Pneumoperitoneum—a review.," *Critical Care Medicine*, vol. 10, no. 7, pp. 476–481, 1982.

[10] E. B. Gottsfried, A. B. Plumser, and M. R. Clair, "Pneumoperitoneum following percutaneous endoscopic gastrostomy. A prospective study," *Gastrointestinal Endoscopy*, vol. 32, no. 6, pp. 397–399, 1986.

[11] M. M. Wojtowycz and J. A. Arata Jr., "Subcutaneous emphysema after percutaneous gastrostomy," *The American Journal of Roentgenology*, vol. 151, no. 2, pp. 311–312, 1988.

[12] G. Stathopoulos, M. A. Rudberg, and J. M. Harig, "Subcutaneous emphysema following PEG," *Gastrointestinal Endoscopy*, vol. 37, no. 3, pp. 374–376, 1991.

[13] M. J. Walker and M. F. Mozes, "Massive subcutaneous emphysema: an unusual presentation of jejunal perforation," *The American Surgeon*, vol. 47, no. 1, pp. 45–48, 1981.

[14] S. A. Thompson, J. S. Harper, and P. Millican, "An unusual case of subcutaneous emphysema," *British Journal of Radiology*, vol. 54, no. 644, pp. 682–683, 1981.

[15] S. N. Rogers, R. Thomson, P. O'Toole, and D. Lowe, "Patients experience with long-term percutaneous endoscopic gastrostomy feeding following primary surgery for oral and oropharyngeal cancer," *Oral Oncology*, vol. 43, no. 5, pp. 499–507, 2007.

[16] G. D. Schapiro and S. A. Edmundowicz, "Complications of percutaneous endoscopic gastrostomy," *Gastrointestinal Endoscopy Clinics of North America*, vol. 6, no. 2, pp. 409–422, 1996.

[17] W. E. Strodel, "Complications of percutaneous gastrostomy," in *Techniques of Percutaneous Endoscopy*, J. L. Ponskyd, Ed., pp. 63–78, Iguku-Shoin, New York, NY, USA, 1988.

[18] A. M. Shah, N. Shah, and J. R. Depasquale, "Replacement gastrostomy tube causing acute pancreatitis: case series with review of literature," *Journal of the Pancreas*, vol. 13, no. 1, pp. 54–57, 2012.

26

Gastric Volvulus and Wandering Spleen: A Rare Surgical Emergency

Georgios Lianos, Konstantinos Vlachos, Nikolaos Papakonstantinou, Christos Katsios, Georgios Baltogiannis, and Dimitrios Godevenos

Division of Surgery, University Hospital of Ioannina, St. Niarchou Avenue, 45110 Ioannina, Greece

Correspondence should be addressed to Georgios Lianos; georgiolianos@yahoo.gr

Academic Editors: J. Griniatsos, G. Rallis, M. Rangarajan, and A. Spinelli

Gastric volvulus is a rare but potentially life-threatening clinical entity due to possible gastric necrosis. A wandering spleen may also be associated with gastric volvulus. Patients presenting with the triad epigastralgia, vomiting followed by retching, and difficulty or inability to pass a nasogastric tube into the stomach are likely to have gastric volvulus. The operating surgeon should include this rare entity in the differential diagnosis when dealing with a patient with such a clinical profile. Herein, we present a case of gastric volvulus associated with a wandering spleen in a 28-year-old Caucasian woman and we provide a brief review of the literature on this issue.

1. Introduction

Gastric volvulus is an extremely rare clinical entity first described by Berti in 1866 [1]. An abnormal rotation (180°) of one part of the stomach around another, potentially leading to obstruction of the gastric cavity is defined gastric volvulus. Volvulus may be organoaxial or mesenteroaxial, occuring around an axis made by two fixed points. When untreated, complete volvulus results in strangulation, which may lead to ischaemia, necrosis, and finally to gastric perforation. Interestingly, mortality rates can achieve levels of 30–50% [2, 3]. Therefore, gastric volvulus is a true and life-threatening surgical emergency if not treated in time. Wandering spleen is also a rare entity characterized by the underdevelopment or complete absence of one or all of the ligaments that hold the spleen in its normal position. Moreover, gastric volvulus and wandering spleen share a common cause, the absence of intraperitoneal visceral ligaments [4, 5]. We hereby present the rare case of a 28-year-old Caucasian woman with gastric volvulus associated with a wandering spleen. We share our experience in successful treatment of this unique case.

2. Case Report

A 28-year-old Caucasian female was admitted to the emergency department of our hospital complaining of severe abdominal pain, nausea, and multiple episodes of bilious vomiting followed by repeating nonproductive retching. Her medical history was unremarkable. Her vital signs showed only mild tachycardia. Upon physical examination the abdominal sounds were present and her abdomen was diffusely tender especially in the upper quadrant. No peptic ulcers or diaphragmatic hernias were included in her family history. Rectal examination showed an empty rectum. The laboratory tests were between normal ranges. There was a significant difficulty in passing a nasogastric tube which finally suctioned out a large amount of gastric fluid. The admission chest X-ray showed an enlarged stomach and an elevated left hemidiaphragm; so a gastrografin swallow was arranged. The latter showed a well-defined "bird beak" sign and a helical trend of the nasogastric tube (Figure 1). Gastroscopy was performed and revealed a large amount of gastric fluid in the stomach and mucosal ischemic lesions. Interestingly, the endoscope failed to intubate the pylorus.

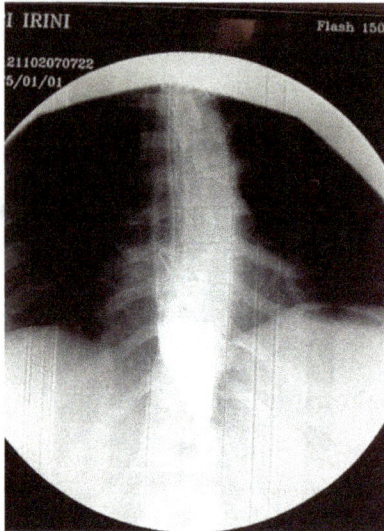

FIGURE 1: "Bird beak" sign and helical trend of the nasogastric tube after gastrografin swallow.

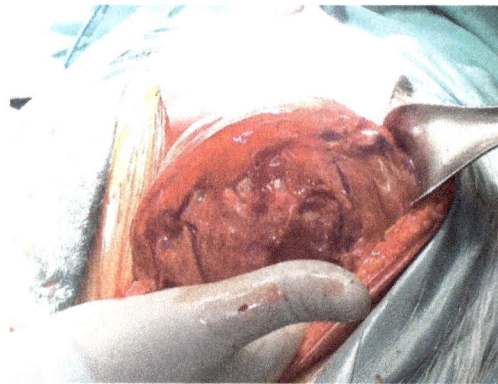

FIGURE 2: Twisted stomach (gastric volvulus).

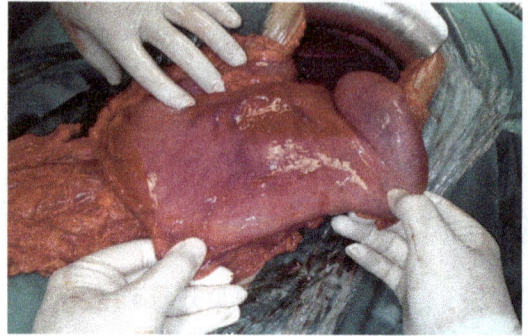

FIGURE 3: The untwisted distended stomach with ischemic mucosal lesions.

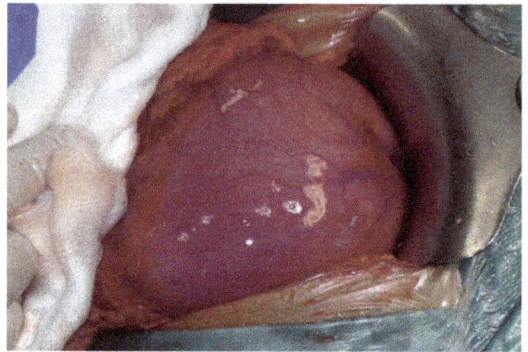

FIGURE 4: The untwisted distended stomach with ischemic mucosal lesions.

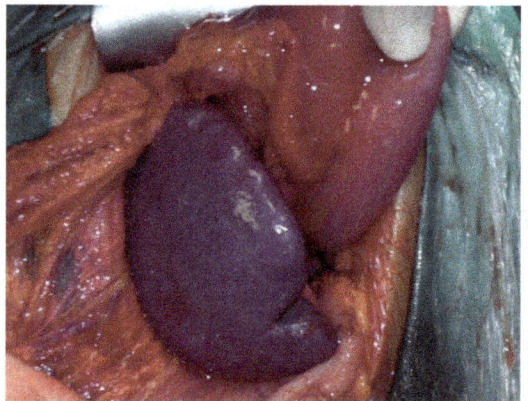

FIGURE 5: The wandering spleen.

An exploratory laparotomy was performed under general anesthesia the day after by midline incision. Intraoperative findings revealed a twisted distended stomach with ischemic lesions. A mesenteroaxial gastric volvulus was identified (Figures 2, 3, and 4). Interestingly, there was a lack of ligaments; so a wandering spleen was observed (Figure 5). The volvulus was untwisted and an approximation of the gastroesophageal junction and pylorus, predisposing to volvulus, was revealed (Figure 6). The stomach was reduced at its anatomic position, as well as the spleen, and an anterior gastropexy was carried out by fixing the greater curvature of the stomach to the anterior abdominal wall (Figure 7). The postoperative period was uneventful and the patient was discharged 10 days later. Two months after the operation, the patient remained asymptomatic.

3. Discussion

Gastric volvulus is a rare entity with difficult diagnosis. The incidence is unknown [6]. An abnormal rotation of one part of the stomach around another of more than 180 degrees is defined gastric volvulus [7]. This infrequent entity is in almost all the cases associated with congenital diaphragmatic hernia and eventration of the diaphragm. Interestingly, there is also a rare association between gastric volvulus and wandering spleen. These entities share a common cause, the absence or laxity of intraperitoneal visceral ligaments. Wandering spleen is a mobile spleen attached only by its vascular pedicle. This spleen can migrate to any part of the abdomen [8]. Gastric volvulus can be acute, chronic, or acute on chronic. Acute gastric volvulus is more rare than chronic.

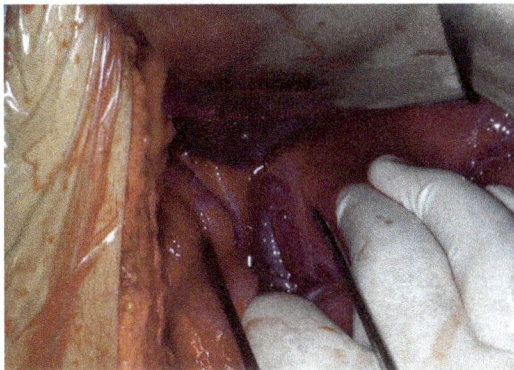

FIGURE 6: The approximation of the gastroesophageal junction and pylorus, leading to gastric volvulus.

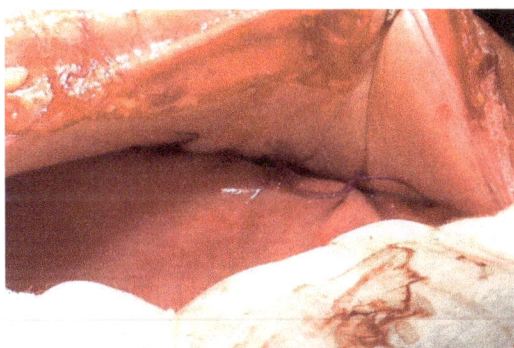

FIGURE 7: Anterior gastropexy.

There are described 3 types of gastric volvulus according to the axis of rotation: organoaxial, mesenteroaxial, and combination. Organoaxial volvulus is the most common and occurs in approximately 59% of cases. Because the duodenum and gastroesophageal (GE) junction are relatively fixed, the stomach rotates around the longitudinal axis extending from the gastroesophageal junction to pylorus. The mesenteroaxial volvulus is presented in 29% of cases. The rotation occurs around the transgastric axis (a line connecting the middle of the lesser curvature with the middle of the greater curvature). It is reported that most cases of chronic gastric volvulus are related to mesenteroaxial rotation. Additionally is described in the literature that a normal stomach cannot rotate more than 180° unless the gastrosplenic or gastrocolic ligaments are divided [9, 10]. The aetiology of gastric volvulus is thought to be secondary to laxity or lack of the gastric (gastrohepatic, gastrosplenic, gastroduodenal, and gastrophrenic) ligaments, allowing approximation of cardiac and pyloric ends when the stomach is full, leading to volvulus, as in our case (Figure 7) [11]. The clinical picture of gastric volvulus may occur as an acute abdominal emergency or as recurrent volvulus. In the literature, the famous Borchardt triad that is present typically in cases of acute gastric volvulus is described. This triad includes severe epigastric pain with distention, vomiting followed by violent, nonproductive retching, and finally difficulty or inability to pass a nasogastric tube into the stomach. Moreover, a missed diagnosis of gastric volvulus may lead

to strangulation, perforation, hemorrhage, ischemia, and gastric necrosis [12]. The mortality rate of gastric volvulus is reported to be up to 42–56%, secondary to gastric ischaemia, perforation, and necrosis [13]. The diagnosis of this rare clinical entity is very challenging. The gold standard method in detecting gastric volvulus is a barium swallow, which has a very high sensitivity and specificity. Additionally, highly suggestive of gastric volvulus is the difficulty during endoscopy to intubate the stomach or the pylorus. As for the treatment, gastric volvulus presenting with acyte symptoms requires immediate surgical intervention. The most approved surgical treatment consists in anterior gastropexy with open or laparoscopic technique. During this method, the greater curvature of the stomach is fixed to the anterior abdominal wall. Subtotal or total gastrectomy is proposed when the stomach appears gangrenous [14, 15].

4. Conclusion

Though rare, gastric volvulus must be always considered in the differential diagnosis when a patient with the Borchardt triad is admitted to the hospital. A missed or delayed diagnosis may result in unfavorable outcomes. It seems that the most important factor in diagnosing gastric volvulus is the awareness of its possibility. The diagnosis is suspected mainly by symptoms and exclusion of other pathologies. Surgical intervention is the optimal treatment. Additionally, gastric volvulus is rarely associated with wandering spleen that may lead to splenic torsion. These entities are potentially life-threatening, if not treated in time.

Authors' Contribution

All authors were actively involved in the preoperative and postoperative care of the patient, read and approved also the final manuscript form.

References

[1] A. Berti, "Singolare attortigliamento dell' esofago col duodeno seguita da rapida morte," *Gazzetta Medica Italiana*, vol. 9, p. 139, 1866.

[2] S. Gourgiotis, V. Vougas, S. Germanos et al., "Acute gastric volvulus: diagnosis and management over 10 years," *Digestive Surgery*, vol. 23, no. 3, pp. 169–172, 2006.

[3] B. Chau and S. Dufel, "Gastric volvulus," *Emergency Medicine Journal*, vol. 24, no. 6, pp. 446–447, 2007.

[4] J. M. Spector and J. Chappell, "Gastric volvulus associated with wandering spleen in a child," *Journal of Pediatric Surgery*, vol. 35, no. 4, pp. 641–642, 2000.

[5] M. E. Zimmermann and R. C. Cohen, "Wandering spleen presenting as an asymptomatic mass," *Australian and New Zealand Journal of Surgery*, vol. 70, no. 12, pp. 904–906, 2000.

[6] N. O. Machado and B. A. Rao, "Gastric volvulus with identifiable cause in adults. Presentation and management," *Saudi Medical Journal*, vol. 25, no. 12, pp. 2032–2034, 2004.

[7] R. Carter, L. A. Brewer, and D. B. Hinshaw, "Acute gastric volvulus: a study of 25 cases," *American Journal of Surgery*, vol. 140, no. 1, pp. 99–106, 1980.

[8] G. Pelizzo, M. A. Lembo, A. Franchella, A. Giombi, F. D'Agostino, and S. Sala, "Gastric volvulus associated with congenital diaphragmatic hernia, wandering spleen, and intrathoracic left kidney: CT findings," *Abdominal Imaging*, vol. 26, no. 3, pp. 306–308, 2001.

[9] L. W. Milne, "Gastric volvulus: two cases and a review of the literature," *Journal of Emergency Medicine*, vol. 12, no. 3, pp. 299–306, 1994.

[10] J. A. Wasselle and J. Norman, "Acute gastric volvulus: pathogenesis, diagnosis, and treatment," *American Journal of Gastroenterology*, vol. 88, no. 10, pp. 1780–1784, 1993.

[11] W. J. Teague, R. Ackroyd, D. I. Watson, and P. G. Devitt, "Changing patterns in the management of gastric volvulus over 14 years," *British Journal of Surgery*, vol. 87, no. 3, pp. 358–361, 2000.

[12] M. Borchardt, "Zur pathologie und therapie des magen volvulus," *Langenbecks Arch Klin Chir Ver Dtsch Z Chir*, vol. 74, pp. 243–260, 1904.

[13] S. Farag, V. Fiallo, S. Nash, and F. Navab, "Gastric perforation in a case of gastric volvulus," *American Journal of Gastroenterology*, vol. 91, pp. 1863–1864, 1996.

[14] A. R. Askew, "Treatment of acute and chronic gastric volvulus," *Annals of the Royal College of Surgeons of England*, vol. 60, no. 4, pp. 326–328, 1978.

[15] C. Palanivelu, M. Rangarajan, A. R. Shetty, and R. Senthilkumar, "Laparoscopic suture gastropexy for gastric volvulus: a report of 14 cases," *Surgical Endoscopy and Other Interventional Techniques*, vol. 21, no. 6, pp. 863–866, 2007.

27

An Extremely Rare Bile Leakage: Aberrant Bile Duct in Left Triangular Ligament (Appendix Fibrosa Hepatis)

İhsan Yıldız ⓘ, Yavuz Savaş Koca ⓘ, and Sezayi Kantar

Department of General Surgery, Suleyman Demirel University Medical School, Isparta, Turkey

Correspondence should be addressed to İhsan Yıldız; drihsanyildiz@gmail.com

Academic Editor: Christophoros Foroulis

Background. The anatomical variability of bile ducts can leave surgeons in very difficult conditions. Ultrasonography, computed tomography, magnetic resonance imaging (MRCP) and endoscopic imaging methods are used in diagnosis. In addition to conservative approaches, endoscopic procedures and laparoscopic or open surgical interventions may be necessary for treatment. In this article, we present a case of aberrant bile duct in left triangular ligament (appendix fibrosa hepatis), which is rarely seen. *Case.* We report the case of a 67-year-old female patient who was operated on due to dumping syndrome symptoms and hiatal hernia. There was a drainage of bile from the left side of the liver which was placed under the cardioesophageal junction. MRCP found bile esophageal in the left triangular ligament of the liver. Aberrant bile ducts were found in the left triangular ligament and ligated. The patient was discharged on the 7th day after operation. *Conclusion.* The anatomical variability of bile ducts can leave surgeons in very difficult conditions. We recommend that the dissected left triangular ligament should be ligated for the aberrant bile duct, especially in female patient.

1. Introduction

The structural anatomy of the bile ducts is highly variable and can be said to have almost no stable anatomy. This variability is more common in women [1]. This situation can often leave the surgeon in difficult situations during surgery on the liver, bile ducts, pancreas, and upper gastrointestinal tract [2].

Therefore, the structure of the bifurcation, especially the anatomy of the biliary tract, should be assessed very well before the operation, and possible ultrasonography, computed tomography, magnetic resonance cholangiopancreatography (MRCP), and endoscopic imaging methods should be used carefully [3, 4]. Nevertheless, after all, there may be bile leakage. Although the gallbladder surgery is performed commonly, bile leakage is seen after upper gastrointestinal system surgery for various reasons [5]. Endoscopic procedures and laparoscopic or open surgical interventions may be necessary, as well as conservative approaches such as waiting for spontaneous abortion of the leakage according to the patient's situation [3, 5, 6].

This patient was presented due to the fact that bile leakage was very extreme and there was only one case in the literature.

2. Case Presentation

A 67-year-old female underwent bilateral truncal vagotomy, cholecystectomy, Billroth-2 gastrectomy, and Roux-en-Y procedure for pyloric stenosis twenty years ago due to early dumping syndrome and sliding-type hiatal hernia. The liver left lobe was mobilized by dissecting the left triangular ligament (appendix fibrosa hepatis) to release the cardioesophageal junction and stomach fundus. The hiatal hernia defect was repaired with a constrictive primary suture. Roux-en-Y anastomosis was externally constricted, and the antidumping procedure was applied. There was no other procedure in the abdomen that could injure the bile ducts such as liver hilar and duodenal stump dissection. A penrose drain was placed under the left lobe of the liver at the level of the cardioesophageal junction. There was a 150 mL bile leak in 24 hours after the first day of surgery. Bile leakage was detected with MRCP on the left side of the left triangular ligament of the liver (Figures 1 and 2). The patient was reoperated, and no pathology was observed except for aberrant bile duct (a 3 mm diameter) with bile leakage at the site where the left liver triangular ligament (appendix fibrosa hepatis) was dissected at the observation by following the drain (Figure 3). The injured bile duct was ligated with the 3/0 prolene suture. On 7 day after the operation, all complaints resolved, and the patient was discharged without any problems in the postoperative period.

3. Discussion

The bile ducts do not have a constant structure, so the surgeons can have undesired surprise during the gastrointestinal system surgery. To avoid these situations, it is necessary to use imaging methods for diagnosis of the biliary tract before surgery, especially in women [2, 3, 5, 6]. It is somewhat more difficult to predict this situation in cases of previous gastric surgery, such as the one described by Iso et al. [6]. This is even more difficult, especially since it is not possible to endoscopically view the anatomy of the bile ducts during Billroth-2 gastrectomy. We have not been able to perform endoscopic imaging because of the presence of Billroth-2 gastrectomy and Roux-en-Y gastrojejunostomy. Today, however, this difficulty can be overcome by MRCP examination [1, 3, 6]. We also used MRCP in this case where endoscopic imaging could not be done, and we diagnosed bile leak with this method.

Conservative approaches for the management of bile leakages and the need for surgical intervention may vary according to the anatomical localization and the amount of the leakage and the clinical condition of the patient [3]. In cases where the bile ducts can be reached by endoscopic method, papillotomy and/or stenting can be used to reduce the intraluminal pressure of the bile ducts and reduce the leakage and stop them completely. However, the bile leak into peritoneum can cause peritonitis even when the drain is placed in the line or not [6]. In these cases, surgical intervention is inevitable. In our case, there was no bile peritonitis because the bile came directly to the drain, and daily diversion of the bile leak was approximately 150–200 mL. In this case, if we had the possibility of performing endoscopic sphincterotomy, we could follow this patient without performing open surgery. However, as mentioned above, the patient did not have a chance to do this operation because he had Billroth-2 gastrectomy and Roux-en-Y gastrojejunostomy. In addition, because of the abdominal surgery performed many times before, intensive intraabdominal adhesions did not allow us to perform laparoscopic procedures and we had to do open surgery. During surgery, aberrant bile ducts and bile leak were observed at the localization of the left triangular ligament (appendix fibrosa hepatis) that was previously detected by MRCP. The leakage was sutured with prolene no. 3/0. Uysal and his colleagues reported that the variations of biliary tracts were seen more frequently in women than in men [1]. It was compatible in this situation that our case was also female. Extrahepatic and intrahepatic variations of the bile ducts are found more frequently on the right side, but the left-settling variations are less and the aberrant biliary tract in the left triangular ligament is an extremely rare case.

We consider that it is important to place a drain to the operation site for early controlling and treatment of bile

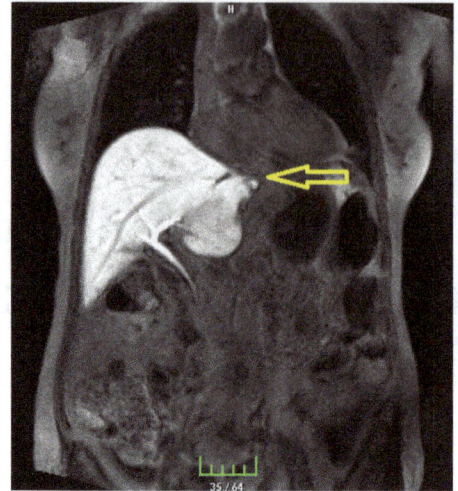

FIGURE 1: MRCP imaging. Bile leakage is shown in the left triangular ligament (appendix fibrosa hepatis).

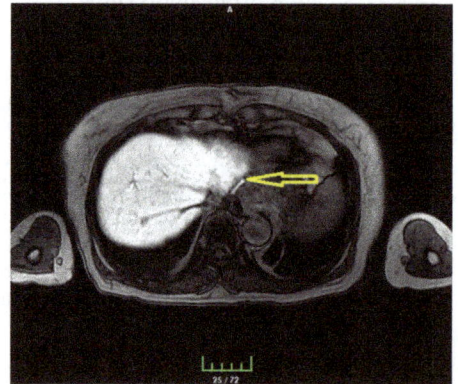

FIGURE 2: MRCP imaging. Bile leakage is shown in the drain.

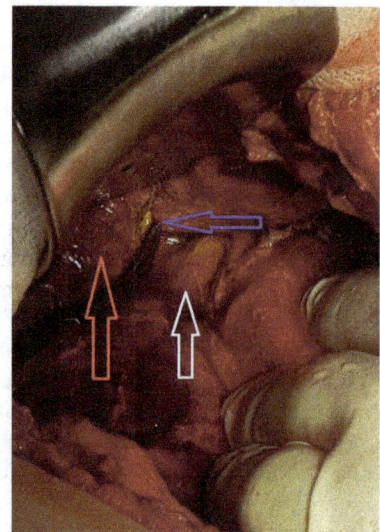

FIGURE 3: Left liver triangular ligament. Blue arrow shows bile leakage, red arrow shows the left triangular ligament, and white arrow shows the cardioesophageal junction.

leakage because of liver, biliary tract, pancreas, and upper gastrointestinal tract surgery, which are likely to encounter undesired surprises such as bile leakage due to the anatomical variations of the bile duct. With this idea, we recommend ligating this region if the left triangular ligament (appendix fibrosa hepatis) is dissected in surgery. In particular, it is necessary to keep in mind the possibility of aberrant bile ducts in the left triangular ligament in female patients with more biliary tract variations.

References

[1] F. Uysal, F. Obuz, A. Uçar, M. Seçil, E. Igci, and O. Dicle, "Anatomic variations of the intrahepatic bile ducts: analysis of magnetic resonance cholangio-pancreatography in 1011 consecutive patients," *Digestion*, vol. 89, no. 3, pp. 194–200, 2014.

[2] R. M. El Gharbawy, L. J. Skandalakis, T. G. Heffron, and J. E. Skandalakis, "Aberrant bile ducts, 'remnant surface bile ducts,' and peribiliary glands: descriptive anatomy, historical nomenclature, and surgical implications," *Clinical Anatomy*, vol. 24, no. 4, pp. 429–440, 2011.

[3] J. Guan, L. Zhang, J. P. Chu, S. C. Lin, and Z. P. Li, "Congenital left intrahepatic bile duct draining into gastric wall mimicking biliary reflux gastritis," *World Journal of Gastroenterology*, vol. 21, no. 11, pp. 3425–3428, 2015.

[4] D. V. Kostov and G. L. Kobakov, "Six rare biliary tract anatomic variations: implications for liver surgery," *Eurasian Journal of Medicine*, vol. 43, no. 2, pp. 67–72, 2011.

[5] H. Shokouh-Amiri, M. K. Fallahzadeh, S. T. Abdehou, M. Sugar, and G. B. Zibari, "Aberrant left main bile duct draining directly into the cystic duct or gallbladder: an unreported anatomical variation and cause of bile duct injury during laparoscopic cholecystectomy," *Journal of the Louisiana State Medical Society*, vol. 166, no. 5, pp. 203–206, 2014.

[6] Y. Iso, I. Kusaba, T. Matsumata et al., "Postoperative bile peritonitis caused by division of an aberrant bile duct in the left triangular ligament of the liver," *American Journal of Gastroenterology*, vol. 91, no. 11, pp. 2428–2430, 1996.

28

Hemophagocytic Lymphohistiocytosis and Gastrointestinal Bleeding: What a Surgeon Should Know

S. Popeskou,[1] **M. Gavillet,**[2] **N. Demartines,**[3] **and D. Christoforidis**[1,4]

[1]*Department of Surgery, Lugano Regional Hospital, Switzerland*
[2]*Department of Hematology, University Hospital of Lausanne, Switzerland*
[3]*Department of Surgery, University Hospital of Lausanne, Switzerland*
[4]*University Hospital of Lausanne, Switzerland*

Correspondence should be addressed to S. Popeskou; salvator10@yahoo.com

Academic Editor: Fernando Turégano

This paper presents to the surgical community an unusual and often ignored cause of gastrointestinal bleeding. Hemophagocytic syndrome or hemophagocytic lymphohistiocytosis (HLH) is a rare medical entity characterized by phagocytosis of red blood cells, leucocytes, platelets, and their precursors in the bone marrow by activated macrophages. When intestinal bleeding is present, the management is very challenging with extremely high mortality rates. Early diagnosis and treatment seem to be the most important factors for a successful outcome. We present two cases and review another 18 from the literature.

1. Introduction

Gastrointestinal (GI) bleeding is a common cause for hospital admission to surgical wards. In westernized countries, the annual incidence of upper GI bleeding is approximately 100 −200/100,000 and for lower GI bleeding 20–30/100,000. The estimated mortality ranges from 6% to 10% for upper GI bleeding and from 2% to 4% for lower GI bleeding [1–4]. Most episodes of lower GI bleeding resolve spontaneously, while others can be treated endoscopically or by interventional radiology. A minority of patients become hemodynamically unstable and require emergency surgery. In such cases, the source of bleeding is not always clear and the surgeon may face the difficult decision to perform extensive colonic resections, at a price of significant mortality rates (up to 25%), without the certitude of controlling the source of bleeding [5–7]. The most frequent causes of lower GI bleeding are diverticulosis and arterial-venous malformations. Other frequent causes are colitis, neoplasms, inflammatory bowel disease, and hemorrhoids [8, 9].

In this paper, we report the dramatic cases of two patients who presented massive lower GI bleeding originating from diffuse GI mucosal ulcerations secondary to acute Epstein Barr virus (EBV) proliferation and hemophagocytic lymphohistiocytosis (HLH) and review the literature for GI bleeding associated with this rare syndrome.

2. Case 1

A 26-year-old male patient, treated for Crohn's disease with azathioprine (150 mg/day) for 3 years, was admitted to the ENT department of a community hospital for treatment of a febrile pharyngitis with 10-day cefuroxime. Lab tests revealed leucopenia (2.7 g/L, 89% neutrophils, 8% monocytes) and a mild elevation of the liver enzymes. Clinically and radiologically, splenomegaly was present. An active EBV infection (IgG and IgM positive) was diagnosed on hospital day 7 and treatment with valacyclovir (1 gr × 3/day) was started. At the same day, the patient presented massive lower GI bleeding requiring admission to the ICU. The initial emergency colonoscopy revealed severe pancolitis with multiple ulcerations which was attributed to a flare of Crohn's colitis. Three days later (day 10), despite multiple transfusions, he became hemodynamically unstable due to continuous bleeding (CRP 121 mg/L, procalcitonin 1.21 mcg/L). The patient was therefore transferred to our University Hospital. Upon arrival, he developed a hypovolemic shock requiring massive blood transfusions and an emergent total colectomy with ileostomy was performed. Broad-spectrum antibiotherapy with piperacillin/tazobactam (4.5 gr × 4/day) and prednisone 50 mg/d was initiated in the immediate postoperative period. A thoracic CT-scan showed bilateral pulmonary infiltrates, which were attributed to transfusion related acute lung injury (TRALI). Blood tests revealed pancytopenia and increasing levels of ferritin (2600 mg/L) thought to be due to the combination of inflammation and azathioprine treatment. Three days later (day 13), the patient was transferred back to the ICU of the first hospital.

There, severe mononucleosis with persistent high EBV viremia despite antiviral treatment was diagnosed. The patient presented multiple episodes of upper GI bleeding that required further repeated transfusions. Upper endoscopy revealed hemorrhagic gastroduodenitis with multiple bleeding ulcers. Blood tests revealed a further increase of ferritin (up to 15,000 μg/L) and LDH (up to 4000 U/L) together with worsening pancytopenia and finally agranulocytosis. Repeated bone morrow biopsies finally revealed HLH with macrophage activation syndrome and hemophagocytosis. The patient was treated with high doses of steroids alone and exhibited transient improvement but eventually expired following multiple organ failure 12 days later. The biopsies from gastric, duodenal, and colonic tissues all revealed an EBV-associated lymphoid proliferation. The autopsy concluded to a generalized EBV infection with lymphoid proliferation of the entire digestive tube and multiple organs, with associated secondary macrophage activation syndrome.

3. Case 2

A 61-year-old male patient in good general health presented with an episode of significant lower GI bleeding. The patient had had a minor similar episode 4 months ago. One month ago, he had felt fatigue and repeated episodes of fever without any other specific symptoms.

Upon primary admission to another hospital, the patient was tachycardic and slightly hypotensive but improved after massive hydration and was transferred to our center. An upper endoscopy revealed only a small Mallory-Weiss type ulcer, which seemed unlikely to have been the source of bleeding. An angio-CT-scan of the abdomen revealed extensive diverticulosis with signs of transverse colitis but without a precise source of bleeding. The patient was treated conservatively but, in the following days, he developed fever and an important inflammatory syndrome (CRP 253 mg/L, normal leucocyte count) with rhabdomyolysis, acute renal failure, and high levels of LDH (1451 U/L) and ferritin (1200 mg/L) along with anemia and progressive thrombocytopenia. Three days after his admission, he once again became hemodynamically unstable due to recurrent massive low GI bleeding. From the time of patient's entry to that point, he had received a total of 10 units of RBC. Emergency laparotomy with intraoperative colonoscopy and enteroscopy was performed. Findings were an important inflammatory status around the transverse colon, a small intestinal perforation at the distal ileum, and 10–20 ulcerated inflammatory lesions in the ileum,

one of which was actively bleeding. A resection of 60 cm of ileum was carried out and the patient was admitted to the ICU for postoperative surveillance. Histopathology of the ileum revealed a high grade NK-T lymphoma Epstein Barr virus (EBV) positive.

Two days after surgery, the patient became septic. A thoracoabdominal CT-scan showed bilateral pleural effusions but no specific septic source. In the absence of radiological signs that would explain the patient's septic status, a "second look" laparotomy was performed but no source of sepsis was identified. Subsequently, the patient's condition deteriorated rapidly. He developed disseminated intravascular coagulation and finally a new episode of GI bleeding. Based on the above listed observations together with ferritin levels at 15000 mcg/L, HLH was suspected and a treatment with CHOP regimen (cyclophosphamide 750 mg/m^2 day 1, doxorubicin 50 mg/m^2/day 1, Oncovin 1.4 mg/m^2/day 1, and prednisone 60 mg/m^2/day 1 to 5) plus etoposide was initiated. No bone marrow biopsies were performed as death due to hemodynamic instability followed the next day. Autopsy revealed a NK-T extranasal EBV + lymphoma with intestinal localization. Bone marrow presented with massive hemophagocytosis without any evidence of tumor infiltration (see Figure 1).

4. Discussion

Hemophagocytic lymphohistiocytosis (HLH) or hemophagocytic syndrome represents a rare pathophysiologic entity characterized by a hyperinflammatory state, cytokine deregulation, impaired function of cytotoxic T-cells (CTL), and natural killer (NK) cells in addition to hemophagocytosis (i.e., phagocytosis by activated macrophages of red blood cells, leucocytes, platelets and their precursors in the blood marrow, spleen, or other lymphoid organs) [23, 24].

There is an inherited or familial form (FHLH) and an acquired or secondary HLH [25]. The FHLH incidence is estimated to be 0.12/100.000 children per year and has its onset under the age of 1 year in the majority (70%–80%) of patients [26]. Patients with inherited immune deficiencies like the Chediak-Higashi syndrome as well as the X-linked proliferative syndrome are also at high risk to develop HLH.

Secondary HLH may occur at all ages [24] and is usually diagnosed in association with malignant (mostly with cutaneous or anaplastic lymphomas), autoimmune, or infectious diseases. Infection associated with HLH is mostly associated with viral infections of the herpes group, in particular EBV and cytomegalovirus (CMV) [23, 25]. EBV induced HLH may mimic or favor T-cell lymphoma and other EBV-linked lymphoproliferative disorders [23]. Other nonviral agents such as bacteria, mycobacteria, protozoa, and fungi can more rarely trigger HLH [24]. Cases of HLH after immunization with measles vaccine, probably in predisposed patients, have also been documented [27].

The dominant clinical characteristics of HLH are persistent fever, usually unresponsive to antibiotics, splenomegaly and/or hepatomegaly, lymphadenopathies, icterus, rash, anorexia, and GI bleeding. Neurological symptoms, such as

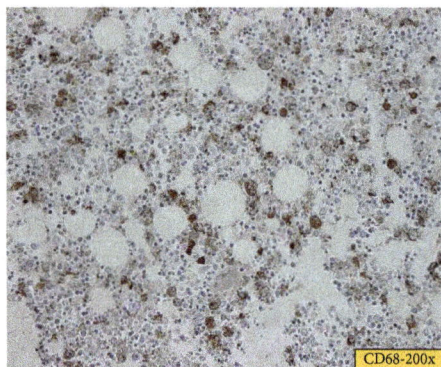

FIGURE 1: Hemophagocytosis in the bone marrow of Case 2.

seizures or cranial nerve palsies, are rare in the acquired form but are found in up to 1/3 of patients with FHLH [25, 28–30].

Laboratory findings include cytopenia, in at least two cell lineages, elevated hemolysis parameters, hypofibrinogenemia (and possibly disseminated intravascular coagulation), hypertriglyceridemia, and hyperferritinemia. Inflammatory markers like the C-reactive protein may be quite high due to the syndrome's inflammatory state. Special markers include increased soluble CD25 (alpha-chain of the interleukin (IL-2) receptor) reflecting increased T lymphocytes activation and turnover and profoundly decreased or absent NK cell activity [24, 29, 31]. The Th1/Th2 biomarker is another recently developed diagnostic tool [32].

Diagnosis in patients with clinical suspicion of HLH requires bone marrow aspiration and biopsy. Positive biopsies reveal normal maturation of all cell lineages, normal or increased cellularity, and infiltration with macrophages/histiocytes associated with hemophagocytosis [25]. However, hemophagocytosis is often initially absent, requiring a repeated exam [24]. Due to the insidious nature of HLH, diagnosis is difficult, needs to be based on a combination of clinical and biological criteria, and is frequently established after the patient's death [22, 25, 33].

Infections must be actively sought as they may be the trigger of the syndrome and represent a treatable cause. Patients should be tested for EBV, CMV, herpes simplex, and adenovirus [24]. Screening for less frequent infectious agents, inherited immune deficiencies, and underlying malignancies should be done according to clinical suspicion.

HLH, whether acquired or familial, is a severe condition and, if left untreated, can lead to rapid deterioration and death. There is no high level evidence to guide treatment; the most widely accepted strategy is aggressive systemic therapy with various combinations of immunosuppressive and chemotherapeutic agents, along with the treatment of the underlying causes, if identified. For the severe forms of the FHLH, hematopoietic stem cell transplantation is currently considered to be the only curative option [32]. FHLH therapies with antithymocyte globulin, steroids, cyclosporin A, and intrathecal methotrexate to pediatric patients have been reported with 73% rapid and complete response [30]. Due to the lack of studies in the adult population, patients

are usually treated with a regimen adapted from pediatric protocols [29]. For adult patients with HLH secondary to pathogens other than EBV, supportive care and treatment of the underlying infection are associated with recovery in 60%–70% [34]. EBV-associated HLH is almost universally fatal if untreated, with death resulting usually from multiorgan failure [31, 35].

The goal of this paper is to raise awareness among surgeons about the rare medical entity of HLH, which may present as a highly life threatening form of GI bleeding. In both cases presented in this paper, the surgeon was faced with a clinical picture of severe GI bleeding. These patients had presented a series of systemic clinical and laboratory findings compatible with HLH (fever unresponsive to antibiotics, splenomegaly, EBV infection, cytopenia, and high ferritin levels) earlier in the course of their illness, but diagnosis of HLH was not suspected until late. Surgical therapy for the GI bleeding was challenging in both cases as the bleeding source had not been localized precisely preoperatively. In the first patient, total colectomy was performed, but bleeding recurred, possibly from the documented coexisting gastroduodenal ulcerations. In the second patient, intraoperative colonoscopy and enteroscopy helped localize the source and guide the extent of the resection, but bleeding recurred as well. The role of surgery cannot be denied in the acute setting of life threatening GI bleeding. However, in these cases, earlier diagnosis and medical treatment of HLH might have prevented fatal recurrence.

The true incidence of GI bleeding in association with HLH is hard to estimate. Guo et al., in a retrospective analysis of 41 children with HLH, reported a rate of 12.2% [36]. In our review of the literature on HLH with associated GI bleeding, we found only a few other case reports (Table 1). Similar to our two cases, mortality was very high (12 deaths out of 18) and almost always secondary to uncontrollable GI bleeding. Of course, the severity of bleeding in this small review may be overrated due to selection and publication bias. The origin of bleeding can be localized throughout the GI tract. Our two patients bled form the colon, the small bowel, and the stomach. The bleeding source can be diffuse or from linear isolated ulcers. These gastrointestinal lesions are secondary to transmural lymphohistiocytic infiltration of macrophages as reported in histological findings [22], which in addition to bleeding may lead to perforation, as in one of our patients. Septic complications may be masked from the underlying hyperinflammatory state caused by HLH. Emergent surgery for intestinal resections or embolization was part of successful treatment in some reports [15, 20, 36]; in others, similar to our patients, it did not help control bleeding definitively [11, 19, 20, 22]. Administration of recombinant activated factor VII seemed to provide short temporary but no definitive control of bleeding in some reports [22, 37].

Hemophagocytic lymphohistiocytosis (HLH) is an elusive medical entity, difficult to diagnose. It may be present as life threatening GI bleeding and pose a challenging clinical problem to the surgeon. Associated cytopenia, high ferritin, and low fibrinogen levels, in combination with symptoms and signs such as fever, hepatosplenomegaly, skin rash, and lymphadenopathies, should raise suspicion early. Viral (EBV,

TABLE 1

Author	n	Age	Concomitant systemic disease	Predominant symptoms and signs	Treatment (surgical/medical)	Outcome
Kanaji et al. [10]	1	25	—	Fever, abdominal pain, and lower GI bleeding	Methylprednisolone (1000 mg/day for 3 consecutive days), g-globulin (0.5 g/day for 3 consecutive days), broad-spectrum antibiotics (PAPM 1 g/day), gabexate mesilate (2500 mg/day), ulinastatin (20×10^4 U/day), and citicoline (1 g/day).	Survived
Eguchi [11]	1	44	Lupus nephritis	Melena, colonic perforation, and peritonitis	CMV immunoglobulin, methyl-prednisolone (1 g/day for three days), prednisolone (60 mg/day), and ganciclovir (dose not specified). Colonoscopic clipping and embolisation of a bleeding sigmoid ulcer	Died
Bhagwati et al. [12]	1	55	—	Fever, abdominal pain, GI bleeding, and acute renal failure	Prednisolone (30 mg/day) and amphotericin and ganciclovir (doses not specified). Multiple transfusions	Died
Koketsu et al. [13]	1	35	—	Lower GI bleeding and fulminant "ulcerative colitis"	Methylprednisolone (1,000 mg/day for 3 consecutive days), subtotal colectomy, and ileostomy with rectal preservation	Survived
Nakase et al. [14]	2	68	—	Massive GI bleeding	https://www.jstage.jst.go.jp/browse/rinketsu/31/2/_contents?	Died
		80	—	Loss of consciousness and MOF	https://www.jstage.jst.go.jp/browse/rinketsu/31/2/_contents?	Died
Ina et al. [15]	1	76	—	Abdominal pain, massive GI bleeding, and jejunal ulcers	Jejunal resection (30 cm) after per operatory endoscopy	Survived
Yashima et al. [16]	1	63	Aplastic anemia	Massive GI bleeding and MOF	Methylprednisolone pulse therapy	Died
Wu et al. [17]	1	23	Hepatitis A and hepatitis C	Fever, jaundice, and massive GI bleeding	Bibliotheque	Died
Takai et al. [18]	1	20	—	Fever, hepatosplenomegaly, and massive GI bleeding	https://www.jstage.jst.go.jp/browse/rinketsu/31/2/_contents?	Died
Hayakawa et al. [19]	1	73	Polyarteritis nodosa	Massive GI bleeding	Methylprednisolone pulse therapy, intravenous immunoglobulin (5,000 mg for 3 days), and weekly intravenous VP-16 (200 mg/day). Embolisation of ileum artery branches	Died
N'Guyen et al. [20]	4	32.2 ± 3.7	Human cytomegalovirus infection present in all 4 patients	Fever, cytopenia, hyperferritinemia, hypertriglyceridemia, and GI bleeding; one patient with pericarditis and tamponade, one with colitis, and one with 2 necrotic gastric ulcers	Corticoids and antiviral therapy (ganciclovir and/or valganciclovir) + anti-TNF	Survived
					Corticoids and antiviral therapy (ganciclovir and/or valganciclovir) + anti-TNF	Survived
					Corticoids and antiviral therapy (ganciclovir and/or valganciclovir) + total colectomy	Survived
					Corticoids and antiviral therapy (ganciclovir and/or valganciclovir). Emergency surgery for 2 gastric ulcer perforations (operation not specified)	Died
Tunç and Ayata [21]	1	4	Visceral leishmaniasis	High fever, malaise, fatigue, massive GI bleeding, and opportunistic infections	Immunoglobulin (IVIG) (400 mg/kg for 5 days), antibiotics (ceftazidime (100 mg/kg/24 h) and amikacin sulfate (15 mg/kg/24 h)), AmBisome (3 mg/kg/day for 5 days), and methylprednisolone (30 mg/kg/day) for 3 consecutive days	Died
Celkan et al. [22]	2	1.5	—	Submandibular lymphadenopathy and hepatomegaly massive lower GI bleeding	Immunoglobulin (0.5 g/kg), steroids (10 mg/m^2), etoposide (150 mg/m^2), cyclosporine (6 mg/kg), and recombinant factor VIIa (rFVIIa) 90 μg/kg (total 4 mg). Resection of 12 cm of Ileum	Died
		4	—	Generalized edema and massive GI bleeding	Recombinant factor VIIa (rFVIIa) 90	Died

MOF: multiorgan failure.

CMV, and herpes simplex virus) and other (*Mycobacterium tuberculosis* and *Mycoplasma pneumonia*) infections should be looked for as they may represent treatable causes. Treatment requires a multidisciplinary approach and surgery may provide a temporary solution for GI bleeding or perforation, but early diagnosis and systemic therapy are the only hope for cure.

References

[1] C. M. Wilcox, B. L. Cryer, H. J. Henk et al., "Mortality associated with gastrointestinal bleeding events: comparing short-term clinical outcomes of patients hospitalized for upper GI bleeding and acute myocardial infarction in a US managed care setting," *Clinical and Experimental Gastroenterology*, vol. 2, pp. 21–30, 2009.

[2] G. F. Longstreth, "Epidemiology of hospitalization for acute upper gastrointestinal hemorrhage: a population-based study," *The American Journal of Gastroenterology*, vol. 90, no. 2, pp. 206–210, 1995.

[3] R. T. Yavorski, R. K. H. Wong, C. Maydonovitch, L. S. Battin, A. Furnia, and D. E. Amundson, "Analysis of 3,294 cases of upper gastrointestinal bleeding in military medical facilities," *The American Journal of Gastroenterology*, vol. 90, no. 4, pp. 568–573, 1995.

[4] D. R. Parker, X. Luo, J. J. Jalbert, and A. R. Assaf, "Impact of upper and lower gastrointestinal blood loss on healthcare utilization and costs: a systematic review," *Journal of Medical Economics*, vol. 14, no. 3, pp. 279–287, 2011.

[5] W. Browder, E. J. Cerise, and M. S. Litwin, "Impact of emergency angiography in massive lower gastrointestinal bleeding," *Annals of Surgery*, vol. 204, no. 5, pp. 530–536, 1986.

[6] I. M. Leitman, D. E. Paull, and G. T. Shires III, "Evaluation and management of massive lower gastrointestinal hemorrhage," *Annals of Surgery*, vol. 209, no. 2, pp. 175–180, 1989.

[7] J. Lee, T. W. Costantini, and R. Coimbra, "Acute lower GI bleeding for the acute care surgeon: current diagnosis and management," *Scandinavian Journal of Surgery*, vol. 98, no. 3, pp. 135–142, 2009.

[8] C. Gayer, A. Chino, C. Lucas et al., "Acute lower gastrointestinal bleeding in 1,112 patients admitted to an urban emergency medical center," *Surgery*, vol. 146, no. 4, pp. 600–607, 2009.

[9] A. M. Vernava III, W. E. Longo, K. S. Virgo, and F. E. Johnson, "A nationwide study of the incidence and etiology of lower gastrointestinal bleeding," *Surgical Research Communications*, vol. 18, no. 2, pp. 113–120, 1996.

[10] S. Kanaji, K. Okuma, Y. Tokumitsu, S. Yoshizawa, M. Nakamura, and Y. Niho, "Hemophagocytic syndrome associated with fulminant ulcerative colitis and presumed acute pancreatitis," *The American Journal of Gastroenterology*, vol. 93, no. 10, pp. 1956–1959, 1998.

[11] K. Eguchi, "Systemic lupus erythematosus complicated by cytomegalovirus-induced hemophagocytic syndrome and colitis," *Internal Medicine*, vol. 41, no. 2, pp. 77–78, 2002.

[12] N. S. Bhagwati, S. J. Oiseth, L. S. Abebe, and P. H. Wiernik, "Intravascular lymphoma associated with hemophagocytic syndrome: a rare but aggressive clinical entity," *Annals of Hematology*, vol. 83, no. 4, pp. 247–250, 2004.

[13] S.-I. Koketsu, T. Watanabe, N. Hori, N. Umetani, Y. Takazawa, and H. Nagawa, "Hemophagocytic syndrome caused by fulminant ulcerative colitis and cytomegalovirus infection: report of a case," *Diseases of the Colon & Rectum*, vol. 47, no. 7, pp. 1250–1253, 2004.

[14] T. Nakase, K. Morita, M. Tomeoku, and M. Katou, "Hemophagocytic syndrome in two elderly men," *Rinsho Ketsueki*, vol. 31, no. 2, pp. 258–259, 1990.

[15] S. Ina, M. Tani, K. Takifuji, S. Yamazoe, Y. Nakatani, and H. Yamaue, "Virus-associated hemophagocytic syndrome and hemorrhagic jejunal ulcer caused by cytomegalovirus infection in a non-compromised host; a case report of unusual entity," *Hepato-Gastroenterology*, vol. 51, no. 56, pp. 491–493, 2004.

[16] A. Yashima, Y. Narigasawa, Y. Ishida et al., "Hemophagocytic syndrome due to miliary tuberculosis in the course of aplastic anemia," *Rinsho Ketsueki*, vol. 39, no. 5, pp. 392–397, 1998.

[17] C.-S. Wu, K.-Y. Chang, P. Dunn, and T.-H. Lo, "Acute hepatitis A with coexistent hepatitis C virus infection presenting as a virus-associated hemophagocytic syndrome: a case report," *American Journal of Gastroenterology*, vol. 90, no. 6, pp. 1002–1005, 1995.

[18] K. Takai, M. Sanada, and H. Shibuya, "Epstein-Barr virus associated natural killer cell leukemia: report of an autopsy case," *Rinsho Ketsueki*, vol. 36, no. 5, pp. 500–505, 1995.

[19] I. Hayakawa, F. Shirasaki, H. Ikeda et al., "Reactive hemophagocytic syndrome in a patient with polyarteritis nodosa associated with Epstein-Barr virus reactivation," *Rheumatology International*, vol. 26, no. 6, pp. 573–576, 2006.

[20] Y. N'Guyen, S. Baumard, J. H. Salmon et al., "Cytomegalovirus associated hemophagocytic lymphohistiocytosis in patients suffering from crohn's disease treated by azathioprine: a series of four cases," *Inflammatory Bowel Diseases*, vol. 17, no. 9, pp. E116–E118, 2011.

[21] B. Tunç and A. Ayata, "Hemophagocytic syndrome: a rare life-threatening complication of visceral leishmaniasis in a young boy," *Pediatric Hematology and Oncology*, vol. 18, no. 8, pp. 531–536, 2001.

[22] T. Celkan, S. Alhaj, M. Civilibal, and M. Elicevik, "Control of bleeding associated with hemophagocytic syndrome in children: an audit of the clinical use of recombinant activated factor VII," *Pediatric Hematology and Oncology*, vol. 24, no. 2, pp. 117–121, 2007.

[23] D. N. Fisman, "Hemophagocytic syndromes and infection," *Emerging Infectious Diseases*, vol. 6, no. 6, pp. 601–608, 2000.

[24] G. E. Janka, "Hemophagocytic syndromes," *Blood Reviews*, vol. 21, no. 5, pp. 245–253, 2007.

[25] R. J. Arceci, "When T cells and macrophages do not talk: the hemophagocytic syndromes," *Current Opinion in Hematology*, vol. 15, no. 4, pp. 359–367, 2008.

[26] J.-I. Henter, G. Elinder, O. Soder, and A. Ost, "Incidence in Sweden and clinical features of familial hemophagocytic lymphohistiocytosis," *Acta Paediatrica*, vol. 80, no. 4, pp. 428–435, 1991.

[27] T. Otagiri, T. Mitsui, T. Kawakami et al., "Haemophagocytic lymphohistiocytosis following measles vaccination," *European Journal of Pediatrics*, vol. 161, no. 9, pp. 494–496, 2002.

[28] J. I. Henter, M. Aricò, G. Elinder, S. Imashuku, and G. Janka, "FHLH. Primary hemophagocytic lymphohistiocytosis," *Hematology/Oncology Clinics of North America*, vol. 12, no. 2, pp. 417–433, 1998.

[29] J.-I. Henter, A. Horne, M. Aricó et al., "HLH-2004: diagnostic and therapeutic guidelines for hemophagocytic lymphohistiocytosis," *Pediatric Blood and Cancer*, vol. 48, no. 2, pp. 124–131, 2007.

[30] N. Mahlaoui, M. Ouachée-Chardin, G. D. S. Basile et al., "Immunotherapy of familial hemophagocytic lymphohistiocytosis with antithymocyte globulins: a single-center retrospective report of 38 patients," *Pediatrics*, vol. 120, no. 3, pp. e622–e628, 2007.

[31] J. Chen, G. Li, J. Lu et al., "A novel type of PTD, common helix-loop-helix motif, could efficiently mediate protein transduction into mammalian cells," *Biochemical and Biophysical Research Communications*, vol. 347, no. 4, pp. 931–940, 2006.

[32] Y.-M. Tang and X.-J. Xu, "Advances in hemophagocytic lymphohistiocytosis: pathogenesis, early diagnosis/differential diagnosis, and treatment," *The Scientific World Journal*, vol. 11, pp. 697–708, 2011.

[33] G. E. Janka, "Familial and acquired hemophagocytic lymphohistiocytosis," *European Journal of Pediatrics*, vol. 166, no. 2, pp. 95–109, 2007.

[34] A. P. Reiner and J. L. Spivak, "Hematophagic histiocytosis. A report of 23 new patients and a review of the literature," *Medicine*, vol. 67, no. 6, pp. 369–388, 1988.

[35] C. Cerboni, A. Zingoni, M. Cippitelli, M. Piccoli, L. Frati, and A. Santoni, "Antigen-activated human T lymphocytes express cell-surface NKG2D ligands via an ATM/ATR-dependent mechanism and become susceptible to autologous NK-cell lysis," *Blood*, vol. 110, no. 2, pp. 606–615, 2007.

[36] X. Guo, Q. Li, and C.-Y. Zhou, "Retrospective analysis of 41 childhood hemophagocytic syndrome," *Zhonghua Xue Ye Xue Za Zhi*, vol. 28, no. 7, pp. 449–453, 2007.

[37] C. G. Millar, M. D. Stringer, I. Sugarman, and M. Richards, "The use of recombinant factor VIIa for bleeding in paediatric practice," *Haemophilia*, vol. 11, no. 2, pp. 171–174, 2005.

29

Multiple Bronchogenic and Gastroenteric Cysts Arising from the Stomach in a Patient with Abdominal Pain

Maykong Leepalao[1] and Jessica Wernberg[2]

[1]*Department of General Surgery, Marshfield Clinic, Marshfield, WI 54449, USA*
[2]*Department of Surgical Oncology, Marshfield Clinic, Marshfield, WI 54449, USA*

Correspondence should be addressed to Maykong Leepalao; leepalao.maykong@marshfieldclinic.org

Academic Editor: Francesco Petrella

Bronchogenic cysts arising from the stomach are uncommon. We discuss a young female patient with presumed enteric duplication cysts who was found to have three bronchogenic and gastroenteric cysts upon pathologic review. We discuss the pathophysiology of bronchogenic cysts and their malignant potential.

1. Introduction

Bronchogenic cysts arising from the stomach are a relatively rare entity. There have been reported cases of intra-abdominal bronchogenic cysts as early as fifty years ago with less than 25 published reports in the literature. This report highlights a rare case of three bronchogenic cysts arising in the gastric wall of an adult patient.

2. Background

A 29-year-old female who had experienced severe left upper quadrant pain during pregnancy presented to our clinic. During her pregnancy, she underwent imaging which demonstrated several large cystic structures felt to be arising from the stomach. These were presumed to be enteric duplication cysts. Due to the symptomatic nature, diagnostic insecurity, and concern over malignant potential of these cysts, resection was recommended.

She did not have any other pertinent medical history. She ran cross country in high school and was healthy. She had no other issues with her prior pregnancies. She was a nonsmoker.

On physical exam, she had palpable fullness in her left upper quadrant but was otherwise nondistended, soft, and nontender. Pertinent preoperative laboratory evaluation revealed no abnormal findings.

CT imaging showed three benign appearing well-demarcated thin-walled simple cystic masses in the left upper abdomen all having a mass effect on the stomach. The cysts measured 9.2 × 6.6 cm, 1.8 × 1.7 cm, and 3.0 × 2.8 cm and were located along the posterior aspect of the upper stomach, anterolateral upper abdomen, and greater curvature of the stomach, respectively (Figures 1 and 2). There had been a slight interval growth from a CT one year earlier.

Patient proceeded to the operating room where she underwent wedge resection via an upper midline incision of all three cysts with no complications. Intraoperatively, the cysts did not communicate with the gastric lumen but arose from the gastric wall. They were all soft and filled with crystalline, particulate-laden fluid.

Pathology demonstrated benign developmental, thin-walled cysts with a smooth muscle wall. These were lined by respiratory ciliated and mucinous glandular epithelium resembling the epithelium of the stomach and respiratory system consistent with bronchogenic and combined bronchogenic/gastroenteric cysts (Figures 3–5).

Given the pathology, a CT chest was completed and showed left lower lobe partial bronchial agenesis. There were no pulmonary cystic lesions. The patient, however, remained asymptomatic with no signs of respiratory difficulty or hypoxia and no further workup was done.

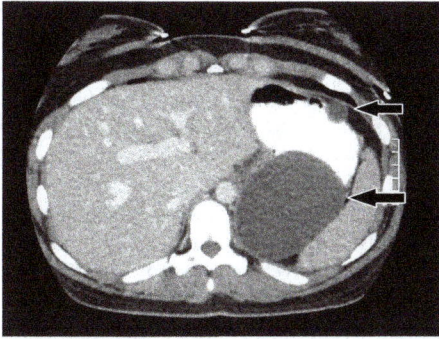

FIGURE 1: Computed tomography of intra-abdominal cysts. Arrows point to multiple cysts arising from the stomach wall (axial).

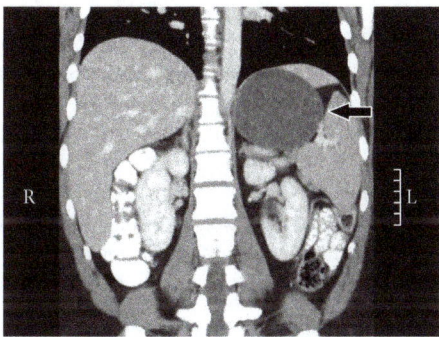

FIGURE 2: Computed tomography of intra-abdominal cysts. Arrow points to bronchogenic cyst arising from the stomach wall (coronal).

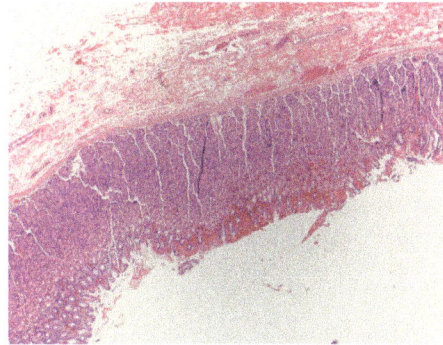

FIGURE 3: Histological H&E stain. Cystic lesion from greater curvature of stomach showing benign developmental cyst with smooth muscle wall and lined by respiratory ciliated epithelium. 40x magnification.

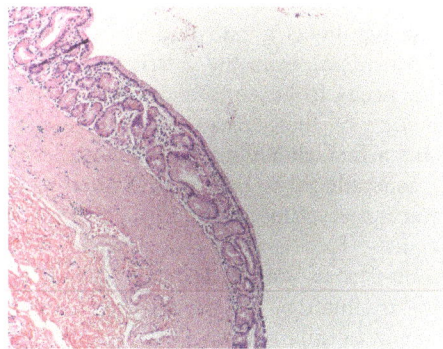

FIGURE 4: Histological H&E stain. Cystic lesion near the greater curvature of the stomach demonstrating benign developmental cyst lined by mucinous glandular epithelium resembling the epithelium of the stomach and respiratory epithelium. 100x magnification.

3. Discussion

There is a paucity of reported cases of intra-abdominal bronchogenic cysts. Our case outlines a unique case of three symptomatic bronchogenic or mixed bronchogenic/enteric gastric cysts. Gensler et al. reported the first case of an intramural gastric cyst in 1966 that was composed of ciliated pseudostratified columnar epithelium with focal squamous metaplasia. Since then, review of the literature reveals less than thirty case reports of single bronchogenic cysts located in the gastric mucosa [1–3].

Bronchogenic cysts typically arise from the foregut during embryological development in the 3rd to 7th week of life [4–10]. Esophageal epithelium undergoes a transient stage of cilia formation during the tenth week of gestation [5, 11] before differentiating into the usual squamous epithelium. This could potentially explain the pathophysiological mechanism for the presence of respiratory epithelium in the proximal gastrointestinal tract [5]. Congenital bronchogenic anomalies are more commonly found in the mediastinum, typically esophagus, or retroperitoneal space [12–16]. Bronchogenic cysts have also been reported to have been found on the skin [17] and diaphragm [18–23] and within the pericardium [24].

Patients have been reported to present with symptoms ranging from reflux to abdominal pain with some having no symptoms at all [6, 25]. Treatment has ranged from observation to aspiration to resection [4, 21, 26]. Patients have

reported recurrence of cysts after aspiration [17]. Regardless, the majority of patients appeared to have undergone resection. The reported patient experienced abdominal pain during pregnancy with resolution after delivery, possibly due to mass effect. A hormonal component could not be excluded.

There have been a few published case reports of bronchogenic cysts involved with adenocarcinoma [26], bronchioloalveolar carcinoma, neuroblastoma [27], and rhabdomyosarcoma; however, there is minimal data in the literature to suggest oncologic potential for bronchogenic cysts [28, 29]. Most bronchogenic cysts are found incidentally and resected at the time. Vazquez et al. describe a case of a bronchogenic cyst that was found at the same time as a neuroblastoma in a pediatric patient. These were resected at separate procedures. They discuss the genetic basis for this association with speculations on oncogene mutations [27]. Sullivan et al. reported a case of adenocarcinoma arising from a retroperitoneal bronchogenic cyst. In that case, ciliated columnar epithelium was not present. Furthermore, some studies have suggested that loss of epithelial lining is associated with malignancy [26]. Our case study did have ciliated respiratory epithelium with no evidence of malignancy. However, the association between malignancy and bronchogenic cysts remains unclear.

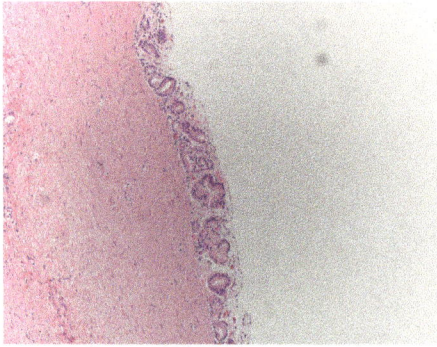

FIGURE 5: Histological H&E stain. Cystic lesion from the gastric cardia showing benign developmental cyst lined by mucinous columnar and respiratory epithelium with smooth muscle in the cyst wall. 100x magnification.

This case highlights a rare finding of multiple bronchogenic cysts arising from the gastric wall. Clearly, more investigation needs to be done to further understand the pathophysiology of these congenital bronchogenic cysts. Symptomatic or incidentally discovered cystic lesions in the foregut are generally felt to be benign. Symptomatic lesions probably warrant resection, especially if there is any diagnostic insecurity. There are occasional reports of bleeding, ulceration, or obstruction [5, 24, 30–34], and, depending on the clinical situation, resection rather than continued observation may be appropriate.

References

[1] H. Ubukata, T. Satani, G. Motohashi et al., "Intra-abdominal bronchogenic cyst with gastric attachment: report of a case," *Surgery Today*, vol. 41, no. 8, pp. 1095–1100, 2011.

[2] C. A. Rubio, A. Orrego, and R. Willén, "Bronchogenic gastric cyst. A case report," *In Vivo*, vol. 19, no. 2, pp. 383–385, 2005.

[3] S. Gensler, B. Seidenberg, H. Rifkin, and B. M. Rubinstein, "Ciliated lined intramural cyst of the stomach: case report and suggested embryogenesis," *Annals of Surgery*, vol. 163, no. 6, pp. 954–956, 1966.

[4] L. Jiang, L. Jiang, N. Cheng, and L. Yan, "Bronchogenic cyst of the gastric fundus in a young woman," *Digestive and Liver Disease*, vol. 42, no. 11, p. 826, 2010.

[5] M. K. Liang and J. L. Marks, "Congenital bronchogenic cyst in the gastric mucosa," *Journal of Clinical Pathology*, vol. 58, article 1344, 2005.

[6] J. Matsubayashi, T. Ishida, T. Ozawa, T. Aoki, Y. Koyanagi, and K. Mukai, "Subphrenic bronchopulmonary foregut malformation with pulmonary-sequestration-like features," *Pathology International*, vol. 53, no. 5, pp. 313–316, 2003.

[7] E. Vlodavsky, B. Czernobilsky, Y. Bar, and B. Lifschitz-Mercer, "Gastric mucosa in a bronchogenic cutaneous cyst in a child: case report and review of literature," *The American Journal of Dermatopathology*, vol. 27, no. 2, pp. 145–147, 2005.

[8] X. Yang and K. Guo, "Bronchogenic cyst of stomach: two cases report and review of the English literature," *Wiener Klinische Wochenschrift*, vol. 125, no. 9-10, pp. 283–287, 2013.

[9] H. Shibahara, T. Arai, S. Yokoi, and S. Hayakawa, "Bronchogenic cyst of the stomach involved with gastric adenocarcinoma," *Clinical Journal of Gastroenterology*, vol. 2, no. 2, pp. 80–84, 2009.

[10] C. Endo, T. Imai, H. Nakagawa, A. Ebina, and M. Kaimori, "Bronchioloalveolar carcinoma arising in a bronchogenic cyst," *Annals of Thoracic Surgery*, vol. 69, no. 3, pp. 933–935, 2000.

[11] H. F. Krous and C. L. Sexauer, "Embryonal rhabdomyosarcoma arising within a congenital bronchogenic cyst in a child," *Journal of Pediatric Surgery*, vol. 16, no. 4, pp. 506–508, 1981.

[12] J. J. Murphy, G. K. Blair, G. C. Fraser et al., "Rhabdomyosarcoma arising within congenital pulmonary cysts: report of three cases," *Journal of Pediatric Surgery*, vol. 27, no. 10, pp. 1364–1367, 1992.

[13] S. M. Sullivan, S. Okada, M. Kudo, and Y. Ebihara, "A retroperitoneal bronchogenic cyst with malignant change," *Pathology International*, vol. 49, no. 4, pp. 338–341, 1999.

[14] R. Castro, M. I. Oliveira, T. Fernandes, and A. J. Madureira, "Retroperitoneal bronchogenic cyst: MRI findings," *Case Reports in Radiology*, vol. 2013, Article ID 853795, 3 pages, 2013.

[15] G. F. Orellana, R. Cárdenas, M. E. Manríquez, H. Ríos, L. Suárez, and D. Videla, "Retroperitoneal bronchogenic cyst: report of one case," *Revista Medica de Chile*, vol. 135, no. 7, pp. 924–931, 2007.

[16] K. H. Kim, J. I. Kim, C. H. Ahn et al., "The first case of intraperitoneal bronchogenic cyst in Korea mimicking a gallbladder tumor," *Journal of Korean Medical Science*, vol. 19, no. 3, pp. 470–473, 2004.

[17] S. Msika, R. Kianmanesh, P. Jouet et al., "Bronchogenic cyst of the right hemidiaphragm mimicking a hydatid cyst of the liver," *Gastroenterologie Clinique et Biologique*, vol. 24, no. 12, pp. 1224–1226, 2000.

[18] H. Cerwenka, M. Uggowitzer, H. Bacher, G. Werkgartner, A. El-Shabrawi, and H. J. Mischinger, "Bronchogenic cyst appearing as a hepatic mass," *Abdominal Imaging*, vol. 25, no. 1, pp. 86–88, 2000.

[19] J. Mouroux, A. Bourgeon, D. Benchimal et al., "Bronchogenic cysts of the esophagus. Classical surgery or video-surgery?" *Chirurgie Paris*, vol. 117, no. 7, pp. 564–568, 1991.

[20] Y. Katayama, H. Kusagawa, T. Komada, S. Shomura, and H. Tenpaku, "Bronchopulmonary foregut malformation," *General Thoracic and Cardiovascular Surgery*, vol. 59, no. 11, pp. 767–770, 2011.

[21] K. Inaba, Y. Sakurai, Y. Umeki, S. Kanaya, Y. Komori, and I. Uyama, "Laparoscopic excision of subdiaphragmatic bronchogenic cyst occurring in the retroperitoneum: report of a case," *Surgical Laparoscopy, Endoscopy and Percutaneous Techniques*, vol. 20, no. 6, pp. e199–e203, 2010.

[22] M. Sato, A. Irisawa, M. S. Bhutani et al., "Gastric bronchogenic cyst diagnosed by endosonographically guided fine needle aspiration biopsy," *Journal of Clinical Ultrasound*, vol. 36, no. 4, pp. 237–239, 2008.

[23] D. A. Hall, R. T. Pu, and Y. Pang, "Diagnosis of foregut and tailgut cysts by endosonographically guided fine-needle aspiration," *Diagnostic Cytopathology*, vol. 35, no. 1, pp. 43–46, 2007.

[24] N. Melo, M. B. Pitman, and D. W. Rattner, "Bronchogenic cyst of the gastric fundus presenting as a gastrointestinal stromal

tumor," *Journal of Laparoendoscopic & Advanced Surgical Techniques, Part A*, vol. 15, no. 2, pp. 163–165, 2005.

[25] S. Y. Song, J. H. Non, S. J. Lee, and H. J. Son, "Bronchogenic cyst of the stomach masquerading as benign stromal tumor," *Pathology International*, vol. 55, no. 2, pp. 87–91, 2005.

[26] B. N. Vazquez, J. Mira, C. Navarro et al., "Neuroblastoma and bronchogenic cyst: a rare association," *European Journal of Pediatric Surgery*, vol. 10, no. 5, pp. 340–342, 2000.

[27] K. K. Nobuhara, Y. C. Gorski, M. P. La Quaglia, and R. C. Shamberger, "Bronchogenic cysts and esophageal duplications: common origins and treatment," *Journal of Pediatric Surgery*, vol. 32, no. 10, pp. 1408–1413, 1997.

[28] M. J. Haddon and A. Bowen, "Bronchopulmonary and neurenteric forms of foregut anomalies. Imaging for diagnosis and management," *Radiologic Clinics of North America*, vol. 29, no. 2, pp. 241–254, 1991.

[29] K. Ohno, T. Miyamoto, H. Murata, K. Kaku, S. Maeda, and K. Yamashita, "Intrapericardial bronchogenic cyst—a report of two surgical cases," *Nihon Kyobu Geka Gakkai Zasshi*, vol. 38, no. 4, pp. 660–666, 1990.

[30] B. Braffman, R. Keller, E. S. Gendal, and S. I. Finkel, "Subdiaphragmatic bronchogenic cyst with gastric communication," *Gastrointestinal Radiology*, vol. 13, no. 4, pp. 309–311, 1988.

[31] M. E. Keohane, I. Schwartz, J. Freed, and R. Dische, "Subdiaphragmatic bronchogenic cyst with communication to the stomach: a case report," *Human Pathology*, vol. 19, no. 7, pp. 868–871, 1988.

[32] E. Anagnostou, V. Soubasi, E. Agakidou, C. Papakonstantinou, N. Antonitsis, and M. Leontsini, "Mediastinal gastroenteric cyst in a neonate containing respiratory-type epithelium and pancreatic tissue," *Pediatric Pulmonology*, vol. 44, no. 12, pp. 1240–1243, 2009.

[33] D. C. Salyer, W. R. Salyer, and J. C. Eggleston, "Benign developmental cysts of the mediastinum," *Archives of Pathology and Laboratory Medicine*, vol. 101, no. 3, pp. 136–139, 1977.

[34] H. Linder, "Intrathoracic gastroenteric cysts," *Surgery*, vol. 25, no. 6, pp. 862–868, 1949.

30

Jejunogastric Intussusception: A Rare Complication of Gastric Surgery

Gokhan Cipe, Fatma Umit Malya, Mustafa Hasbahceci, Yeliz Emine Ersoy, Oguzhan Karatepe, and Mahmut Muslumanoglu

Bezmialem Vakıf University, Department of General Surgery, 34093 Istanbul, Turkey

Correspondence should be addressed to Fatma Umit Malya; fumitm@gmail.com

Academic Editors: N. Nissen and Y. Takami

Jejunogastric intussusception is a rare complication of gastric surgery. It usually presents with severe epigastric pain, vomiting, and hematemesis. A history of gastric surgery can help in making an accurate and early diagnosis which calls forth an urgent surgical intervention. Only reduction or resection with revision of the previously performed anastomosis is the choice which is decided according to the operative findings. We present a case of JGI in a patient with a history of Billroth II operation diagnosed by computed tomography. At emergent laparotomy, an efferent loop type JGI was found. Due to necrosis, resection of the intussuscepted bowel with Roux-en-Y anastomosis was performed. Postoperative recovery was uneventful.

1. Introduction

Jejunogastric intussusception (JGI) is a rare complication of gastrectomy with an incidence of 0.1% [1]. It is thought that it can occur any time after several types of the gastric operations including gastrojejunostomy and Billroth II resection [2–4]. A mortality rate of 10% and even as high as of 50% has been reported if surgical intervention has been delayed [5, 6], therefore, early diagnosis of this condition is mandatory. Although a history of gastric surgery may help in making such a diagnosis, preoperative awareness of this condition has been reported to be difficult in most of the cases.

In this paper, we aim to report a case of JGI with regard to its presentation, diagnosis, and surgical treatment.

2. Case Report

A 63-year-old male patient was admitted to the hospital with severe colicky epigastric pain followed by hematemesis. There was a past history of gastric surgery (Billroth II operation), which had been performed 23 years previously for peptic ulcer disease. On physical examination, there was a mildly distended abdomen, epigastric tenderness, and a vague feeling of an epigastric mass on deep palpation.

The usual laboratory investigation was unremarkable. A computed tomography showed a distended stomach containing a nonhomogeneous mass (Figure 1). The diagnosis of JGI was established, and an emergent laparotomy was performed. At laparotomy, an ischemic efferent loop was found to be intussuscepted in a retrograde manner into the gastric lumen (Figures 2 and 3). Following reduction of this jejunal segment, resection with Roux-en-Y anastomosis was performed due to ongoing necrosis (Figure 4). The patient was discharged at the fifth postoperative day without any complaint.

3. Discussion

The term retrograde intussusception (invagination) was first introduced by John Hunter to define an invagination of the intussusceptum in an antiperistaltic or proximal direction as opposed to the usual peristaltic or distal direction [7]. Intussusception is an uncommon condition that may arise at any age. It is usually seen in childhood, and only 5% of cases occur in adults [8]. Jejunogastric intussusception is a rare complication of gastrojejunostomy, Billroth II gastrectomy, and Roux-en-Y anastomosis. There were less than 200 published cases since its first description in 1914 by Bozzi in a patient with gastrojejunostomy [3]. In 1922, Lundberg

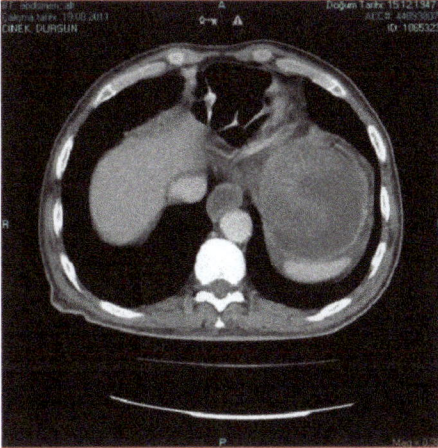

FIGURE 1: Emergency CT scan of the abdomen. Dilated stomach with intragastric nonhomogeneous mass compatible with bowel loops.

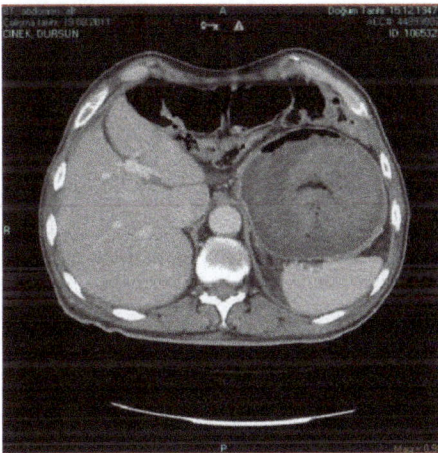

FIGURE 2: Emergency CT scan of the abdomen. Another section showing a dilated stomach with intragastric nonhomogeneous mass compatible with bowel loops.

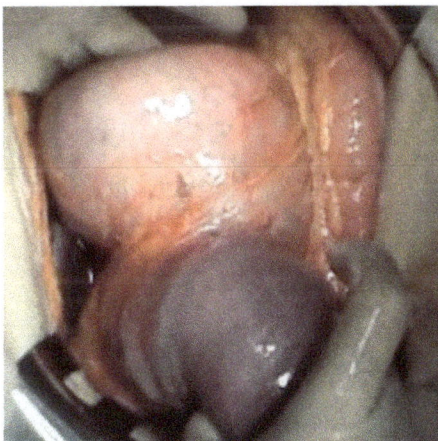

FIGURE 3: Invagination of the efferent loop to the stomach.

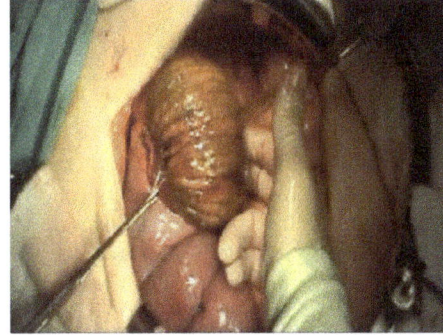

FIGURE 4: Another view of invagination of the efferent loop to the stomach.

reported a case of JGI in a patient with a history of Billroth II resection [4]. According to the type of intussuscepted loop, JGI is classified into three types: type I, antegrade or afferent loop intussusception; type II, retrograde or efferent loop intussusception; and type III, combined form [5]. Efferent loop JGI is seen in 80% of the cases as in the present case, while others account for the remaining 20% [5]. The exact mechanism of JGI is still not well understood. Long afferent loop, jejunal spasm with abnormal motility, increased mobility of the efferent loop, and adhesions leading to the intussusception of a more mobile segment into a fixed segment may be the underlying causes [1]. It is also postulated that increased intra-abdominal pressure, a dilated atonic stomach especially after vagotomy, and retrograde peristalsis may be responsible for the development of JGI [1].

Two different forms of JGI have been described according to its clinical presentation [9]. In the acute form, incarceration and strangulation of the intussuscepted loop causing acute severe epigastric pain, vomiting, and subsequently, hematemesis generally occur. However, spontaneous reduction is usual in the chronic type. A palpable abdominal mass can be observed in almost half of the cases [1, 10]. It should be kept in mind that a sudden onset of epigastric pain, vomiting and subsequent hematemesis, and a palpable epigastric mass in a patient with a previous gastric surgery can be important diagnostic clues for JGI [1]. Therefore, carefully taken history with good physical examination helps to suspect this rare condition in a gastrectomized patient as in this case.

Early diagnosis of the acute form is of paramount importance. The first specific diagnostic study should be an emergent endoscopy which is carried out by endoscopists aware of JGI and its endoscopic picture. Computed tomography allows the differentiation of the distinct stages of the disease. It shows a dilated stomach with intragastric filling by the bowel loops. In spite of the endoscopic and imaging findings, most reported cases of JGI were diagnosed at surgery [9].

Surgical options include only reduction or resection of the compromised bowel with revision of the anastomosis depending on the conditions found during the operation [6]. It could not be possible to prevent necrosis in the intussuscepted jejunal bowel despite early diagnosis and immediate surgical intervention. Therefore, resection with revision of the previous anastomosis can be the most appropriate surgical method in a patient with acute JGI.

4. Conclusions

JGI is a rare life-threatening complication of gastric surgery which is often diagnosed at surgery. Although endoscopy and computed tomography may be helpful during preoperative evaluation, laparotomy is usually required for the correct diagnosis. Early surgical intervention is the most important factor for prevention of morbidity and mortality.

References

[1] J. O. Waits, R. W. Beart Jr., and J. W. Charboneau, "Jejunogastric intussusception," *Archives of Surgery*, vol. 115, no. 12, pp. 1449–1452, 1980.

[2] E. F. Conklin and A. M. Markowitz, "Intussusception, a complication of gastric surgery," *Surgery*, vol. 57, no. 3, pp. 480–488, 1965.

[3] E. Bozzi, "Annotation," *Bulletin of Academy of Medicine*, vol. 122, pp. 3–4, 1914.

[4] S. Lundberg, "Retrograde Dunndarminvagination nach Gastroenterostomie," *Acta Chirurgica Scandinavica*, vol. 54, pp. 423–433, 1922.

[5] R. Shackman, "Jejunogastric intussusception," *British Journal of Surgery*, vol. 27, pp. 475–480, 1940.

[6] W. L. Sibley, "Chronic intermittent intussusception through the stoma of a previous gastro-enterostomy," *Proceedings of the Staff Meetings. Mayo Clinic*, vol. 9, pp. 364–365, 1934.

[7] L. B. Mason, "Retrograde jejunogastric intussusception following gastrectomy," *Archives of Surgery*, vol. 81, pp. 485–491, 1960.

[8] L. C. Dawes, R. Hunt, J. K. Wong, and S. Begg, "Multiplanar reconstruction in adult intussusception: case report and literature review," *Australasian Radiology*, vol. 48, no. 1, pp. 74–76, 2004.

[9] H. Tokue and Y. Tsushima, "Jejunogastric intussusception: life-threatening complication occuring 55 years after gastrojejunostomy," *Internal Medicine*, vol. 48, no. 18, pp. 1657–1660, 2009.

[10] D. G. Foster, "Retrograde jejunogastric intussusception-a rare cause of hematemesis," *AMA Archives of Surgery*, vol. 73, pp. 1009–1017, 1956.

31

Gastric Duplication Cyst: Two Case Reports and Review of the Literature

Jai P. Singh, Heena Rajdeo, Kalyani Bhuta, and John A. Savino

Department of Surgery, Westchester Medical Center, New York Medical College, Valhalla, NY 10595, USA

Correspondence should be addressed to Jai P. Singh; drjp04@gmail.com

Academic Editors: G. Santori and E. Xenos

Background. Duplication of the alimentary tract is a rare congenital anomaly. Gastric duplication cysts (GDCs) represent 4% of all alimentary tract duplications, and approximately 67% manifest within the first year of life. Duplication cysts in adults are generally encountered as incidental findings at endoscopy or laparotomy. Herein, we report two rare cases of symptomatic GDC presenting in adults. *Case 1.* A 27-year-old male presented with a five-month history of back pain. Exam revealed mild epigastric tenderness with a vague palpable mass in left upper abdomen. CT scan showed $8 \times 7.4 \times 6$ cm homogenous, nonseptated cystic mass posterosuperior to pancreatic tail. On laparotomy, a cystic mass measuring 11×8 cm was found, which was densely adherent to posterior wall of stomach suggestive of GDC. *Case 2.* A 28-year-old woman presented with epigastric pain associated with vomiting for 2 months. Exam revealed mild epigastric tenderness. CT scan showed four cystic lesions in the medial wall of distal stomach measuring approximately one cm each suggestive of duplication cysts. Exploratory laparotomy with antrectomy and truncal vagotomy with Billroth II reconstruction were performed. Pathology in both patients was diagnostic of GDC. *Conclusion.* GDC is a rare anomaly, and its presentation in adults is even rarer.

1. Introduction

Duplication of the alimentary tract is a relatively rare congenital anomaly. It can affect any part of the gastrointestinal tract with ileum being the most common site [1, 2]. These malformations are believed to be congenital, formed before the differentiation of epithelial lining, and therefore named for the organ with which they are associated [3]. Duplication cysts of the stomach represent four per cent of all alimentary tract duplications. Approximately 67 per cent of gastric duplication cysts (GDCs) are identified within the first year of life [4]. Duplication cysts in adults are generally asymptomatic and encountered as incidental findings at endoscopy or laparotomy [4]. Herein, we report two rare cases of symptomatic duplication cysts of stomach presenting in adults.

2. Case Reports

2.1. Case 1. A 27-year-old male presented with a five-month history of progressively increasing back pain associated with mild epigastric discomfort and loss of appetite. Review of systems revealed weight loss of approximately 25 pounds with occasional nausea. He denied vomiting and alteration of bowel habits. Family history was significant for the fact that his mother had been previously treated for benign cystic neoplasm of pancreas. Past medical history was not significant. Physical examination revealed mild epigastric tenderness with a vague palpable mass in the epigastric and left subcostal regions measuring approximately 7×5 cm.

MRI and CT scans of the abdomen demonstrated $8 \times 7.4 \times 6$ cm homogenous, nonseptated cystic mass posterosuperior to pancreatic tail (Figure 1). Left adrenal gland was not clearly identified. Pancreatic and biliary ducts were not dilated, and there was no evidence of any other mass or lymphadenopathy.

Since it was not clear whether the mass was arising from adrenal or pancreas, a complete adrenal workup was done including 24-hour urinary cortisol, urinary VMA, metanephrine level, serum aldosterone, and renin, which did not reveal any evidence of functional adrenal tumor.

On exploratory laparotomy pancreas and left adrenal appeared normal; however there was a soft cystic mass measuring approximately 11×8 cm, which was densely adherent to posterior wall of stomach close to the greater curvature.

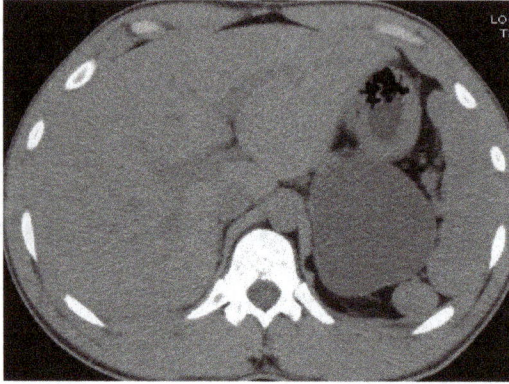

FIGURE 1: CT scan showing 8 × 7.4 × 6 cm homogenous, nonseptated cystic mass posterosuperior to pancreatic tail.

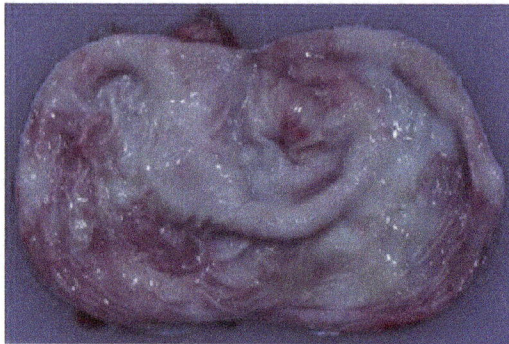

FIGURE 2: Inner surface of specimen was smooth and white-pink in color with a 1.5 × 1.2 cm rough area.

Excision of cystic mass along with resection of adjoining stomach was performed for a presumed gastric duplication cyst.

Surgical specimen measured 10 × 7 cm. Cut surface of specimen revealed a light yellowish gelatinous material. The inner surface was smooth and white-pink in color with 1.5 × 1.2 cm rough area (Figure 2). There was no communication between cyst and resected gastric segment.

Patient's postoperative course was uneventful. He was discharged on postoperative day 4 and has been asymptomatic since then.

On microscopy, cyst wall was composed of mucosa, submucosa, and muscularis propria with myenteric plexus. The mucosa was predominantly gastric body type consisting of parietal, chief, and mucus cells with patchy intervening areas of simple columnar epithelium containing apical mucus and cilia seen in embryonic intestinal epithelium (Figure 3).

2.2. Case 2. A 28-year-old woman was transferred from community hospital for evaluation of recurrent, nonradiating epigastric pain associated with nausea and occasional nonbilious vomiting for two months. She denied any change in bowel habits and weight loss. Her medical history was significant for lumbar herniated disc and recurrent shoulder

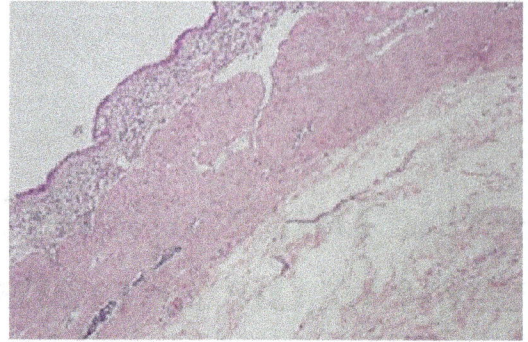

FIGURE 3: Photomicrograph: cyst wall was composed of mucosa, submucosa, and muscularis propria. The mucosa was predominantly a gastric body type with patchy intervening areas of simple columnar epithelium containing apical mucus and cilia seen in embryonic intestinal epithelium.

dislocation. Physical exam was unremarkable except for mild epigastric tenderness.

Diagnostic work up included abdominal CT scan, which demonstrated four cystic lesions in the medial wall of distal antrum and pylorus measuring approximately one cm each, suggestive of duplication cysts (Figure 4).

Upper GI endoscopy showed bulging of the gastric antrum and pylorus by an external compression without any mucosal abnormality. Endoscopic ultrasound showed multiple intramural cystic lesions measuring 3.5 × 2.5 cm in total dimension. The cysts appeared to be lined by mucosal layer with surrounding muscularis propria suggestive of duplication cysts. Fine needle aspiration was attempted but failed.

An exploratory laparotomy with antrectomy and truncal vagotomy with billroth II reconstruction were performed.

Patient's postoperative course was uneventful. She was discharged on postoperative day 10 and has been asymptomatic since then.

Cut surface of specimen revealed two cysts filled with clear mucinous fluid measuring 2 cm and 1.3 cm in the greatest dimension. The inner surface of cysts was lined by pink-tan epithelium, and wall thickness was approximately 0.6 cm. There was no communication between the cysts and gastric segment. On microscopy, cyst wall was composed of mucosa, submucosa, and muscularis propria. Mucosa was predominantly of gastric type with small islands of pancreatic acini (Figure 5).

3. Discussion

Gastrointestinal duplication is a relatively rare anomaly that may occur at any level from oral cavity to rectum with ileum being the most common site. Duplication cysts of the stomach are quite rare, and most of them have been reported in children [1, 5, 6]. Duplication cysts of ileum are usually located on mesenteric border [7], whereas the usual location for gastric duplication cysts is along the greater curvature

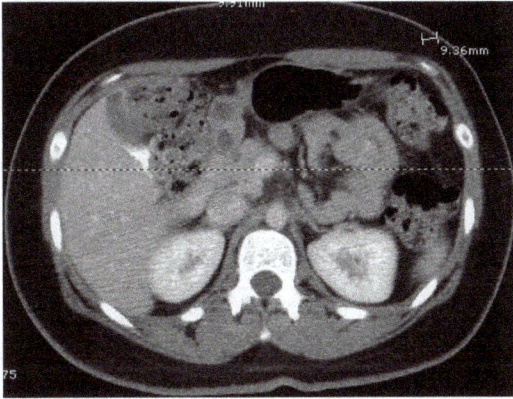

FIGURE 4: CT scan demonstrated four cystic lesions in the medial wall of distal antrum and pylorus measuring approximately one cm each, suggestive of duplication cysts.

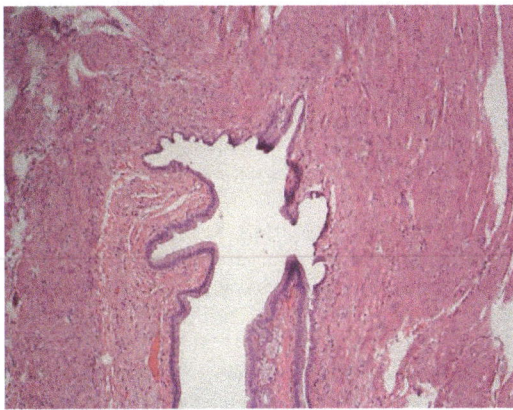

FIGURE 5: Photomicrograph: cyst wall was composed of mucosa, submucosa, and muscularis propria. Mucosa was predominantly of gastric type with small islands of pancreatic acini.

[4, 6, 7]. The duplication cyst is entirely separated from the adjacent bowel but shares a common wall [8].

The essential criteria for diagnosis of a gastric duplication cyst are (a) the wall of the cyst is contiguous with the stomach wall; (b) the cyst is surrounded by smooth muscle, which is continuous with the muscle of the stomach; and (c) the cyst wall is lined by epithelium of gastric or any other type of gut mucosa [1, 4, 9].

Our present cases fulfilled these criteria excluding other diagnoses.

Gastric duplication cysts comprise 4% of all gastrointestinal duplications. Various other congenital anomalies such as alimentary tract duplications, esophageal diverticulum, or spinal cord abnormalities are encountered in up to 50% patients [8].

These malformations are believed to be congenital, formed before the differentiation of epithelial lining, and therefore named for the organ with which they are associated [3, 10]. Duplications result from the disturbances in embryonic development, and various theories have been proposed for the actual mechanism. Bremer proposed the

theory of errors of recanalization and fusion of longitudinal folds. He suggested that duplication cysts originated from the fusion of longitudinal folds allowing the passage of a bridge of submucosa and muscle at the second and third month of intrauterine life [5]. McLetchie suggested that adhesion of notochord and embryonic endoderm might not elongate as quickly as its surrounding structures, causing traction diverticulum leading to duplication cyst formation [5]. Other theories of enteric duplication include abortive twinning, persistent embryological diverticula, and hypoxic or traumatic events [5]. There is no single theory that is satisfactory for all types of duplications [5].

Greater than 80% of gastric duplications are cystic and do not communicate with lumen of the stomach. The remainders are tubular with some communication [5]. The structure is defined as tubular when the lumen is contiguous and cystic when the lumen is not contiguous with stomach lumen [6]. The mucosal lining of duplication may be histologically similar to the segment of gut to which it is topographically related. However, some duplications may include lining from other segment of alimentary or respiratory tract. The presence of respiratory epithelium in the cysts of thorax, tongue, liver, and stomach suggests that the undifferentiated epithelium of foregut might undergo transition to differentiated specialized epithelium during embryonic period [5].

Gastric duplications typically become symptomatic during childhood. 67% are diagnosed within the first year of life, and less than 25% are discovered after age 12 [4]. The duplication cysts of the stomach are usually diagnosed intraoperatively in adults [10]. In our first patient, the preoperative CT and MRI findings were interpreted as being most consistent with a pancreatic neoplasm, and diagnosis of GDC was suspected only during surgery.

The clinical presentation of gastric duplication cysts can be highly variable and nonspecific ranging from vague abdominal pain to nausea, vomiting, epigastric fullness, weight loss, anemia, dysphagia, dyspepsia with abdominal tenderness and epigastric mass on physical examination [4, 10]. Because most cases occur along the greater curvature of the stomach, the cysts can potentially compress the adjacent organs such as pancreas, kidney, spleen, and adrenal gland. Accordingly, the differential diagnosis would include lesions arising from these organs [2]. The cysts may also be manifested by complications such as infection, gastrointestinal bleeding, perforation, ulceration, fistula formation, obstruction, compression, or carcinoma arising in the cysts [7, 8]. Up to 10% of gastric duplications may contain ectopic pancreatic tissue which may lead to pancreatitis and mimic a pancreatic pseudocyst [3, 8].

Because of the rarity of adult gastric duplications, it is difficult to outline their natural history with certainty. As with the native gastric mucosa, the cyst lining may undergo erosions, ulceration, and regenerative changes. In noncommunicating cysts, increased fluid production may result in pressure-induced necrosis of the mucosa. These changes may lead to bleeding into the cyst or perforation into the peritoneal cavity.

Duplication cysts have the potential for neoplastic transformation. The production of oncofetal antigens raises the problem of a precancerous condition in long standing intestinal duplications [8]. Out of 11 reported cases of malignancy arising within the duplication cysts, 8 were adenocarcinomas [4]. Five of the carcinomas originated from gastric duplications. Adenomyoma arising from a gastric duplication has also been reported [4]. Malignancies arising from duplication cysts are likely to be present at advanced stages because of their unusual symptoms and difficulty of diagnosis [4].

Although it is difficult to diagnose GDC preoperatively, recent imaging modalities have provided some informative findings. CT scan and endoscopic ultrasound (EUS) are the best ways to identify GDC [8]. Classically, radiographic studies show an intramural filling defect indenting the gastric contour [8]. Contrast-enhanced CT scan typically demonstrates GDC as a thick-walled cystic lesion with enhancement of the inner lining [2]. Calcification is occasionally observed on CT. These findings are of diagnostic significance for GDCs [2]. However, since mucinous cystic tumors of the pancreas also show similar radiological features, GDCs adjoining the pancreas are indistinguishable from pancreatic mucinous cystic tumors based on these CT findings. Moreover, because the wall is sometimes thin, enhancement of the inner cyst wall is not always demonstrated. Generally, MRI can provide additional information about the cyst content compared to CT scan. However, the nature of the fluid in the GDC was reported to differ in each case according to bleeding, chronic inflammation, or infection. Therefore, MRI seems to be of less significance than expected in diagnosing GDCs [2]. EUS is useful in distinguishing between the intramural and extramural lesions of the stomach. When EUS demonstrates a cyst with an echogenic internal mucosal layer and a hypoechoic intermediate muscular layer, the diagnosis of GDC is highly likely [2]. The role of EUS-guided FNA in GDC is uncertain because (a) the cytological features of GDC may closely resemble those of mucinous pancreatic neoplasms, and (b) GDCs with elevated levels of CEA and CA19-9 have been reported, mimicking mucinous pancreatic neoplasms [4, 8, 11].

Complete removal is the treatment choice to avoid the risk of possible complications such as obstruction, torsion, perforation, hemorrhage, and malignancy [9, 10]. A noncommunicating GDC is classically treated by complete excision of the cyst and resection of the shared wall between stomach and the duplication cyst [8]. Communicating GDC usually requires no intervention when both gastric lumens are patent [8]. Drainage and marsupialization of the cyst have been suggested. However, marsupialization into the stomach exposes the unprotected mucosa of the cyst to gastric contents with the risk of ulceration [4]. Drainage procedures such as cystojejunostomy may be complicated by stenosis of the anastomosis or blind loop syndrome and therefore discouraged [4]. Furthermore, leaving the cyst in place is ill-advised given the potential for malignant transformation [4].

4. Conclusion

In summary, this unusual developmental anomaly should be included in the differential diagnosis of cystic masses of the gastrointestinal tract, and the possibility of malignancy should also be considered. While the diagnosis of gastrointestinal tract duplications may be suggested by imaging studies, more often the correct diagnosis is not established prior to surgery. Due to the risk of malignant transformation and other complications, GDCs should be treated surgically by complete resection.

Acknowledgment

The authors would like to acknowledge with gratitude the contribution of Dr Judy Sarungbam, M. D. from the Department of Pathology, Westchester Medical Center, New York Medical College for pathological analysis.

References

[1] K. Kuraoka, H. Nakayama, T. Kagawa, T. Ichikawa, and W. Yasui, "Adenocarcinoma arising from a gastric duplication cyst with invasion to the stomach: a case report with literature review," *Journal of Clinical Pathology*, vol. 57, no. 4, pp. 428–431, 2004.

[2] H. Maeda, T. Okabayashi, I. Nishimori et al., "Diagnostic challenge to distinguish gastric duplication cyst from pancreatic cystic lesions in adult," *Internal Medicine*, vol. 46, no. 14, pp. 1101–1104, 2007.

[3] T. Theodosopoulos, A. Marinis, K. Karapanos et al., "Foregut duplication cysts of the stomach with respiratory epithelium," *World Journal of Gastroenterology*, vol. 13, no. 8, pp. 1279–1281, 2007.

[4] J. Johnston, G. H. Wheatley, H. F. El Sayed, W. B. Marsh, E. C. Ellison, and M. Bloomston, "Gastric duplication cysts expressing carcinoembryonic antigen mimicking cystic pancreatic neoplasms in two adults," *American Surgeon*, vol. 74, no. 1, pp. 91–94, 2008.

[5] D. H. Kim, J. S. Kim, E. S. Nam, and H. S. Shin, "Foregut duplication cyst of the stomach," *Pathology International*, vol. 50, no. 2, pp. 142–145, 2000.

[6] S. Murakami, H. Isozaki, T. Shou, K. Sakai, and H. Toyota, "Foregut duplication cyst of the stomach with pseudostratified columnar ciliated epithelium," *Pathology International*, vol. 58, no. 3, pp. 187–190, 2008.

[7] R. D. Laraja, R. E. Rothenberg, J. Chapman, Imran-Ul-Haq, and M. T. Sabatini, "Foregut duplication cyst: a report of a case," *American Surgeon*, vol. 61, no. 9, pp. 840–841, 1995.

[8] X. B. D'Journo, V. Moutardier, O. Turrini et al., "Gastric duplication in an adult mimicking mucinous cystadenoma of the pancreas," *Journal of Clinical Pathology*, vol. 57, no. 11, pp. 1215–1218, 2004.

[9] G. Horne, C. Ming-Lum, A. W. Kirkpatrick, and R. L. Parker, "High-grade neuroendocrine carcinoma arising in a gastric duplication cyst: a case report with literature review," *International Journal of Surgical Pathology*, vol. 15, no. 2, pp. 187–191, 2007.

[10] K. Mardi, V. Kaushal, and S. Gupta, "Foregut duplication cysts of stomach masquerading as leiomyoma," *Indian Journal of Pathology and Microbiology*, vol. 53, no. 1, pp. 160–161, 2010.

[11] B. Wang, W. J. Hunter, S. Bin-Sagheer, and C. Bewtra, "Rare potential pitfall in endoscopic ultrasound-guided fine needle aspiration biopsy in gastric duplication cyst," *Acta Cytologica*, vol. 53, no. 2, pp. 219–222, 2009.

An Ulcerated Ileal Gastrointestinal Stromal Tumor Disguised as Acute Appendicitis

Ashish Lal Shrestha [ID][1] **and Girishma Shrestha**[2]

[1]Department of General Surgery, United Mission Hospital, Tansen, Palpa, Nepal
[2]Department of Pathology, Patan Academy of Health Sciences, Lagankhel, Kathmandu, Nepal

Correspondence should be addressed to Ashish Lal Shrestha; butchgrunty@yahoo.com

Academic Editor: Boris Kirshtein

Background. Gastrointestinal stromal tumor (GIST) of the ileum is not a common differential to consider in the management of acute right iliac fossa (RIF) pain and tenderness. Finding of a normal-looking appendix intraoperatively should arouse the surgeon to explore further and look for other unanticipated pathologies. We present a case, clinically diagnosed as acute appendicitis and intraoperatively found to be an ulcerated ileal GIST. *Case Presentation.* A 28-year-old female without previous comorbidities presented to the emergency unit with sudden pain around the umbilicus that later migrated and localized to the RIF for one day. There was associated intermittent fever and anorexia without urinary symptoms. Abdominal examination revealed guarding and rebound tenderness at RIF. Examination by 2 senior surgeons at different points of time, the same day, made a clinical diagnosis of acute appendicitis. Ultrasonogram (USG) was inconclusive. At laparotomy through Lanz incision, the appendix was found to be normal and no other pathology was identified on walking bowel up to 3 ft proximal to ileocecal junction (ICJ). Just when closure was thought of, an ulcerated lesion could be seen through the medial aspect of the incision. On further exploration, a 7×5 cm ulcerated lesion arising from the antimesenteric border of the ileum was noted with localized interloop hemoperitoneum and inflammatory exudates. Ileal segmental resection anastomosis was done with peritoneal toileting. The lesion was subsequently reported to be an ulcerated malignant GIST. *Conclusion.* The commonest cause of RIF pain with localized peritonitis is an acutely inflamed appendix. Dilemma arises when the appendix is found to look normal. Further exploration is indicted to not miss other findings.

1. Introduction

The term "GIST" was first introduced by Mazur and Clark in 1983 to include the nonepithelial tumors of digestive tract that lack ultrastructure of smooth muscle cells and immunohistochemical properties of Schwann cells. GISTs are known to arise from the interstitial cells of Cajal that are regarded as the pacemaker cells, constituting a part of the autonomic nervous system of the gut and controlling intestinal peristalsis [1]. GISTs may vary in presentation and sometimes mimic other commoner conditions. We report an interesting case of an ulcerated small bowel GIST that behaved clinically like acute appendicitis. The clinical presentation, investigative findings, and management are discussed along with relevant literatures.

2. Case Presentation

A 28-year-old female with insignificant past medico surgical history presented with one day of acute onset pain in the periumbilical region that later migrated and confined to the RIF. She had associated intermittent fever, nausea, and loss of appetite. She did not have any urinary symptoms, bowel irregularities, or gynecological complaints. Abdominal examination was performed by two senior surgeons at two different occasions; the same day had findings of guarding and rebound tenderness at RIF. Hematological tests showed polymorphonuclear leukocytosis with left shift. Biochemical tests and urinalysis were normal. Urinary pregnancy test was negative. Abdominal radiographs were unremarkable. USG could not visualize appendix and was inconclusive except for probe tenderness in RIF. CT scan of the abdomen could not be done due to unavailability. A clinical diagnosis of acute appendicitis was made assigning an Alvarado score of 9/10. Laparotomy was performed using the Lanz incision in RIF. Intraoperatively appendix was found to be normal without evidence of inflammation or infection in RIF. In view of symptoms and signs, a possibility of other pathology was thought. Walking the bowel proximally up to 3 feet (1 m) did not show a Meckel's diverticulum or any other small bowel lesions. There were no obvious mesenteric lymph nodal enlargement and pelvic organs looked pristine. Approaching closure, just when the medial edge of the incision was retracted superomedially, a hemorrhagic lesion seemed to appear little deeper in the mid abdomen. Therefore, the incision was extended transversely from the medial edge to explore further. Entire bowel was explored and this revealed an ulcerated lesion measuring 7 × 5 cm arising from the antimesenteric border of the ileum 8 feet (2.5 m) from ICJ with localized interloop hemoperitoneum and inflammatory exudates as shown in Figure 1. Resection of ileal segment containing the lesion was performed followed by restoration of bowel continuity and peritoneal toileting. The lesion was subsequently reported to be an ulcerated malignant ileal GIST.

Histopathologically, gross examination confirmed the operative findings, and the cut section revealed a nodular lesion protruding out of the serosal surface measuring 7 × 5 cm along with 2 lymph nodes each measuring 2 × 1 cm.

Microscopically, the growth from the ileum had villous lining epithelium with focal ulceration. The submucosal region had a circumscribed nodule with proliferation of loosely cohesive spindle cells; some of which were arranged in vague storiform pattern and others in long fascicles. There were areas with epitheloid cells forming small anastomosing nests and cords. The areas in between these showed skenoid fibers along with focal areas of hemorrhage, infarction, and congestion as shown in Figure 2. The mitotic figures were seen (8/50 high-power field). The lymph nodes were microscopically identified to be reactive, and the resected margins of the ileum were free of tumor.

Based on tumor size and mitotic activity, possibility of a malignant GIST was suggested along with immunohistochemical analysis (CD117 and CD34) for further confirmation. The patient had an uneventful recovery and was discharged on the 8th postoperative day. She was advised to review a week later at the outpatients but failed to report. All possible contacts were used to trace her, but she remained inaccessible and lost to follow-up.

3. Discussion

It is a common clinical situation to have a patient presenting with periumbilical pain subsequently localizing to the RIF associated with vomiting with or without nausea and fever. The classical symptom complex called Murphy's triad is often observed and tends to occur in the same sequential order [2]. The findings of guarding at the RIF with McBurney's point tenderness are suspicious of acute appendicitis along with various named signs [3]. Leukocytosis

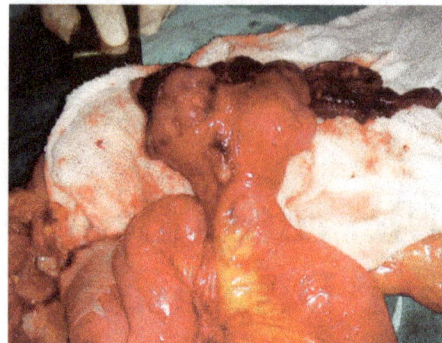

FIGURE 1: The intraoperative image of the ulcerated ileal GIST arising from the antimesenteric border with interloop hemoperitoneum and inflammatory exudates.

and neutrophilic left shift added to the USG findings of a noncompressible blind tube > 6 mm in RIF with probe tenderness strongly impress upon the surgeon to wait no further before embarking on an emergency appendectomy. The usual finding is that of an inflamed appendix with or without associated complications (gangrene, perforation, or periappendicular collection). Figure 3 shows an uncomplicated appendicitis in a different patient.

The annual global incidence of appendicitis is reported to be 11 cases per 10,000 population [4]. In one study, the sensitivity and specificity of clinical examination to diagnose appendicitis were 99% and 76% and the same for USG were 99% and 91%, respectively [5]. Various scoring systems have also been devised to aid accurate preoperative diagnosis, for example, Alvarado, Ohhmann, Eskelinen, and RIPASA, and report a wide range of variability in sensitivity, specificity, and predictive validity in different comparative studies [6]. Despite our long-term experience in treating this condition, there have been several incidences of finding an unanticipated pathology intraoperatively and the "On Table Surprise" does not stop to amaze us even now. In most series, a negative appendectomy rate of 10–20% is considered acceptable though newer studies quote an even lesser rate [7, 8]. A normal-looking appendix certainly arouses the surgeon to suspect something sinister and thence the usual tendency to look for conditions like an inflamed Meckel's diverticulum, the incidence of which is said to be 2%. The other pathologies that may be encountered are mesenteric lymphadenitis, large or small bowel diverticulitis, right ureteric pathology, and a wide variety of gynecological ailments like ruptured ovarian follicle with midcycle ovulatory bleeding (Mittelschmerz's), ovarian torsion, salpingitis, and ruptured ectopic pregnancy especially in women of child bearing age [9]. But a ruptured small bowel GIST is certainly not the prime suspect under usual circumstances. GISTs are known to us since the time they were first reported by Mazur and Clark in 1983. They have constantly made their presence felt in various case reports globally when they were not recognized preoperatively. Refractory peptic ulcer disease, gastrointestinal bleeding, pneumomediastinum, acute diffuse peritonitis, abdominal abscesses, and sudden perforation with hemoperitoneum have all been the various modes of presentation of GISTs [10–15]. One similar incidence of a GIST mimicking

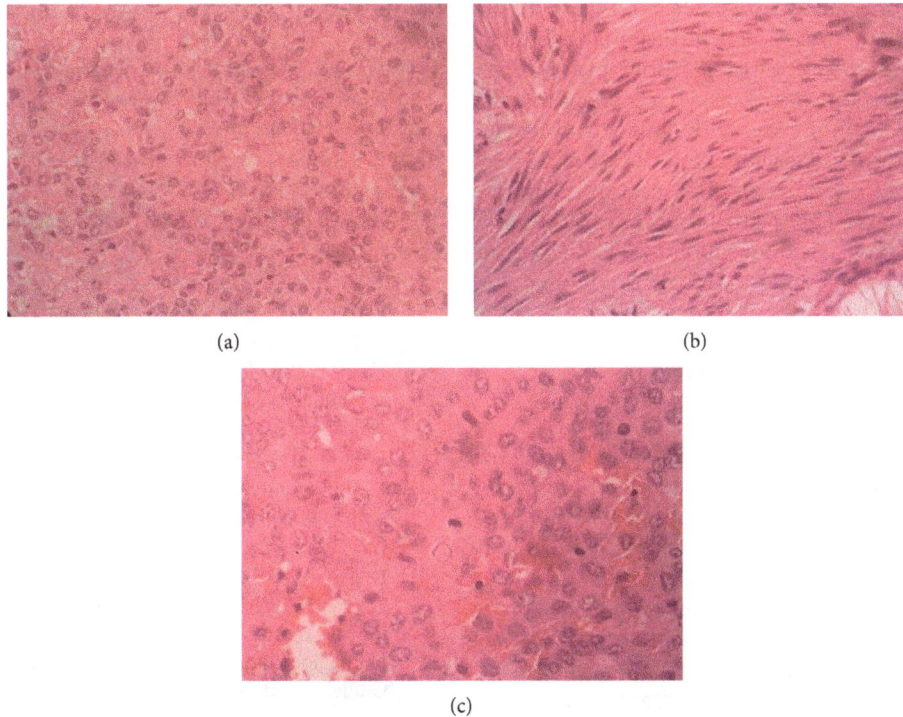

(a)

(b)

(c)

FIGURE 2: Microscopic appearance of the ileal malignant GIST (stained with eosin/hematoxylin stain) under high-power magnification showing mitotic figures. (a) Tumor cells exhibiting epithelioid morphology (H&E; 20x). (b) Spindle cells in fascicles (H&E; 20x). (c) Areas with frequent mitotic activity (H&E; 40x).

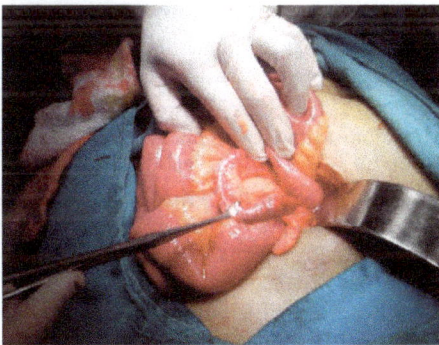

FIGURE 3: An uncomplicated appendicitis in a different patient.

appendicitis was found reportedly from the jejunum; however, ours was one from the ileum [16]. The usual age of presentation of GIST is 40 to 60 years and the common sites of origin are the stomach and followed by small bowel and colorectum and rarely esophagus. Although many are diagnosed incidentally, some with advanced disease present with symptoms that include nonspecific abdominal pain and large abdominal masses. Occasionally, luminal erosion of a highly vascular GIST may present with a life-threatening gastrointestinal hemorrhage, while on account of luminal narrowing, the other forms of presentation may be obstruction and perforation. Tumor rupture in this regard seems to be more dreadful condition; in that, it carries risks of tumor dissemination that can be difficult to treat apart from hemoperitoneum and acute abdomen. Some may even present with

metastasis to the liver and peritoneum and very rarely to the lungs. Also of note are local spread to adjacent viscera like the intestine, omentum, and diaphragm. Cross-sectional imaging with a CT scan is helpful in identifying the extent of lesion and studying the characters like necrosis, ulceration, calcification, ascites, and local and distant metastasis that denote the aggressive nature of primary lesion to plan a subsequent operative therapy. PET scan is considered an important adjunct to CT in evaluation and in order to assess response to chemotherapy [1]. In an acute setting, and in a peripheral set up like ours, both these modalities are only of theoretical value. Similarly, endoscopic ultrasound and FNAC are invaluable in preoperative tissue diagnosis in centers where the expertise is available. Definitive diagnosis is possible with histopathological examination of the tissue aided by immunohistochemistry (IHC); the current panel of which includes CD117, smooth muscle actin, CD34, desmin, and S-100. Unfortunately, in our case, it was unavailable and had to be sent to a tertiary care center on receiving the histopathological report. Since the patient did not follow up in the postoperative period, it could not be done. An extensive search in PubMed, Medline, and Google in reference to GIST misdiagnosed as appendicitis was done from 2000 till now. Only 4 cases were found to have been reported worldwide of which 1 was in the stomach, 2 were in the jejunum, and 1 was in the ileum [16–19]. This was the second report of similar presentation of GIST in the ileum. In all the cases, treatment approach was surgical with laparoscopic resection in 1 and open resection in the rest. Our patient underwent open resection with an uneventful recovery.

Had she returned for follow-up, she should have been evaluated for metastatic disease and further management. But since that was not possible, we could neither plan further treatment nor prognosticate her disease. In general, prognosis of GIST depends upon the size of the tumor and to the mitotic rate: tumors > 10 cm or with a mitotic rate of >5 per 50 HPF having higher risk of recurrence, metastatic spread, and a poorer prognosis. Other prognostic factors include tumor-free surgical margins, tumor rupture, and c-kit mutation [17]. The IHC and other molecular studies could not be done in our patient.

4. Conclusion

In essence, an ulcerated malignant GIST of the ileum masquerading as acute appendicitis is a common presentation of an uncommon diagnosis. Disproportionate symptoms and signs inconsistent with a normal-looking appendix on table should alert the surgeon to suspect other possible causes no matter how remote. Negative appendectomy should not be taken lightly and mandates thorough exploration of the entire length of bowel. Definitive diagnosis is possible on histopathological evaluation aided by IHC. Resection with negative margins and further therapy based on IHC panel forms the backbone of management. The awareness of the clinical presentation and good pathological expertise are important adjuncts in the diagnosis. Surgery is the mainstay of treatment in the acute presentation.

Abbreviations

GIST: Gastrointestinal stromal tumor
RIF: Right iliac fossa
USG: Ultrasonogram
ICJ: Ileocecal junction
CT: Computed tomography
IHC: Immunohistochemistry.

Authors' Contributions

Ashish Lal Shrestha participated in the surgical and perioperative management of the patient and conception and design of the report and wrote the paper. Girishma Shrestha performed the histopathological analysis of the report. Both have been involved in the diagnosis and patient care. Both authors read and approved the final paper. Both the authors were involved in planning, analysis of the case, and writing of the paper.

Acknowledgments

The authors would like to thank the ward staff of the hospital for providing support and helping in management of the patient.

References

[1] M. Zinner and S. Ashley, *Maingot's Abdominal Operations*, McGraw-Hill Professional, New York, NY, USA, 11th edition, 2006.

[2] R. S. Lawson, "Murphy's triad," *British Medical Journal*, vol. 1, no. 5745, pp. 401-402, 1971.

[3] A. Sachdeva and A. K. Dutta, *Advances in Pediatrics*, JP Medical Ltd, 2012.

[4] A. Petroianu, "Diagnosis of acute appendicitis," *International Journal of Surgery*, vol. 10, no. 3, pp. 115–119, 2012.

[5] J. S. Park, J. H. Jeong, J. I. Lee, J. H. Lee, J. K. Park, and H. J. Moon, "Accuracies of diagnostic methods for acute appendicitis," *The American Surgeon*, vol. 79, no. 1, pp. 101–106, 2013.

[6] H. Erdem, S. Çetinkünar, K. Daş et al., "Alvarado, Eskelinen, Ohhmann and Raja Isteri Pengiran Anak Saleha appendicitis scores for diagnosis of acute appendicitis," *World Journal of Gastroenterology*, vol. 19, no. 47, pp. 9057–9062, 2013.

[7] D. Papeš, S. Sršen Medančić, A. Antabak, I. Sjekavica, and T. Luetić, "What is the acceptable rate of negative appendectomy? Comment on prospective evaluation of the added value of imaging within the Dutch National Diagnostic Appendicitis Guideline - do we forget our clinical eye?," *Digestive Surgery*, vol. 32, no. 3, pp. 181-182, 2015.

[8] M. Colson, K. A. Skinner, and G. Dunnington, "High negative appendectomy rates are no longer acceptable," *The American Journal of Surgery*, vol. 174, no. 6, pp. 723–727, 1997.

[9] D. J. Humes and J. Simpson, "Acute appendicitis," *BMJ*, vol. 333, no. 7567, pp. 530–534, 2006.

[10] M. Mokhtare, T. Taghvaei, and H. Tirgar Fakheri, "Acute bleeding in duodenal gastrointestinal stromal tumor," *Middle East Journal of Digestive Diseases*, vol. 5, no. 1, pp. 47–51, 2013.

[11] M. Sugimoto, T. Hikichi, Y. Shioya et al., "A case of gastrointestinal storomal tumor with pneumomediastinum," *Fukushima Journal of Medical Science*, vol. 59, no. 2, pp. 97–101, 2013.

[12] P. Rubini and F. Tartamella, "Primary gastrointestinal stromal tumour of the ileum pre-operatively diagnosed as an abdominal abscess," *Molecular and Clinical Oncology*, vol. 5, no. 5, pp. 596–598, 2016.

[13] J. D. Jones, S. Oh, C. Clark, and R. Pawa, "A bleeding duodenal GIST masquerading as refractory peptic ulcer disease," *ACG Case Reports Journal*, vol. 3, no. 4, article e189, 2016.

[14] S. Ulusan, Z. Koc, and F. Kayaselcuk, "Spontaneously ruptured gastrointestinal stromal tumor with pelvic abscess: a case report and review," *Gastroenterology Research*, vol. 2, no. 6, pp. 361–363, 2009.

[15] W. Attaallah, Ş. Coşkun, G. Özden, H. Mollamemişoğlu, and C. Yeğen, "Spontaneous rupture of extraluminal jejunal gastrointestinal stromal tumor causing acute abdomen and hemoperitoneum," *Turkish Journal of Surgery*, vol. 31, no. 2, pp. 99–101, 2015.

[16] M. Ajduk, D. Mikulić, B. Sebecic et al., "Spontaneously ruptured gastrointestinal stromal tumor (GIST) of the jejunum mimicking acute appendicitis," *Collegium Antropologicum*, vol. 28, no. 2, pp. 937–941, 2004.

[17] E. Elangovan, "A rare case of jejunal GIST presenting as acute abdomen," *University Journal of Surgery and Surgical Specialities*, vol. 3, no. 2, 2017.

Transvaginal Small Bowel Evisceration following Abdominoperineal Resection

Enver Kunduz, Huseyin Bektasoglu ⓘ, Samet Yigman, and Huseyin Akbulut

Department of General Surgery, Faculty of Medicine, Bezmialem Vakif University, Istanbul, Turkey

Correspondence should be addressed to Huseyin Bektasoglu; hkbektasoglu@yahoo.com

Academic Editor: Gabriel Sandblom

Abdominoperineal resection (APR) is one of the surgical techniques performed for the distal rectal cancer. The perineal herniation is one of the complications of APR surgery. In this report, we aim to demonstrate a rare case of small bowel evisceration and strangulation secondary to the transvaginal herniation evolved in the late stage after perineal hernia repair following laparoscopic APR.

1. Introduction

Abdominoperineal resection (APR) is one of the techniques performed in the surgical treatment of the distal rectal cancer [1]. The perineal herniation is one of the complications seen after APR operations [2]. The perineal herniation after APR was described for the first time at the end of the 1930s, and it is not presented in the literature as a series but rather as a presentation of cases [3]. Various techniques such as synthetic patch, reconstruction with the muscle flap, and biomedical patch repair are recommended in the literature to prevent more frequent herniation due to a large perineal defect in the extralevator APR operations [4]. The perineal herniation after classical APR is restored by posterior or abdominal approaches [5]. The vaginal reconstruction is needed in cases of posterior vaginal wall resection due to the posterior wall invasion of the tumor, but the reconstructive techniques are not recommended for vagina in classical APR [6]. Although there have been several reports about the transvaginal herniation following hysterectomy or trauma, we could not find any report of the transvaginal herniation and evisceration following the abdominoperineal resection and the perineal hernia repair in English literature. This article aims to present a case of transvaginal evisceration and small bowel strangulation in a patient who underwent perineal hernia repair after laparoscopic APR.

2. Case Report

A 67-year-old female patient with a locally advanced distal rectal adenocarcinoma (cT3N+) underwent laparoscopic abdominoperineal resection after short-term radiotherapy. A vaginal resection or repair was not required for the patient as she did not have any intraoperative problems. The patient with the pathology test result of pT2N0 received adjuvant chemotherapy. No complication was observed in the third and sixth month controls; however, the perineal hernia was detected at the ninth month. The abdominal computed tomography (CT) imaging taken without valsalva maneuver revealed no pathological findings except perineal hernia (Figure 1). The patient was, then, scheduled for follow-up, since she had no complaints. However, surgery was decided for the perineal hernia in the first postoperative year upon the growth of hernia and the restriction of daily activities due to the hernia.

The patient was placed on a Jackknife position. The perineal defect was revealed by dissecting the hernia vesicle through posterior approach. After the hernia content was reduced into the abdomen, the double-sided synthetic patch was placed over the defect and fixed to the levator ani muscle laterally, the vagina anteriorly, and the coccyx posteriorly with the 2/0 polyprolene sutures. The patient was discharged without any complication.

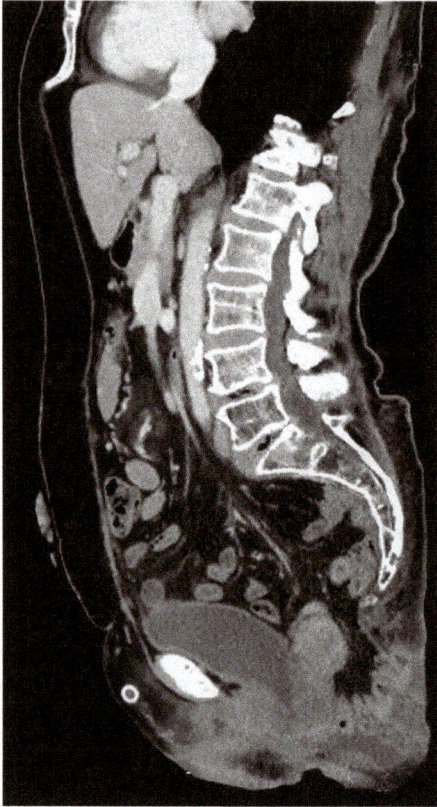

FIGURE 1: Herniated small bowel segments through the pelvis in CT scan.

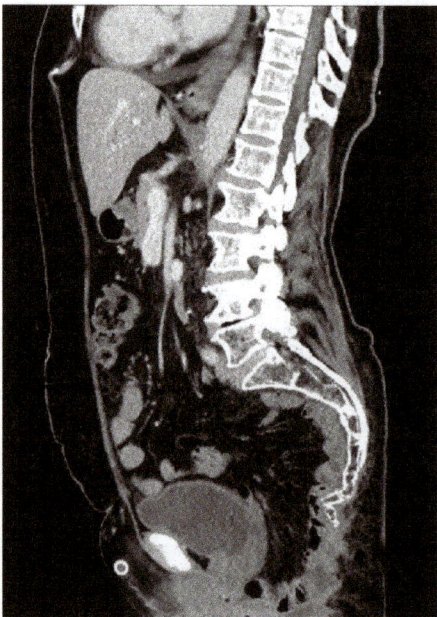

FIGURE 2: The sagittal image of the pelvis after perineal hernia repair.

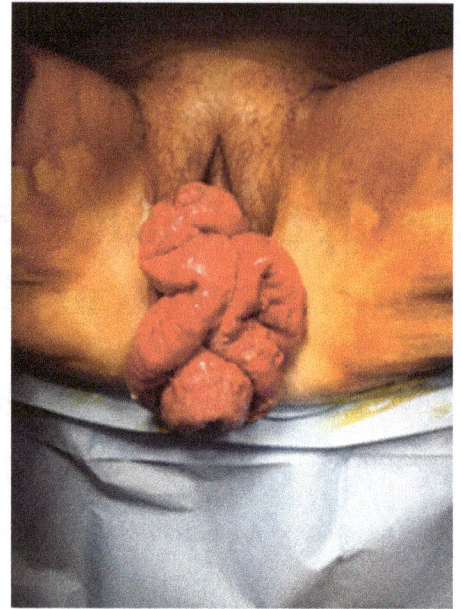

FIGURE 3: Vaginal evisceration of the small bowels.

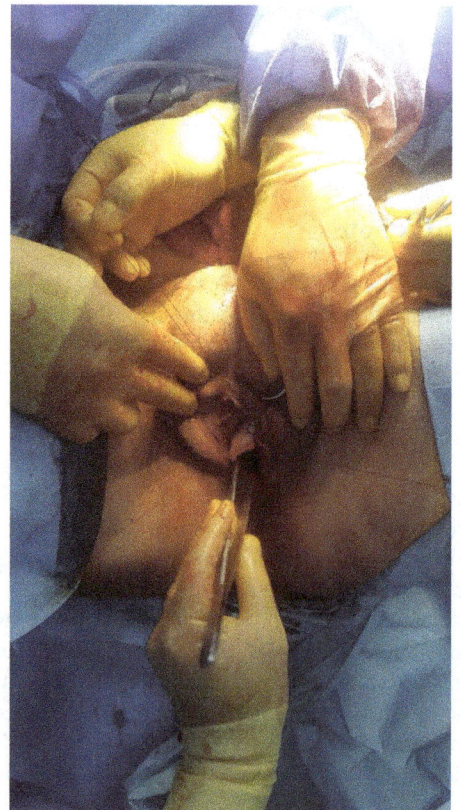

FIGURE 4: Repair of the vaginal defect with primary sutures.

The patient had no complaints related to the perineal hernia during the follow-up using CT imaging (Figure 2). The patient who was followed in the oncology clinic without problem was admitted to the emergency department with the complaint of prolapsed intestines from the vagina 12 months after the repair of the perineal hernia. During the examination, the small intestines were observed to be freely prolapsed from the vagina and several local ischemic changes were detected (Figure 3). In the emergency laparotomy, the terminal ileum revealed a herniation out of the posterior vaginal wall of the 110 cm ileum segment from the 10th cm of caecum. The ischemic areas were observed to be developed locally in the ileum. Following the withdrawal of the small intestine into the abdomen, a functional side-by-side ileocolic anastomosis was performed by resecting the ischemic segment with the caecum. The formerly placed mesh material was explored and seen as intact (no folding or detachment) and well placed below the levator ani muscle. As the formerly placed mesh material was located below levator ani muscle level, it was not covering the posterior vaginal wall. Instead, the previous mesh was only anchored to vagina anteriorly below the levator level. The vaginal defect was reconstructed with interrupted sutures by using the 3/0 polydioxanone (Figure 4). A new double-sided mesh material with antiadhesion barrier site facing the viscera was placed over the pelvic brim and fixed to the pubic bone anteriorly, the sacral promontory posteriorly, and the pelvic wall laterally by using the 2/0 polypropylene sutures. The patient was uneventfully discharged on the postoperative day 4; the wound sites were observed to be healed at three months, and no herniation finding was observed.

3. Discussion

The perineal herniation has been reported as 1–13% after the classical APR surgery [7]. The large pelvis, the previous hysterectomy, the radiation treatment, the excessive length of the small bowel mesentery, and the perineal infection are reported as the risk factors [8]. In addition, the dissection of Denonvilliers' fascia in men and the rectovaginal septum in women is thought to cause herniation [9]. Akatsu at al. speculated that the laparoscopic surgery may facilitate the small bowels sliding down to the pelvis due to the fewer intra-abdominal adhesions and may result in herniation [10].

The perineal herniation may be reconstructed through transabdominal or transperineal approach. Although the transperineal approach is a less invasive procedure, there are some disadvantages such as the poor exposure, the inadequate mobilization of the muscles, and the difficulty in competing with the adhesions compared with the transabdominal approach [11]. In addition, local, regional, or distal pedunculated muscle flaps may be used in reconstruction of the perineal defects. The vertical rectus abdominis myocutaneous flap (VRAM) is a common technique used in reconstruction of the perineal defects. VRAM flap has advantages such as long pedicle, large volume and surface area, and low incidence of necrosis [12].

In this case, a recurrent perineal herniation through vagina has occurred, and a portion of the small intestine eviscerated and strangulated after one year of the transperineal hernia repair following the abdominoperineal resection. It may be claimed that the transvaginal herniation occurred due to the chronic protrusion of the abdominal viscera to the weakened vaginal wall due to the loosening of the pelvic structures, the advanced age, and the previous surgeries. The intraoperative findings such as well-placed previous mesh material far from

current vaginal defect and no relevant intra-abdominal adhesions may support the reason mentioned above. However, the anchoring suture placed in the vagina in the former perineal repair may be another reason for transvaginal herniation.

References

[1] F. Mauvais, C. Sabbagh, O. Brehant et al., "The current abdominoperineal resection: oncological problems and surgical modifications for low rectal cancer," *Journal of Visceral Surgery*, vol. 148, no. 2, pp. e85–e93, 2011.

[2] T. G. Lee and S. J. Lee, "Mesh-based transperineal repair of a perineal hernia after a laparoscopic abdominoperineal resection," *Annals of Coloproctology*, vol. 30, no. 4, pp. 197–200, 2014.

[3] M. Mjoli, D. A. Sloothaak, C. J. Buskens, W. A. Bemelman, and P. J. Tanis, "Perineal hernia repair after abdominoperineal resection: a pooled analysis," *Colorectal Disease*, vol. 14, no. 7, pp. e400–e406, 2012.

[4] H. Sumrien, P. Newman, C. Burt et al., "The use of a negative pressure wound management system in perineal wound closure after extralevator abdominoperineal excision (ELAPE) for low rectal cancer," *Techniques in Coloproctology*, vol. 20, no. 9, pp. 627–631, 2016.

[5] G. Dapri, L. Gerard, L. Cardinali et al., "Laparoscopic prosthetic parastomal and perineal hernia repair after abdominoperineal resection," *Techniques in Coloproctology*, vol. 21, no. 1, pp. 73–77, 2017.

[6] S. W. Bell, N. Dehni, M. Chaouat, J. C. Lifante, R. Parc, and E. Tiret, "Primary rectus abdominis myocutaneous flap for repair of perineal and vaginal defects after extended abdominoperineal resection," *British Journal of Surgery*, vol. 92, no. 4, pp. 482–486, 2005.

[7] G. D. Musters, C. J. Buskens, W. A. Bemelman, and P. J. Tanis, "Perineal wound healing after abdominoperineal resection for rectal cancer: a systematic review and meta-analysis," *Diseases of the Colon & Rectum*, vol. 57, no. 9, pp. 1129–1139, 2014.

[8] F. G. de Campos, A. Habr-Gama, S. E. Araújo et al., "Incidence and management of perineal hernia after laparoscopic proctectomy," *Surgical Laparoscopy, Endoscopy & Percutaneous Techniques*, vol. 15, no. 6, pp. 366–370, 2005.

[9] D. Stamatiou, J. E. Skandalakis, L. J. Skandalakis, and P. Mirilas, "Perineal hernia: surgical anatomy, embryology, and technique of repair," *American Surgeons*, vol. 76, no. 5, pp. 474–479, 2010.

[10] T. Akatsu, S. Murai, S. Kamiya et al., "Perineal hernia as a rare complication after laparoscopic abdominoperineal resection: report of a case," *Surgery Today*, vol. 39, no. 4, pp. 340–343, 2009.

[11] J. Li and W. Zhang, "How we do it: repair of large perineal hernia after abdominoperineal resection," *Hernia*, vol. 21, no. 6, pp. 957–961, 2017.

[12] M. Mughal, R. J. Baker, A. Muneer, and A. Mosahebi, "Reconstruction of perineal defects," *Annals of the Royal College of Surgeons of England*, vol. 95, no. 8, pp. 539–544, 2013.

34

Cholecystectomy of an Intrahepatic Gallbladder in an Ectopic Pelvic Liver: A Case Report

Rachel Mathis,[1] Joshua Stodghill,[1] Timothy Shaver,[2] and George Younan[2]

[1]*Department of Surgery, Inova Fairfax Hospital, Fairfax, VA, USA*
[2]*Virginia Surgery Associates, Fairfax, VA, USA*

Correspondence should be addressed to George Younan; grg.younan@gmail.com

Academic Editor: Tahsin Colak

Introduction. Ectopic pelvic liver is an exceedingly rare condition usually resulting after repair of congenital abdominal wall defects. Intrahepatic gallbladder is another rare condition predisposing patients to cholelithiasis and its sequelae. We describe a cholecystectomy in a patient with an intrahepatic gallbladder in a pelvic ectopic liver. *Presentation of Case.* A 33-year-old woman with a history of omphalocele repair as an infant presented with signs and symptoms of symptomatic cholelithiasis and chronic cholecystitis, however, in an unusual location. After extensive workup and symptomatic treatment, cholecystectomy was recommended and performed via laparotomy and hepatotomy using microwave technology for parenchymal hepatic transection. *Discussion.* Given the rare combination of an intrahepatic gallbladder and an ectopic pelvic liver, advanced surgical techniques must be employed for cholecystectomies, in addition to involvement of hepatobiliary experienced surgeons due to the distortion of the biliary and hepatic vascular anatomy. *Conclusion.* Cholecystectomy by experienced hepatobiliary surgeons is a safe and effective treatment for cholecystitis in patients with intrahepatic gallbladders in ectopic pelvic livers.

1. Introduction

Ectopic or wandering liver is exceedingly rare outside of the pediatric population and is generally confined to colonic interposition into the right upper quadrant or epigastric region [1–3]. Few reports exist in the literature about a pelvic location of the liver in adults [4, 5]. Intrahepatic gallbladder—one that is partially or completely surrounded by the liver parenchyma—is slightly more common, though also rare [6]. An intrahepatic gallbladder often exhibits impaired function, which may lead to stasis and gallstone formation [7]. Thus, patients with intrahepatic gallbladders are more prone to complications of cholelithiasis, such as cholecystitis. To the knowledge of the authors of this paper, there are only two prior case reports of intrahepatic gallbladders in pelvic livers; both associated with previous omphalocele repair in infancy [8]. Herein, we describe a case of successful surgical treatment of chronic cholecystitis in a woman with a history of omphalocele repair as an infant with an intrahepatic gallbladder in an ectopic pelvic liver.

2. Case Presentation

A 33-year-old African American woman with a history of omphalocele repair as an infant presented to the general surgery clinic with left upper and lower quadrant abdominal pain that radiates to the back, nausea related to fatty food ingestion, bloating, diarrhea, and subjective fevers. She had undergone an extensive workup with her gastroenterologist and was found to have cholelithiasis. Her past medical history included gastroesophageal reflux disease, anxiety, depression, and kidney stones. Past surgical history was significant for repair of an omphalocele shortly after birth. Her social history was negative for smoking or alcohol use.

On physical examination, she was hemodynamically normal, and the only pertinent finding was tenderness to palpation in her midabdomen. All blood tests were within normal limits including a white blood cell count and liver function tests. Abdominal ultrasound demonstrated cholelithiasis and sludge in an intrahepatic gallbladder located in her ectopic liver, but no evidence of gallbladder wall

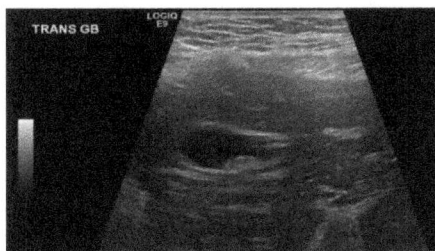

FIGURE 1: Transabdominal ultrasound demonstrated sludge and stones in a contracted gallbladder.

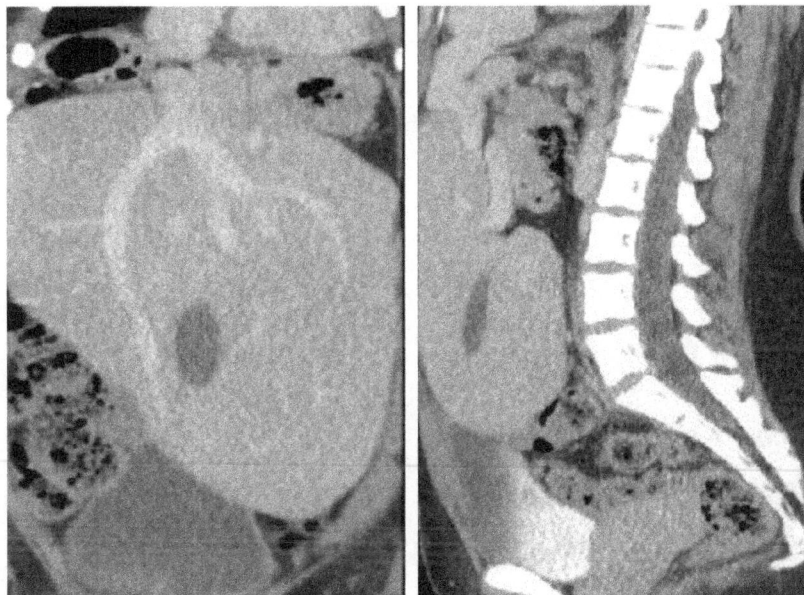

FIGURE 2: Coronal and sagittal computed tomography pictures showing the pelvic location of the liver and the intrahepatic location of the gallbladder.

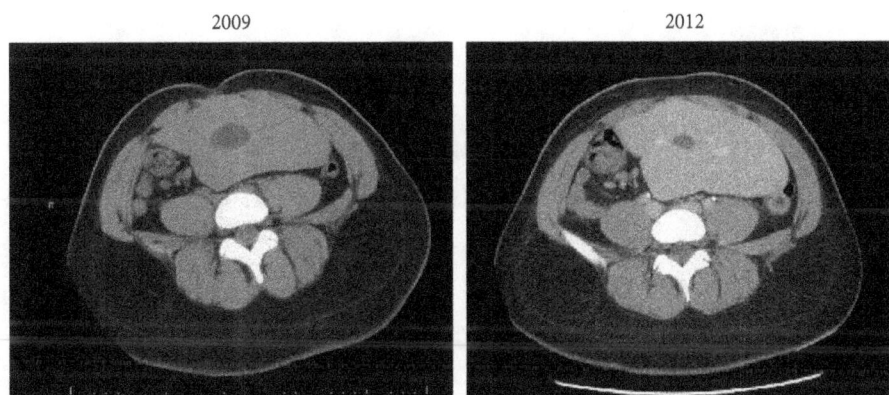

FIGURE 3: Axial computed tomography pictures showing contracture of the gallbladder from 2009 to 2012.

thickening or pericholecystic fluid (Figure 1). Previous computed tomography (CT) scans demonstrated an ectopic liver located in the pelvis as well as an intrahepatic gallbladder and interval contracture of the gallbladder in subsequent scans (Figures 2 and 3). Magnetic resonance cholangiopancreatography (MRCP) demonstrated a relatively decompressed intrahepatic gallbladder in the pelvis joining the hepatic duct more superiorly with the common bile duct emptying into the duodenum, which has its usual right upper quadrant location (Figure 4). As the patient had been symptomatic for several months and her clinical status did not improve during a period of observation and trial of ursodiol, cholecystectomy was recommended. The patient was consented for open cholecystectomy due to her unusual anatomy and likely need for hepatotomy to access the gallbladder.

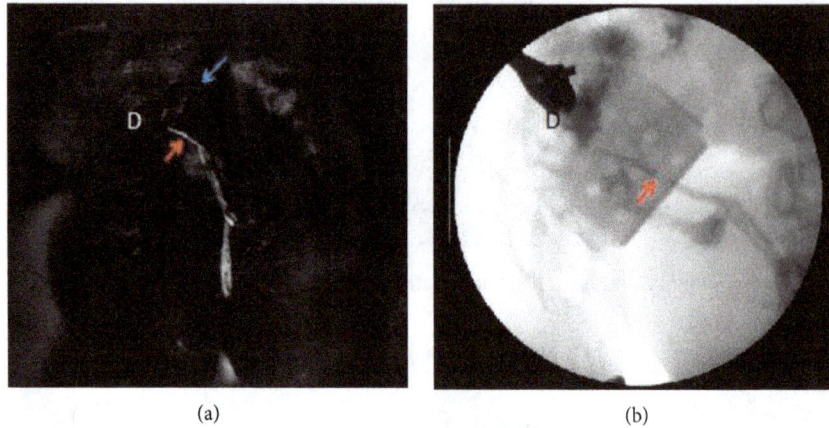

(a)   (b)

FIGURE 4: MRCP shown in (a) and intraoperative cholangiogram in (b) depicting the biliary tree with the gallbladder inferiorly. The hepatic ducts join to form the common hepatic and bile ducts (red arrow) that empty into the duodenum which has its usual right upper quadrant location. The pancreatic duct is depicted by the blue arrow. D = duodenum.

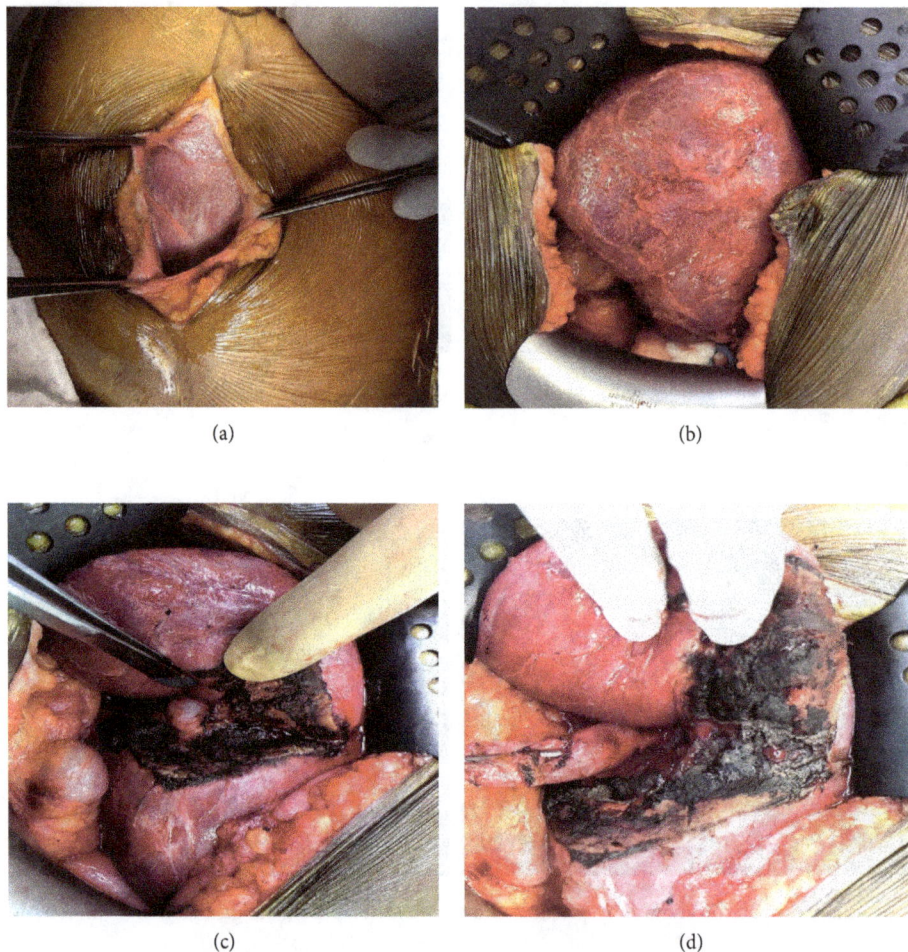

(a)   (b)

(c)   (d)

FIGURE 5: Midline laparotomy incision demonstrating the ectopic liver with adhesions (a, b). Hepatotomy exposing the intrahepatic gallbladder inferior to forceps (c) and dissected free of the surrounding parenchyma and retracted left laterally (d).

At laparotomy, the liver was encountered just beneath the fascia in the lower abdomen and was adhesed to the anterior abdominal wall and into the pelvis. A small portion of the gallbladder infundibulum was identified in a cleft on the underside of the liver once it was rotated right to left and cranially. The cleft was extended to the edge of the liver and down to the gallbladder with a recently introduced microwave ablation technology for hepatic parenchymal pretransection coagulation, to expose the gallbladder, which was then separated from the surrounding liver parenchyma (Figure 5). The cystic artery was identified, ligated, and divided. The cystic duct was identified, and a stone was found to be lodged in the cystic duct, which was then manipulated up into the fundus. The cystic duct was then ligated and divided, and a cholangiogram was performed via the cystic duct stump. The right and left hepatic ducts were visualized, as well as a long common bile duct, which traveled cranially to the right upper quadrant, where contrast was visualized within the duodenum (Figure 4). Ultrasound of the whole liver was then performed. There were no abnormal lesions noted. The patient recovered without major events and was discharged to home on postoperative day three. Final pathology revealed chronic cholecystitis with cholelithiasis.

3. Discussion

Intrahepatic gallbladder results from failure of the gallbladder to move from its intrahepatic position in the first trimester of gestation [9–12]. Intrahepatic gallbladders do not completely empty, leading to impaired function, contributing to stasis and cholelithiasis [13]. Patients with intrahepatic gallbladders, therefore, are susceptible to cholecystitis and other complications of cholelithiasis [14]. To our knowledge, this is the first report in the literature that describes a planned cholecystectomy for cholecystitis in an adult patient with an intrahepatic gallbladder in an ectopic pelvic liver. There are only two case reports in the literature of an intrahepatic gallbladder in a pelvic liver [8, 15]. Both of these patients had their aberrant anatomy discovered incidentally, and both had omphalocele repairs in infancy. Of note, in all three cases, the right and left hepatic duct joined to form the common bile duct that took a cranial course to enter the duodenal ampulla in the usual location. As patients after omphalocele repair are living longer, the existence of abnormal anatomy should be considered in these patients [16]. As care for patients with omphalocele improves, these patients are living longer. The existence of cholecystitis in pelvic intrahepatic gallbladders may become a more prevalent issue presented to surgeons. When evaluating these patients, planning MRCP in addition to intraoperative cholangiograms to study the "upside-down" biliary anatomy is a major benefit, allowing tracing and avoiding injury of the extrahepatic biliary tree.

In the case of the patient presented here, the use of ursodiol did not relieve her symptoms or cholecystitis. A review of literature has revealed varied efficacy of ursodiol in the nonsurgical treatment of chronic cholecystitis with return of symptoms in at least 50% of patients [17, 18]. Therefore, surgery remains the mainstay treatment for diseases of the gallbladder. Due to the rarity of this combination of intrahepatic gallbladder and ectopic liver, which causes an abnormal orientation of biliary anatomy, involving an experienced hepatobiliary surgeon is recommended.

Advances in surgical techniques and technology now allow preoperative recognition of aberrant anatomy and improved surgical planning. Multiple strategies are

described and now used for parenchymal liver transection in hepatectomies, and while no method has been found to be superior, we elected to use a new approach for our hepatotomy in order to access the intrahepatic location of the gallbladder [19]. In recent years, microwave technology has been used with good results in pretransection coagulation of liver tissue prior to performing hepatotomy. This method, while not proven in large studies as superior to other methods, provides a fast and efficient way to hepatic parenchymal transection, minimizing blood loss and bile leaks [20–22].

There is no published data on risk of malignancy in pelvic livers. In this case, intraoperative ultrasound of the entire liver was completed to rule out any further abnormal anatomy or lesion. With no abnormal anatomy or lesion identified, no biopsy of the liver was taken.

4. Conclusion

As patients with a prior history of omphalocele are living longer, the existence of intrahepatic pelvic gallbladders is expected to be increasingly reported [16]. Gallbladder disease occurring in intrahepatic gallbladders poses an additional surgical risk to patients and adds to the complexity of the cholecystectomy procedure especially if the gallbladder is located in an ectopic pelvic liver. Obtaining preoperative planning MRCP and intraoperative cholangiogram is recommended. Expert hepatobiliary surgeon involvement is recommended as the combination of intrahepatic gallbladder and ectopic pelvic liver distorts the normal biliary and hepatic vascular anatomy. The use of microwave technology for pretransection coagulation of liver tissue during hepatectomy is a safe and effective method to employ during the above described procedures [20–22].

References

[1] M. T. B. Siddins and R. J. Cade, "Hepatocolonic vagrancy: wandering liver with colonic abnormalities," *Australian and New Zealand Journal of Surgery*, vol. 60, no. 5, pp. 400–403, 1990.

[2] F. Al-Ali, R. I. Macpherson, H. B. Othersen, and K. Chavin, "A "wandering liver" in an infant," *Pediatric Radiology*, vol. 27, no. 3, p. 287, 1997.

[3] B. Newman, A. Bowen, and K. D. Eggli, "Recognition of malposition of the liver and spleen: CT, MRI, nuclear scan and fluoroscopic imaging," *Pediatric Radiology*, vol. 24, no. 4, pp. 274–279, 1994.

[4] N. Leone, S. Saettone, P. De Paolis et al., "Ectopic livers and related pathology: report of three cases of benign lesions," *Digestive Diseases and Sciences*, vol. 50, no. 10, pp. 1818–1822, 2005.

[5] D. W. D'Amato, H. R. Balon, and P. J. Arpasi, "An "upside-down" liver and gallbladder discovered on hepatobiliary scan," *Clinical Nuclear Medicine*, vol. 24, no. 2, pp. 140–142, 1999.

[6] A. W. Castleberry, D. A. Geller, and A. Tsung, "The pineapple upside-down liver cake," *Hepatology*, vol. 49, no. 6, pp. 2113–2114, 2009.

[7] J. J. Guiteau, M. Fisher, R. T. Cotton, and J. A. Goss, "Intrahepatic gallbladder," *Journal of the American College of Surgeons*, vol. 209, no. 5, p. 672, 2009.

[8] K. Puthenpurayil, A. Blachar, and J. V. Ferris, "Pelvic ectopia of the liver in an adult associated with omphalocele repair as a neonate," *American Journal of Roentgenology*, vol. 177, no. 5, pp. 1113–1115, 2001.

[9] C. Lusink and A. Sali, "Intrahepatic gallbladder and obstructive jaundice," *Medical Journal of Australia*, vol. 142, no. 1, pp. 53–54, 1985.

[10] H. Ando, "Embryology of the biliary tract," *Digestive Surgery*, vol. 27, no. 2, pp. 87–89, 2010.

[11] T. Roskams and V. Desmet, "Embryology of extra- and intrahepatic bile ducts, the ductal plate," *Anatomical Record*, vol. 291, no. 6, pp. 628–635, 2008.

[12] A. Dhulkotia, S. Kumar, V. Kabra, and H. S. Shukla, "Aberrant gallbladder situated beneath the left lobe of liver," *Hepato Pancreato Biliary*, vol. 4, no. 1, pp. 39–42, 2002.

[13] S. Agarwal, B. B. Lal, D. Rawat, A. Rastogi, K. G. Bharathy, and S. Alam, "Progressive familial intrahepatic cholestasis (PFIC) in Indian children: clinical spectrum and outcome," *Journal of Clinical and Experimental Hepatology*, vol. 6, no. 3, pp. 203–208, 2016.

[14] S. W. Lobo, R. G. Menezes, S. Mamata et al., "Ectopic partial intrahepatic gall bladder with cholelithiasis–a rare anomaly," *Nepal Medical College Journal*, vol. 9, no. 4, pp. 286–288, 2007.

[15] S. Shakir, A. Razzak, and S. M. Malik, "Wrong turn from right quadrant," *Gastroenterology*, vol. 146, no. 1, pp. 323–324, 2014.

[16] J. C. Dunn and E. W. Fonkalsrud, "Improved survival of infants with omphalocele," *American Journal of Surgery*, vol. 173, no. 4, pp. 284–287, 1997.

[17] G. Salen, "Gallstone dissolution therapy with ursodiol. Efficacy and safety," *Digestive Diseases and Sciences*, vol. 34, no. 12, pp. 39S–43S, 1989.

[18] J. J. Hyun, H. S. Lee, C. D. Kim et al., "Efficacy of magnesium trihydrate of ursodeoxycholic acid and chenodeoxycholic acid for gallstone dissolution: a prospective multicenter trial," *Gut and Liver*, vol. 9, no. 4, pp. 547–555, 2015.

[19] V. Pamecha, K. S. Gurusamy, D. Sharma, and B. R. Davidson, "Techniques for liver parenchymal transection: a meta-analysis of randomized controlled trials," *Hepato Pancreato Biliary*, vol. 11, no. 4, pp. 275–281, 2009.

[20] E. Moggia, B. Rouse, C. Simillis et al., "Methods to decrease blood loss during liver resection: a network meta-analysis," *Cochrane Database of Systematic Reviews*, vol. 10, p. CD010683, 2016.

[21] J. C. Weber, G. Navarra, L. R. Jiao, J. P. Nicholls, S. L. Jensen, and N. A. Habib, "New technique for liver resection using heat coagulative necrosis," *Annals of Surgery*, vol. 236, no. 5, pp. 560–563, 2002.

[22] K. Tan, X. Du, J. Yin et al., "Microwave tissue coagulation technique in anatomical liver resection," *Biomedical Reports*, vol. 2, no. 2, pp. 177–182, 2014.

35

Coexistence of Primary GEJ Adenocarcinoma and Pedunculated Gastric Gastrointestinal Stromal Tumor

Aroub Alkaaki,[1] **Basma Abdulhadi,**[1] **Murad Aljiffry,**[1] **Mohammed Nassif ⓘ,**[1]
Haneen Al-Maghrabi ⓘ,[2] **and Ashraf A. Maghrabi ⓘ**[1]

[1]*Department of Surgery, Faculty of Medicine, King Abdulaziz University, Jeddah, Saudi Arabia*
[2]*Department of Pathology, King Faisal Specialist Hospital and Research Center, Jeddah, Saudi Arabia*

Correspondence should be addressed to Ashraf A. Maghrabi; ashrafmaghrabi@gmail.com

Academic Editor: Neil Donald Merrett

Gastrointestinal stromal tumors (GISTs) are the most common mesenchymal tumors of the digestive system, although they account for only 0.1–3% of all gastrointestinal (GI) malignancies. They can arise anywhere along the GI tract with gastric predominance. Concurrent occurrence of GIST and gastroesophageal junction (GEJ) neoplasm is rare. We report a 55-year-old gentleman presenting with a polyp at the GEJ and a synchronous, large, and pedunculated gastric mass at the greater curvature. Those were treated with a wedge resection of the gastric pedunculated mass with negative margins along with transgastric submucosal resection of the GEJ polyp. Pathological examination confirmed synchronous invasive GEJ adenocarcinoma and a high-grade gastric GIST.

1. Introduction

Gastrointestinal stromal tumors (GIST) are the most common mesenchymal tumors of the gastrointestinal (GI) tract predominantly involving the stomach [1, 2]. Concurrent occurrence of GIST and gastroesophageal junction neoplasms has rarely been reported in the literature [3]. We report a case of a 55-year-old gentleman with an incidental finding of a synchronous pedunculated gastric GIST and a polyp containing adenocarcinoma at the gastroesophageal junction.

2. Case Report

A 55-year-old gentleman, ex-smoker, presented to our hospital complaining of mild epigastric pain, regurgitation, and heartburn. On top of that, he has a long-standing history of gastroesophageal reflux disease (GERD), which was managed by proton pump inhibitors. His past medical history was significant for hypertension. He was previously diagnosed

with a liver hemangioma based on abdominal ultrasound two years before the presentation. He had no relevant family history. Physical examination revealed mild epigastric tenderness with no palpable abdominal mass. Laboratory data showed no anemia but positive stool occult blood test. Tumor markers including AFP, CEA, and CA 19-9 were all within normal range. Upper GI endoscopy revealed mild esophagitis, Los Angles grade A along with Barrett's esophagus without dysplasia and a 1 cm polyp at the GEJ. A sample was sent for histopathology; the rest of the stomach and duodenum were normal. The patient did not have a previous endoscopy prior to this one.

Infused computed tomography (CT) of the abdomen and chest showed mild GEJ thickness with no evidence of mediastinal or celiac lymphadenopathy and no signs of metastasis. It also demonstrated a large heterogeneously enhancing mass about 6×9.5 cm with central necrosis in the upper abdomen that appears to be originating from the gastric antrum (greater curve). The mass was highly suggestive of GIST based on CT; it was the same mass that was previously

(a)   (b)

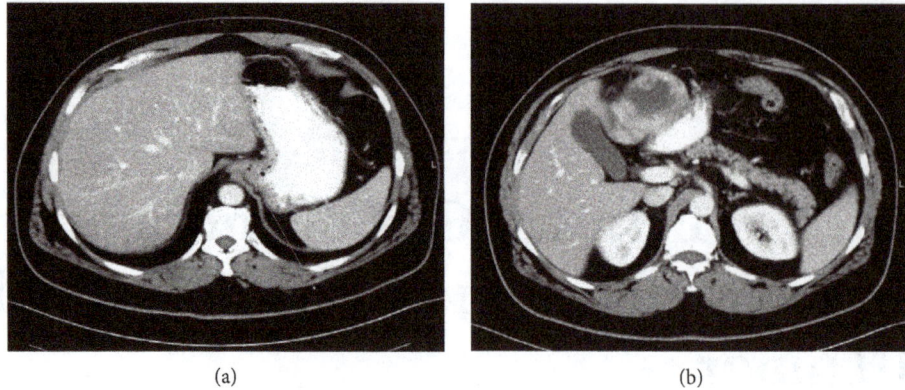

FIGURE 1: Infused CT of the abdomen. (a) Circumferential thickening of the lower esophagus. (b) A large mass with peripheral enhancement and central necrosis most likely representing gastric GIST.

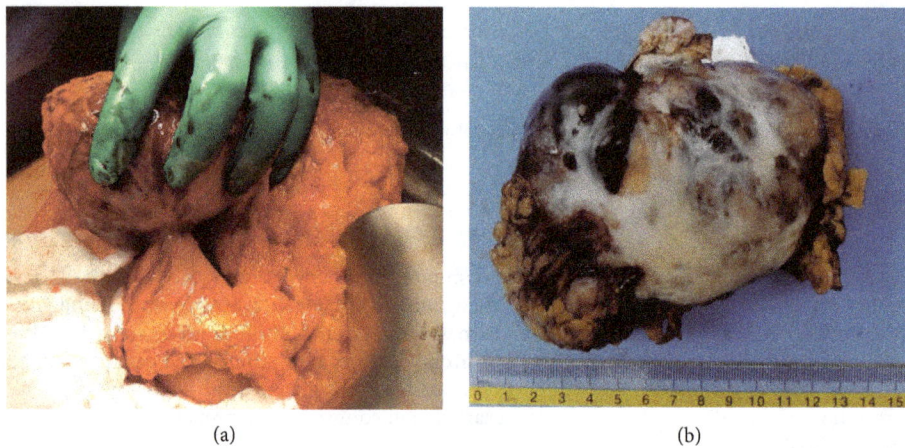

(a)   (b)

FIGURE 2: (a) Intraoperative photography of pedunculated gastric mass. (b) Gross examination of the mass, measures around $10 \times 7 \times 6$ cm.

misdiagnosed as a liver hemangioma (Figure 1). Endoscopic ultrasound confirmed the previous findings. However, no biopsy was attempted due to the risk of bleeding.

Histopathological examination of the GEJ polyp revealed tubulovillous adenoma with elements of adenocarcinoma in situ. The patient was admitted with a provisional diagnosis of early-stage adenocarcinoma of GEJ along with the incidental finding of enlarging gastric GIST. A trial of endoscopic mucosal resection of GEJ polyp was attempted but failed because of the polyp location that created a technical difficulty. Therefore, the patient was taken to the operating room with a plan to perform a wedge resection of the gastric mass and a submucosal resection of GEJ polyp through the same gastric opening. We planned to use frozen section (FS) to document negative margin resection and determine the need for a formal esophagectomy. Intraoperatively; a large ($10 \times 7 \times 6$ cm), extraluminal pedunculated mass was found at the posterior wall of the greater curvature of the stomach (Figure 2). Wedge resection of the gastric mass with negative margins was achieved along with a transgastric submucosal resection of the GEJ polyp. Fortunately, the FS examination of the polyp showed negative margins as well with no evidence of deep invasion. Postoperatively, the patient had a smooth course and was discharged home in a stable

condition. The final pathological examination revealed a GEJ polyp around $1.7 \times 1.4 \times 0.6$ cm. Microscopically, there was a focus of invasive adenocarcinoma involving the superficial submucosa of the polypoid lesion, negative margins, and no lymphovascular invasion (T1a NxM0). Furthermore, the gastric wall mass measured around $10 \times 7 \times 6$ cm with a 2×1.5 cm stalk. Histopathology revealed encapsulated high-grade epithelioid GIST tumor with negative margins (pT3). The mitotic rate of 6/50 HPF and immunohistochemical stains were positive for DOG1 and CD34 but negative for CD117 (c-Kit) (Figure 3).

The final diagnosis was synchronous early-stage GEJ adenocarcinoma and a high-grade gastric GIST. Therefore, the patient was started on adjuvant imatinib treatment, along with endoscopic surveillance every six months and proton pump inhibitors.

3. Discussion

The term GIST was first coined by Mazur and Clark [4]. Although they account for only 0.1–3% of all GI malignancies, GISTs are the most common mesenchymal tumors of the GI tract. They can arise anywhere along the GI tract with a preferred gastric location in about 60% of the cases,

(a)

(b)

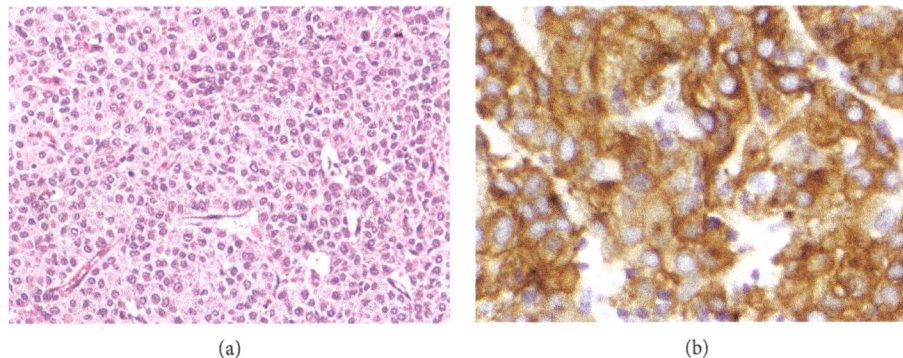

FIGURE 3: Microscopic examination of the gastric mass. (a) Epithelioid GIST of the stomach with rounded nuclei and a clear cytoplasm. (b) Epithelioid GIST strongly staining for DOG1.

followed by the small bowel (25–35%), colon and rectum (5–10%), and esophagus (<5%). They originate from the intestinal cells of Cajal or their precursors [1, 2]. GISTs are composed of either spindle (70%) or epithelioid (20%) cells or mixed. They are usually positive for c-Kit (CD117), CD34, and DOG1 immunostaining [5]. DOG1 was discovered in 2004 and showed strong positivity in different histological types of GIST [6]. It is a highly sensitive and specific marker for detecting GISTs of gastric origin, those of epithelioid morphology and those harboring PDGFRA mutation [6, 7]. Lopes et al. found that DOG1 was positive in 87–94%, while CD117 and CD34 were positive in 74–95% and 60–70% of the examined GIST cases, respectively [8].

GISTs usually arise from the stomach wall and extend inward toward the mucosa or outward toward the serosa, while pedunculated GIST is a unique pattern of growth that has rarely been reported [9, 10]. Many GISTs are diagnosed after the onset of clinical symptoms including abdominal mass, pain, and bleeding [11]. However, occasionally they are discovered incidentally during the evaluation of other clinical entities [12]. GIST and other primary GI tract neoplasms are distinct tumors originating from different cell layers. Synchronous development of such carcinomas is uncommon [13]. The percentage of GIST with other diagnosed neoplasms has been reported to range between 3 and 33% [14]. Most cases involve adenocarcinomas, lymphomas, carcinoids, or leiomyosarcomas of the stomach [15].

Concurrent occurrence of GIST and GEJ neoplasms is rare; only a few cases have been reported in the literature [3]. Spinelli et al. reported a case with squamous cell carcinoma of the lower third of the esophagus with an incidental pathologic diagnosis of a concomitant GIST in the thoracic tract [11].

Similarly, Hsiao et al. reported a 75-year-old man who had a concurrent GIST and adenocarcinoma at the GEJ [3], in addition to a case series by Chan et al. who documented 4 cases with coexistence of GEJ adenocarcinomas and gastric GISTs [16].

Synchronous occurrence of gastric epithelial and stromal tumor raises the question whether such an occurrence is a simple coincidence or the two lesions are related to a certain etiology [17]. Various hypotheses have been proposed regarding this simultaneous presentation, including

gene mutation such as c-Kit mutations, expression of metallothioneins, and *H. pylori* infection that may promote proliferation of different cell lines, while other authors considered the possibility of sporadic occurrence especially in countries that exhibit a high incidence of gastric cancer, such as Japan. Currently, there is no strong data to support such hypotheses [3, 5, 17].

Surgery has been so far the most effective treatment modality for GIST. Resection is usually accomplished with a wedge resection of the stomach, whereas formal gastric resection is occasionally required for larger and difficultly located GISTs [13]. High-grade GISTs, recurrent cases, metastatic diseases, and unresectable tumors can be treated with tyrosine-kinase inhibitors, such as imatinib [18]. While surgical resection remains the mainstay of treatment of resectable GIST, neoadjuvant imatinib may be preferred in a potentially resectable tumor if a reduction in tumor size would significantly decrease the morbidity of surgery. However, proof of the survival and effectiveness of neoadjuvant imatinib has not been sufficiently justified. Tumor biopsy should be performed to confirm the diagnosis and tumor genotype before establishing a neoadjuvant treatment [19].

Most of the GISTs that have been reported with simultaneous neoplasms were small with low mitotic count and very low risk of invasion [5, 14, 16]. Our case seems to be unique in that the GIST was the larger lesion and it was composed of a high-grade epithelioid component with a high mitotic rate. Although the GIST was large, wedge resection of the stomach was enough to achieve negative margins. This was due to its pedunculated nature. Transgastric submucosal resection of the GEJ polyp was accomplished through the same stomach incision, with negative surgical margins. In our case, the GEJ polyp could not be resected endoscopically due to technical difficulties. Laparoscopic surgery would be an option but we decided to proceed with an open surgery because of the large GIST tumor and the difficult position of the GEJ polyp. There was no role for neoadjuvant therapy as the tumor was resectable and no preoperative biopsy was performed. Since the GEJ polyp was an early-stage adenocarcinoma and the GIST a high-risk tumor, therefore the patient was started on adjuvant imatinib treatment along with endoscopic surveillance every six months and proton pump inhibitors.

4. Conclusion

We report a rare case of synchronous gastric GIST and a GEJ polypoid adenocarcinoma. Further studies are needed to analyze the correlation between the simultaneous occurrence of GISTs and other primary GI neoplasms.

Disclosure

An earlier version of this work was presented at the Canadian Surgery Forum, 2016.

References

[1] R. Kaur, S. Bhalla, S. Nundy, and S. Jain, "Synchronous gastric gastrointestinal stromal tumor (GIST) and other primary neoplasms of gastrointestinal tract: report of two cases," *Annals of Gastroenterology*, vol. 26, no. 4, pp. 356–359, 2013.

[2] M. Miettinen and J. Lasota, "Gastrointestinal stromal tumors–definition, clinical, histological, immunohistochemical, and molecular genetic features and differential diagnosis," *Virchows Archiv*, vol. 438, no. 1, pp. 1–12, 2001.

[3] H. H. Hsiao, S. F. Yang, Y. C. Liu, M. J. Yang, and S. F. Lin, "Synchronous gastrointestinal stromal tumor and adenocarcinoma at the gastroesophageal junction," *The Kaohsiung Journal of Medical Sciences*, vol. 25, no. 6, pp. 338–341, 2009.

[4] M. T. Mazur and H. B. Clark, "Gastric stromal tumors. Reappraisal of histogenesis," *The American Journal of Surgical Pathology*, vol. 7, no. 6, pp. 507–520, 1983.

[5] R. Cai, G. Ren, and D. B. Wang, "Synchronous adenocarcinoma and gastrointestinal stromal tumors in the stomach," *World Journal of Gastroenterology*, vol. 19, no. 20, pp. 3117–3123, 2013.

[6] W. Swalchick, R. Shamekh, and M. M. Bui, "Is DOG1 immunoreactivity specific to gastrointestinal stromal tumor?," *Cancer Control*, vol. 22, no. 4, pp. 498–504, 2015.

[7] B. Guler, F. Ozyilmaz, B. Tokuc, N. Can, and E. Tastekin, "Histopathological features of gastrointestinal stromal tumors and the contribution of DOG1 expression to the diagnosis," *Balkan Medical Journal*, vol. 32, no. 4, pp. 388–396, 2015.

[8] L. F. Lopes, R. B. West, L. M. Bacchi, M. van de Rijn, and C. E. Bacchi, "DOG1 for the diagnosis of gastrointestinal stromal tumor (GIST): comparison between 2 different antibodies," *Applied Immunohistochemistry & Molecular Morphology*, vol. 18, no. 4, pp. 333–337, 2010.

[9] G. Cavallaro, A. Sadighi, A. Polistena et al., "Pedunculated giant GISTs of the stomach with exophytic growth: report of two cases," *International Journal of Surgery*, vol. 6, no. 6, pp. e80–e82, 2008.

[10] J. L. Pugh, T. Jie, and A. K. Bhattacharyya, "Pedunculated gastrointestinal stromal tumor (GIST) of the stomach presenting as pancreatic mucinous cystadenocarcinoma: a case report," *Journal of Clinical & Experimental Pathology*, vol. 3, no. 1, 2013.

[11] G. P. Spinelli, E. Miele, F. Tomao et al., "The synchronous occurrence of squamous cell carcinoma and gastrointestinal stromal tumor (GIST) at esophageal site," *World Journal of Surgical Oncology*, vol. 6, no. 1, p. 116, 2008.

[12] S. Ulusan, Z. Koc, and F. Kayaselcuk, "Gastrointestinal stromal tumours: CT findings," *The British Journal of Radiology*, vol. 81, no. 968, pp. 618–623, 2008.

[13] Y. Zhou, X. D. Wu, Q. Shi, and J. Jia, "Coexistence of gastrointestinal stromal tumor, esophageal and gastric cardia carcinomas," *World Journal of Gastroenterology*, vol. 19, no. 12, pp. 2005–2008, 2013.

[14] L. Liszka, E. Zielińska-Pająk, J. Pająk, D. Gołka, and J. Huszno, "Coexistence of gastrointestinal stromal tumors with other neoplasms," *Journal of Gastroenterology*, vol. 42, no. 8, pp. 641–649, 2007.

[15] S. Nakamura, K. Aoyagi, S. Iwanaga, T. Yao, M. Tsuneyoshi, and M. Fujishima, "Synchronous and metachronous primary gastric lymphoma and adenocarcinoma: a clinicopathological study of 12 patients," *Cancer*, vol. 79, no. 6, pp. 1077–1085, 1997.

[16] C. H. F. Chan, J. Cools-Lartigue, V. A. Marcus, L. S. Feldman, and L. E. Ferri, "The impact of incidental gastrointestinal stromal tumours on patients undergoing resection of upper gastrointestinal neoplasms," *Canadian Journal of Surgery*, vol. 55, no. 6, pp. 366–370, 2012.

[17] A. Maiorana, R. Fante, A. Maria Cesinaro, and R. Adriana Fano, "Synchronous occurrence of epithelial and stromal tumors in the stomach: a report of 6 cases," *Archives of Pathology & Laboratory Medicine*, vol. 124, no. 5, pp. 682–686, 2000.

[18] U. I. Chaudhry and R. P. DeMatteo, "Advances in the surgical management of gastrointestinal stromal tumor," *Advances in Surgery*, vol. 45, no. 1, pp. 197–209, 2011.

[19] T. Ishikawa, T. Kanda, H. Kameyama, and T. Wakai, "Neoadjuvant therapy for gastrointestinal stromal tumor," *Translational gastroenterology and hepatology*, vol. 3, p. 3, 2018.

36

Gallbladder Volvulus in a Patient with Type I Choledochal Cyst: A Case Report and Review of the Literature

George Younan, Max Schumm, Fadwa Ali, and Kathleen K. Christians

Division of Surgical Oncology, Department of Surgery, Milwaukee, WI, USA

Correspondence should be addressed to Kathleen K. Christians; kchristi@mcw.edu

Academic Editor: Marcello Picchio

Introduction. Gallbladder volvulus is a rare, potentially fatal condition unless diagnosed and treated early. Choledochal cysts are rare congenital malformations of the biliary tree predisposing to different pathologies and posing the risk of degradation into cholangiocarcinoma and gallbladder cancer. Dealing with both diseases at once has not been published yet in the literature. *Presentation of Case.* We report a case of gallbladder volvulus in an elderly female who happened to have a concomitant type I choledochal cyst. Treatment was achieved with a cholecystectomy and observation and follow-up of the choledochal cyst. *Discussion.* Prompt diagnosis and surgical management of gallbladder volvulus is important to avoid the morbidity and mortality of gangrenous cholecystitis and biliary peritonitis in a frail old population of patients. Precise clinical diagnosis, supplemented with specific imaging clues, helps in the diagnosis. Management of choledochal cysts is also surgical; however the timing of surgery is still a matter of debate. *Conclusion.* We describe in this report the first case of gallbladder volvulus in a patient with a choledochal cyst and propose a management algorithm of a very rare biliary tree pathology combination.

1. Introduction

Gallbladder volvulus is a rare, difficult-to-diagnose clinical condition that presents as acute abdomen and often leads to significant morbidity due to the delay in diagnosis and surgical treatment. Since first reported by Wendel in 1898 as a "floating gallbladder," more than five hundred cases have been reported in the literature with an incidence of approximately 1 in 365,000 hospital admissions [1, 2]. Volvulus of the gallbladder usually presents in elderly frail women in their seventh or eighth decade of life [3]. With prompt surgical intervention, the potential for gallbladder gangrene and perforation can be averted and an excellent prognosis is achieved [4–6]. Choledochal cysts are also uncommon pathological dilations of the biliary tree, first reported in [7]. While being associated with multiple congenital anomalies of the hepatobiliary and pancreatic systems, they have not been reported to increase the likelihood of gallbladder volvulus. Herein we describe a case of successful surgical treatment of gallbladder volvulus in an elderly woman with concomitant Todani type IC choledochal cyst, shedding the light on the

perioperative management of an extremely rare biliary tree disease combination [8].

2. Case Presentation

A 92-year-old woman presented to the emergency room with acute onset of right upper quadrant pain, nausea, and vomiting. She was previously in her usual state of health with minimal medical or surgical comorbidities with the exception of a minor weight loss. Her past medical history is significant for gastroesophageal reflux, history of peptic ulcer disease, and osteoarthritis. She has had cataract surgery in the past in addition to colonic polypectomy for benign polyps a few years prior to her presentation. Her family history was significant for uterine cancer in her mother, without known genetic predisposition. On physical examination, she was hemodynamically normal and the only pertinent finding was tenderness to palpation in her right upper and lower abdominal quadrants. All blood tests were within normal limits including a white blood cell count and liver function

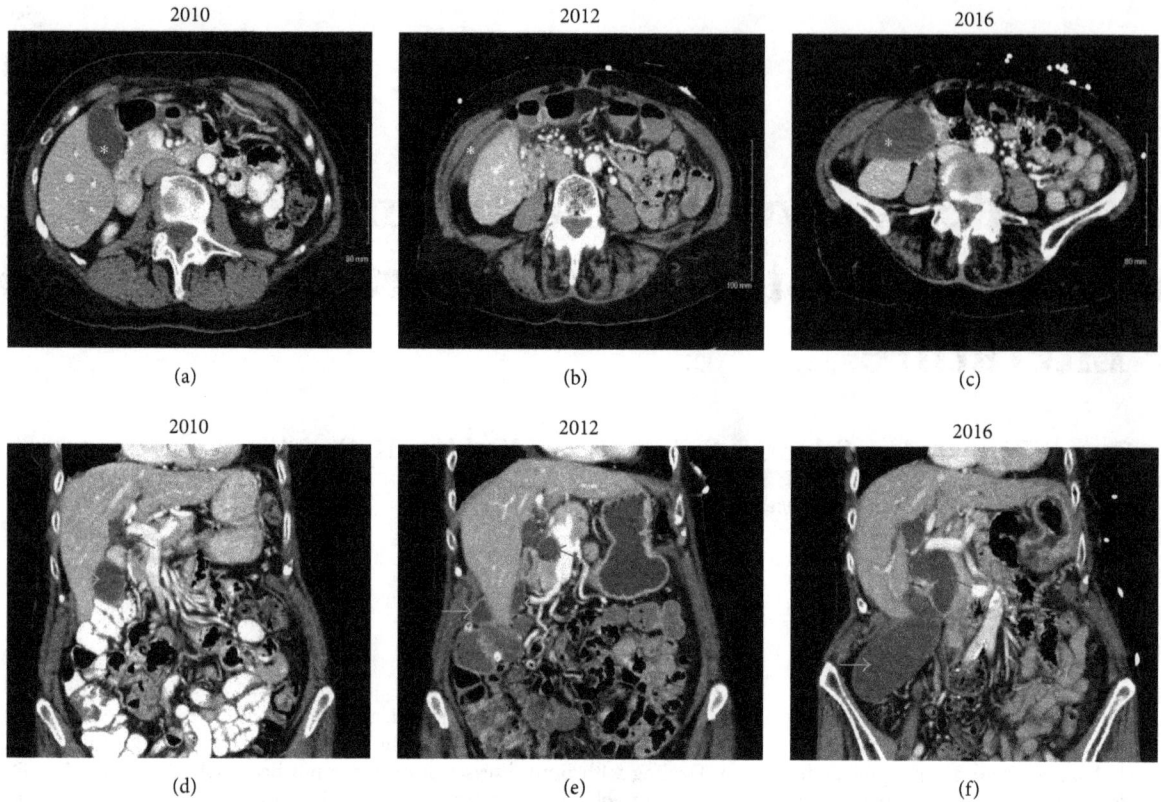

FIGURE 1: (a), (b), and (c) show computed tomography axial images of the abdomen with the gallbladder marked by (∗). Notice the different anatomical positions of the gallbladder over a six-year period. (d), (e), and (f) show computed tomography coronal images of the abdomen showing changes in the anatomical position of the gallbladder (blue arrow); the choledochal cyst (red arrow) is shown to be increasing in size over the same period.

tests. A right upper quadrant ultrasound demonstrated gallbladder distention with mild gallbladder wall thickening, but no evidence of gallstones, sludge, or pericholecystic fluid. A computed tomography (CT) scan demonstrated a markedly dilated extrahepatic biliary ductal system (intrapancreatic common bile duct > 2.5 cm) and a markedly distended gallbladder (Figure 1). The patient was admitted to the hospital for treatment of acute cholecystitis including bowel rest and antibiotics. Given the marked dilation of the intra- and extrahepatic bile ducts an obstructing mass at the head of the pancreas or the distal bile duct had to be ruled out. Magnetic resonance cholangiopancreatography (MRCP) demonstrated a distended gallbladder with wall thickening, edema, and pericholecystic fluid confirming acalculous cholecystitis, with a mention of focal narrowing and wall thickening of the cystic duct. The extrahepatic bile duct had a fusiform dilation measuring 27 mm in the largest dimension (Figure 2). Endoscopic retrograde cholangiopancreatography (ERCP) and an endoscopic ultrasound (EUS) failed to show a pancreatic head mass or distal common bile duct stricture; however the cystic duct did not opacify, suggesting an obstruction in the absence of gallstones. The patient's clinical status did not improve during a short period of observation; she developed increasing abdominal pain and leukocytosis

to 13.5 $e^3/\mu L$. After reviewing of previous CT scans spanning several years, the gallbladder was noted to be located in several different locations adding suspicion for gallbladder torsion to the differential diagnosis (Figure 1). The patient was consented for open cholecystectomy due to the extremely large size of her gallbladder, her concomitant small body habitus, and a relative delay in diagnosis.

At laparotomy, a gangrenous, necrotic gallbladder was identified in the right lower quadrant and was nonadherent to the liver bed. The gallbladder was completely torsed (360 degrees) around the cystic duct and cystic artery. The gallbladder was so mobile that it could be brought out onto the abdominal wall and detorsed; a blood clot was visible in the gallbladder mesentery at the point of torsion. The gallbladder was readily removed following simple ligation of the cystic artery and duct (Figure 3). The choledochal cyst was not addressed given her advanced age and lack of malignancy seen on axial imaging, ERCP, and EUS. Inspection of the specimen revealed significant gallbladder wall thickening and absence of gallstones (Figure 3). The patient recovered without major events and was discharged to a rehabilitation facility on postoperative day four. Final pathology revealed severe acute cholecystitis with transmural necrosis and acute serositis.

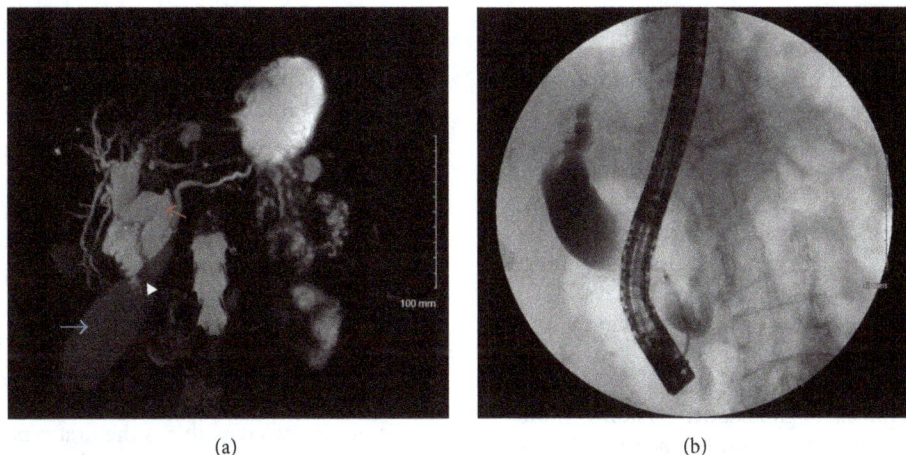

(a) (b)

FIGURE 2: An MRCP image is shown in (a), demonstrating the type 1C choledochal cyst (red arrow), in addition to the distended, torsed gallbladder (blue arrow). Notice the severe narrowing of the gallbladder infundibulum as it joins the dilated bile duct (arrowhead). (b) is an ERCP cholangiogram demonstrating the choledochal cyst without distal common bile duct stricture or stone. The gallbladder did not opacify with contrast due to cystic duct obstruction.

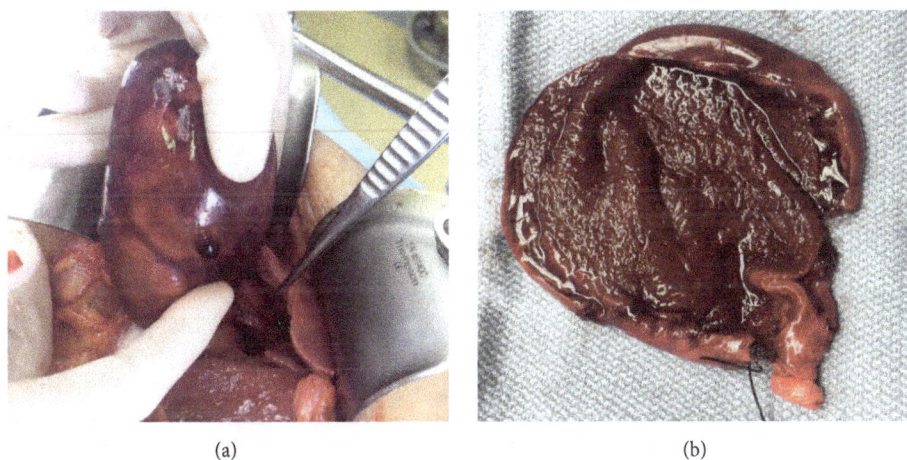

(a) (b)

FIGURE 3: An intraoperative photograph showing the severe distention and discoloration of the gallbladder. This was observed upon entry into the abdomen, the gallbladder was found to be torsed around the cystic duct and cystic artery (shown next to the instrument tip), and there was no other attachment between the gallbladder and the liver. Figure 2(b) shows the gallbladder after it was opened on the back table; no gallstones were found. There was a significant gallbladder wall thickening and necrosis.

3. Discussion

Gallbladder volvulus or torsion occurs when the gallbladder rotates either clockwise or counterclockwise around its mesentery along the axis of the cystic duct and cystic artery causing complete obstruction of blood flow and biliary drainage resulting in acute gangrenous cholecystitis [3]. This condition is extremely rare; it occurs in less than 0.1% patients who undergo urgent cholecystectomies for presumed acute cholecystitis [4]. The incidence of gallbladder volvulus increases with age and peaks in subjects between sixty and eighty years of age. It is more common in women, with a female : male ratio of 3-4 : 1 [2].

The etiology of gallbladder torsion is unknown. Anatomic anomalies, such as an abnormally long mesentery or abnormal fixation of the gallbladder to the liver, can result in a suspended gallbladder allowing it to freely float from the liver bed [3]. It is thought to occur more commonly in the elderly due to the loss of visceral fat, liver atrophy, and increased elasticity that allows the gallbladder to freely hang or "float." Significant peristaltic movements of the stomach, duodenum, and nearby colon, in addition to mechanical predisposition caused by kyphoscoliosis, have been cited in the literature as predisposing factors for gallbladder torsion [9, 10]. Gallstones are considered incidental rather than causative when found in patients with gallbladder volvulus. They are only present in 25–50% of patients with gallbladder torsion, and thus they are unlikely to be the underlying etiology [10].

Patients with gallbladder torsion present with symptoms similar to biliary colic or acute cholecystitis including acute onset of right upper quadrant pain. The acuteness of the presentation depends on whether the volvulus is partial or complete; a partial torsion is followed by spontaneous detorsion and resolution of symptoms, thus presenting like biliary colic, whereas a complete torsion (typically of more than 180°) presents with acute cholecystitis-type symptoms with worsening over the ensuing hours to days [11]. As in our patient, laboratory investigations typically show a normal to elevated white blood cell count. Liver function tests are normal as the common bile duct remains unobstructed [9]. Preoperative diagnosis of gallbladder torsion is difficult since clinical features overlap with other acute gallbladder conditions [12]. The distinction between torsion and acute calculous cholecystitis is important; while cholecystitis can initially be treated conservatively, delay in intervention could prove fatal in the setting of gallbladder torsion. Torsion of the gallbladder has a mortality rate of 6%; none of the reported deaths occurred in patients diagnosed preoperatively [13]. Thus, early diagnosis and prompt intervention can reduce the mortality associated with this condition [13–15].

In the past, gallbladder torsion was typically diagnosed intraoperatively. However, advancements in diagnostic imaging as well as the increased use of imaging in the workup of patients with acute abdomen have led to an increase in preoperative diagnosis [16]. Ultrasonography and computed tomography are the main imaging modalities used for diagnosis, although they are often nonspecific [12]. These imaging approaches may reveal a floating gallbladder without stones, nonadherent to the liver bed, and outside of the usual anatomic fossa [3]. Previous reports have identified computed tomography criteria for identifying gallbladder torsion including (1) fluid collection between the gallbladder and its fossa, (2) the presence of horizontal rather than vertical axis of the gallbladder, (3) the presence of a cystic duct located on the right side of the gallbladder, and (4) the "whirl sign" of a twisted cystic artery with medial deviation of the extrahepatic bile duct [17]. A hepatobiliary iminodiacetic acid (HIDA) scan theoretically shows a characteristic, though not sensitive, "bull's eye" appearance of the torsed gallbladder [18]. T2-weighted MRI images are useful for evaluating necrosis of the gallbladder wall as in cases of torsion [19, 20]. More recent reports have suggested the use of chronological and sequential diagnostic imaging as a means of diagnosing gallbladder torsion [21]. The present case illustrates the usefulness of comparing imaging from prior admissions in order to make the preoperative diagnosis of gallbladder torsion, which can be appreciated retrospectively (Figure 1). Computed tomography axial images from four and six years priorly illustrate the mobile and floating nature of our patient's gallbladder; these can be helpful when patients present with atypical symptoms, poor response to antibiotics, or acalculous cholecystitis.

Early diagnosis and prompt surgical intervention with detorsion and cholecystectomy are important to avoid complications of perforation and bilious peritonitis [22]. The use of transhepatic cholecystostomy tube for management of gallbladder volvulus is not recommended due to the extrahepatic location of the gallbladder and the necrotic gallbladder wall, both of which increase the likelihood of bile spillage and peritonitis. While laparoscopic detorsion and cholecystectomy is effective in the management of gallbladder torsion, we chose open cholecystectomy due to the very large size of the gallbladder reaching a pelvic location in a patient with an extremely small body habitus (no room for laparoscopic instrumentation/visualization) [23, 24]. Laparoscopic cholecystectomy and dissection of the critical view of safety in gallbladder torsion patients id usually straightforward given the lack of a cystic plate attaching the gallbladder to the liver [12, 23].

To our knowledge, this is the first report in the literature that describes the presence of gallbladder torsion in a patient with a choledochal cyst. Choledochal cysts have been associated with other anomalies within the pancreaticobiliary tree including multiseptated gallbladder, heterotopic pancreas, and pancreatic divisum, but they have not been reported to predispose to volvulus of the gallbladder [8, 25]. Choledochal cysts are classified into five types based on the Alonso-Lej modification of the initial Todani classification [26]. Our patient had a type I choledochal cyst which is the most common cyst type [7]. The presence of a choledochal cyst is considered an indication for surgical resection as many of these become symptomatic, presenting with recurrent cholangitis or pancreatitis and harbor a risk of synchronous cholangiocarcinoma [27, 28]. In a large, multi-institutional western study that included 394 patients, cyst excision to include extrahepatic bile duct resection and hepaticoenterostomy was the standard of surgical care and completed in 80.3% of patients [7]. Malignancy was found in 9.1% and at follow-up, 3.3% of patients had cancer recurrence with a median survival of 3.5 years [7]. This study reconfirmed prophylactic surgical resection of choledochal cysts.

Due to the rarity of this combination of gallbladder torsion and choledochal cyst, a hepatobiliary surgeon should be involved from the outset. Prompt gallbladder detorsion and cholecystectomy is the standard of care for gallbladder volvulus regardless of the timing of diagnosis (pre- or intraoperatively). Extrapolation from common surgical practice precludes excision of the choledochal cyst and construction of a hepaticoenterostomy in the setting of an acutely inflamed and potentially infected field; thus laparoscopic cholecystectomy should be done first. The patient can then be brought back electively for choledochal cyst resection. In cases of acute cholecystitis without gallbladder torsion, conservative management of cholecystitis can be attempted with antibiotics with or without percutaneous cholecystostomy drainage which may then allow for a one-stage procedure (cholecystectomy and choledochal cyst resection). We suggest an algorithm extrapolated from literature data suggesting a plan of action when a gallbladder volvulus is encountered in a patient with choledochal cysts (Figure 4). It is based on the patient's clinical status and the chronicity of the volvulus in addition to the cyst type, as the procedures needed to treat choledochal cysts vary from a simple ERCP/sphincterotomy

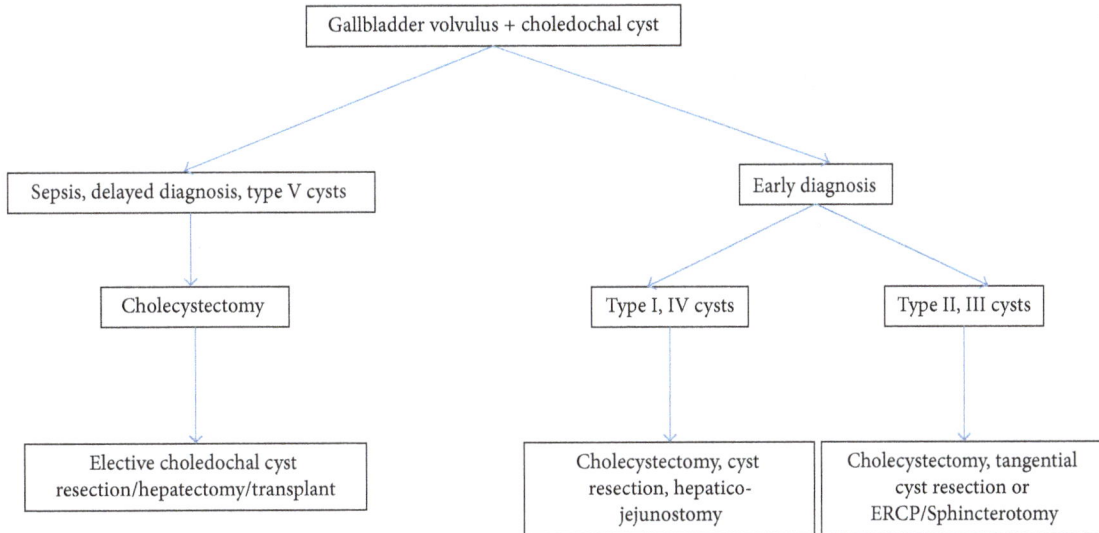

FIGURE 4: Algorithm for treatment of gallbladder volvulus in patients with concomitant choledochal cysts.

in choledochoceles (Todani type III cysts), reaching liver transplant in Caroli's disease (Todani type V cysts).

4. Conclusion

Gallbladder volvulus and choledochal cysts are two very rare entities of the biliary tree. Volvulus should be considered in the elderly female patients with symptoms suggestive of sudden onset of acute acalculous cholecystitis with imaging characteristics pointing towards a free-floating gallbladder. While gallbladder volvulus requires a high index of suspicion and early surgical intervention to avoid significant morbidity and mortality in a frail patient population, choledochal cysts can be dealt with electively taking into account their symptoms and risk for malignancy relative to age.

References

[1] A. V. Wendel, "VI. A case of floating gall-bladder and kidney complicated by cholelithiasis, with perforation of the gall-bladder," *Annals of Surgery*, vol. 27, no. 2, pp. 199–202, 1898.

[2] D. J. Reilly, G. Kalogeropoulos, and D. Thiruchelvam, "Torsion of the gallbladder: a systematic review," *HPB*, vol. 14, no. 10, pp. 669–672, 2012.

[3] N. J. Mouawad, B. Crofts, R. Streu, R. Desrochers, and B. C. Kimball, "Acute gallbladder torsion—a continued pre-operative diagnostic dilemma," *World Journal of Emergency Surgery*, vol. 6, no. 1, article 13, 2011.

[4] A. Nakao, T. Matsuda, S. Funabiki et al., "Gallbladder torsion: case report and review of 245 cases reported in the Japanese literature," *Journal of Hepato-Biliary-Pancreatic Surgery*, vol. 6, no. 4, pp. 418–421, 1999.

[5] S. Y. Kim and J. T. Moore, "Volvulus of the gallbladder: laparoscopic detorsion and removal," *Surgical Endoscopy*, vol. 17, no. 11, p. 1849, 2003.

[6] H. A. Amarillo, E. D. Pirchi, and M. E. Mihura, "Complete gallbladder and cystic pedicle torsion. Laparoscopic diagnosis and treatment," *Surgical Endoscopy*, vol. 17, no. 5, pp. 832–833, 2003.

[7] K. C. Soares, Y. Kim, G. Spolverato et al., "Presentation and clinical outcomes of choledochal cysts in children and adults: a multi-institutional analysis," *JAMA Surgery*, vol. 150, no. 6, pp. 577–584, 2015.

[8] T. Todani, Y. Watanabe, M. Narusue, K. Tabuchi, and K. Okajima, "Congenital bile duct cysts: classification, operative procedures, and review of thirty-seven cases including cancer arising from choledochal cyst," *The American Journal of Surgery*, vol. 134, no. 2, pp. 263–269, 1977.

[9] P. C. Garciavilla, J. F. Alvarez, and G. V. Uzqueda, "Diagnosis and laparoscopic approach to gallbladder torsion and cholelithiasis," *Journal of the Society of Laparoendoscopic Surgeons*, vol. 14, no. 1, pp. 147–151, 2010.

[10] A. C. Stieber and J. J. Bauer, "Volvulus of the gallbladder," *The American Journal of Gastroenterology*, vol. 78, no. 2, pp. 96–98, 1983.

[11] A. A. Shaikh, A. Charles, S. Domingo, and G. Schaub, "Gallbladder volvulus: report of two original cases and review of the literature," *The American Surgeon*, vol. 71, no. 1, pp. 87–89, 2005.

[12] E. A. Boonstra, B. van Etten, T. R. Prins, E. Sieders, and B. L. van Leeuwen, "Torsion of the gallbladder," *Journal of Gastrointestinal Surgery*, vol. 16, no. 4, pp. 882–884, 2012.

[13] M. S. Vedanayagam, I. Nikolopoulos, G. Janakan, and A. El-Gaddal, "Gallbladder volvulus: a case of mimicry," *BMJ Case Reports*, vol. 2013, 2013.

[14] G. Janakan, A. A. Ayantunde, and H. Hoque, "Acute gallbladder torsion: an unexpected intraoperative finding," *World Journal of Emergency Surgery*, vol. 3, no. 1, article 9, 2008.

[15] G. C. Christoudias, "Gallbladder volvulus with gangrene. Case report and review of the literature," *Journal of the Society of Laparoendoscopic Surgeons*, vol. 1, no. 2, pp. 167–170, 1997.

[16] E. Hinoshita, T. Nishizaki, K. Wakasugi et al., "Pre-operative imaging can diagnose torsion of the gallbladder: report of a case," *Hepato-Gastroenterology*, vol. 46, no. 28, pp. 2212–2215, 1999.

[17] Y. Tajima, N. Tsuneoka, T. Kuroki, and T. Kanematsu, "Gallbladder torsion showing a 'whirl sign' on a multidetector computed tomography scan," *American Journal of Surgery*, vol. 197, no. 1, pp. e9–e10, 2009.

[18] G. J. Wang, M. Colln, J. Crossett, and R. A. Holmes, "'Bulls-eye' image of gallbladder volvulus," *Clinical Nuclear Medicine*, vol. 12, no. 3, pp. 231–232, 1987.

[19] M. Fukuchi, K. Nakazato, H. Shoji, H. Naitoh, and H. Kuwano, "Torsion of the gallbladder diagnosed by magnetic resonance cholangiopancreatography," *International Surgery*, vol. 97, no. 3, pp. 235–238, 2012.

[20] M. Usui, S. Matsuda, H. Suzuki, and Y. Ogura, "Preoperative diagnosis of gallbladder torsion by magnetic resonance cholangiopancreatography," *Scandinavian Journal of Gastroenterology*, vol. 35, no. 2, pp. 218–222, 2000.

[21] T. Koyanagi and K. Sato, "Complete gallbladder torsion diagnosed with sequential computed tomography scans: a case report," *Journal of Medical Case Reports*, vol. 6, article 289, 2012.

[22] B. J. Pottorf, L. Alfaro, and H. W. Hollis, "A clinician's guide to the diagnosis and management of gallbladder volvulus," *The Permanente Journal*, vol. 17, no. 2, pp. 80–83, 2013.

[23] Y. K. Sunder, S. P. Akhilesh, G. Raman, S. Deborshi, and M. H. Shantilal, "Laparoscopic management of a two staged gall bladder torsion," *World Journal of Gastrointestinal Surgery*, vol. 7, no. 12, pp. 403–407, 2015.

[24] T. Nguyen, A. Geraci, and J. J. Bauer, "Laparoscopic cholecystectomy for gallbladder volvulus," *Surgical Endoscopy*, vol. 9, no. 5, pp. 519–521, 1995.

[25] K. C. Soares, D. J. Arnaoutakis, I. Kamel et al., "Choledochal cysts: presentation, clinical differentiation, and management," *Journal of the American College of Surgeons*, vol. 219, no. 6, pp. 1167–1180, 2014.

[26] F. Alonso-Lej, W. B. Rever Jr., and D. J. Pessagno, "Congenital choledochal cyst, with a report of 2, and an analysis of 94, cases," *International Abstracts of Surgery*, vol. 108, no. 1, pp. 1–30, 1959.

[27] P. A. Lipsett, H. A. Pitt, P. M. Colombani, J. K. Boitnott, and J. L. Cameron, "Choledochal cyst disease: a changing pattern of presentation," *Annals of Surgery*, vol. 220, no. 5, pp. 644–652, 1994.

[28] B. H. Edil, K. Olino, and J. L. Cameron, "The current management of choledochal cysts," *Advances in Surgery*, vol. 43, no. 1, pp. 221–232, 2009.

37

Multiple Gastric Gastrointestinal Stromal Tumors in a Patient with Neurofibromatosis Type 1

Makoto Tomatsu,[1] Jun Isogaki,[1] Takahiro Watanabe,[1] Kiyoshige Yajima,[1] Takuya Okumura,[1] Kimihiro Yamashita,[1] Kenji Suzuki,[1] Akihiro Kawabe,[1] Akira Komiyama,[2] and Seiichi Hirota[3]

[1]*Department of Surgery, Fujinomiya City General Hospital, 3-1 Nishiki-cho, Fujinomiya, Shizuoka 418-0076, Japan*
[2]*Department of Diagnostic Pathology, Fujinomiya City General Hospital, 3-1 Nishiki-cho, Fujinomiya, Shizuoka 418-0076, Japan*
[3]*Department of Surgical Pathology, Hyogo College of Medicine, 1-1 Mukogawa-cho, Nishinomiya, Hyogo 663-8501, Japan*

Correspondence should be addressed to Makoto Tomatsu; tomatsumakoto@gmail.com

Academic Editor: Tahsin Colak

Gastrointestinal stromal tumors (GISTs) are relatively common in neurofibromatosis type 1 (NF 1) patients. Approximately 90% of GISTs associated with NF 1 are located in the small intestine, while sporadic GISTs are most commonly located in the stomach. Here we report an extremely rare case of an NF 1 patient with multiple gastric GITs (90 or more) but without multiple small intestinal tumors. A 63-year-old female patient who had a history of NF 1 underwent surgery for a gastric neuroendocrine tumor and gastric submucosal tumor (SMT). During the operation, multiple small nodules were identified on the serosal surface of the upper stomach. SMT and multiple nodules on the serosal surface were diagnosed as GISTs consisting of spindle cells positive for KIT, CD34, and DOG-1. Both GIST and the normal gastric mucosa showed no mutations not only in the c-*kit* gene (exons 8, 9, 11, 13, and 17) but also in the *PDGFRA* gene (exons 12, 14, and 18). This patient is being followed up without the administration of a tyrosine kinase inhibitor.

1. Introduction

Neurofibromatosis type 1 (NF 1) is one of the most common autosomal dominant traits, with a rate of occurrence of approximately 1 in 4000 in the general population [1]. The cause of NF 1 is a mutation in the *NF 1* gene that encodes neurofibromin. Because neurofibromin inhibits Ras oncogene activity, the loss of neurofibromin function results in Ras activation and subsequent tumor formation [2].

Gastrointestinal stromal tumors (GISTs) are relatively common with prevalences estimated to vary from 5% to 30% in NF 1 patients [1]. Approximately 90% of GISTs associated with NF 1 are located in the small intestine, and only 5.4% are located in the stomach [3].

In this paper, an extremely rare case of multiple gastric GISTs in an NF 1 patient is reported.

2. Case Report

A 63-year-old female was examined for dysphagia. She and her father had a history of NF 1. The patient presented with multiple neurofibromas and some cafe-au-lait spots all over her body (Figure 1(a)).

Upper gastrointestinal endoscopy revealed a neuroendocrine tumor (NET) located on the posterior side of the upper gastric wall and a submucosal tumor (SMT) located on the greater curvature of the middle gastric wall (Figures 1(b) and 1(c)). Computed tomography (CT) indicated only SMT, which was approximately 30 mm in diameter and had a smooth surface (Figure 1(d)). CT did not show NET or any other lesion.

Preoperative diagnosis was a gastric NET in combination with a gastric SMT suspected to be GIST. Laparoscopic

(a)

(b)

(c)

(d)

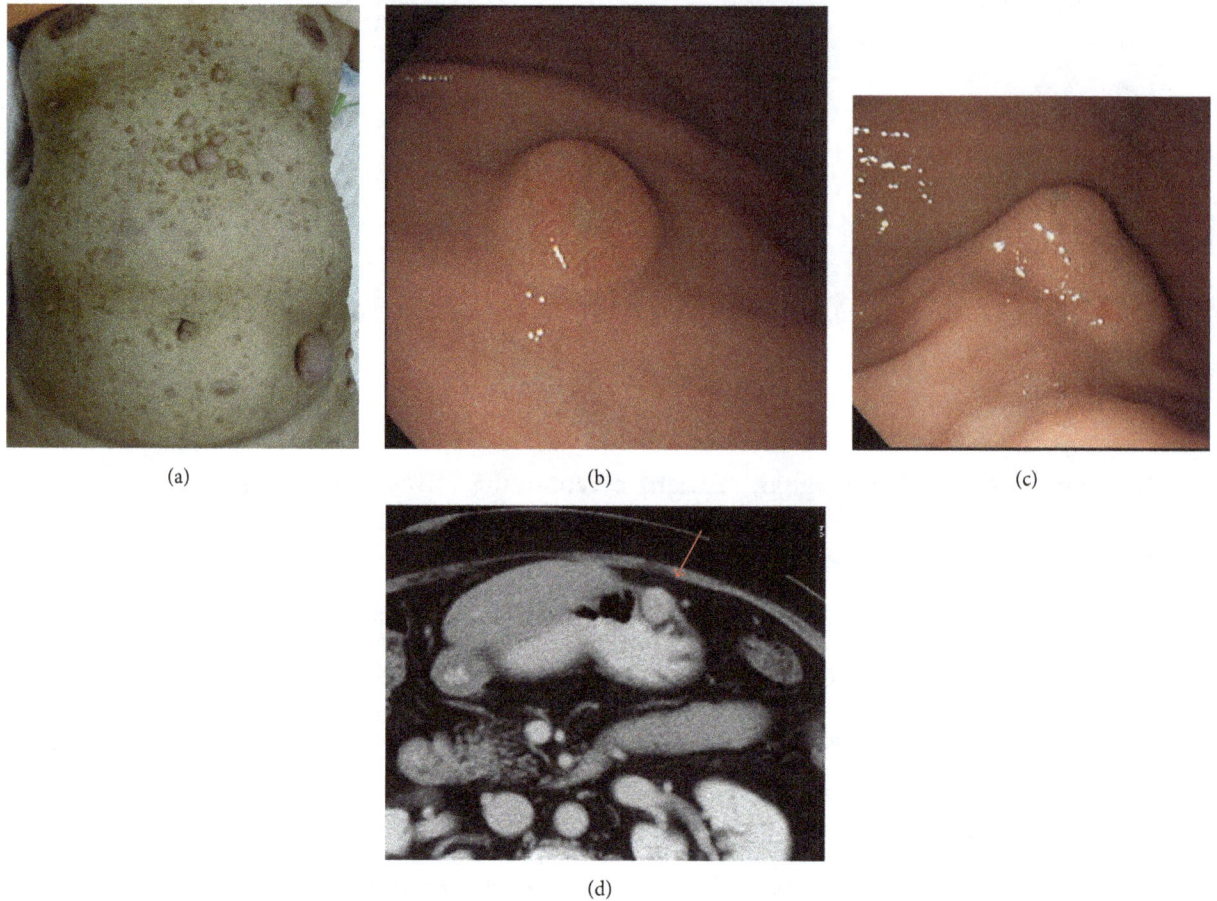

FIGURE 1: (a) There are multiple neurofibromas and some cafe-au-lait spots all over the body skin. (b) Upper gastrointestinal endoscopy shows neuroendocrine tumor located on posterior side of upper gastric wall. The size was about 10 mm. (c) And submucosal tumor located on greater curvature side of middle gastric wall. The size was about 30 mm. (d) Computed tomography showed only a SMT (arrow); the size was about 30 mm and the surface was smooth. Other lesions could not be pointed out.

proximal gastrectomy with D1+ lymph node dissection for NET and partial gastrectomy for SMT were planned.

During the operation, multiple small nodules were identified on the serosal surface of the upper stomach (Figure 2). Most nodules were resected by proximal gastrectomy. There were no apparent abnormalities on the serosal surface of the small intestine or colorectum.

The result of a histopathological examination of the upper gastric lesion was consistent with NET G1; the MIB-1 index was 2%, without any lymph node metastases. In contrast, SMT of the middle gastric wall contained two intramural lesions (1.4 × 1.2 cm and 0.8 × 0.6 cm). These SMTs were compatible with GISTs; three mitotic figures in 50 HPF were seen. There were no findings indicating tumor rupture in these two lesions (Figure 3(a)). There were 90 or more small nodules on the gastric serosal surface, which were diagnosed as GISTs. These consisted of spindle cells positive for KIT (CD117), CD34, and DOG-1 (Figures 3(b) and 4). All these small nodules located under the serosa confirm that they were not a peritoneal metastasis.

Analyses of the c-kit gene and platelet-derived growth factor receptor α (PDGFRA) gene were performed in one

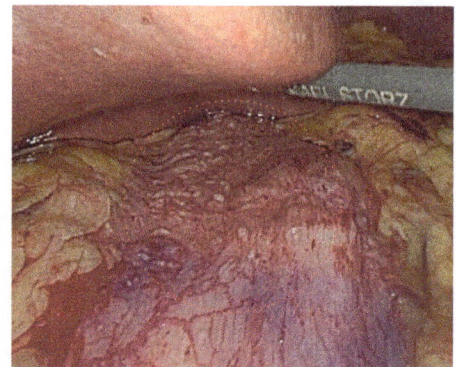

FIGURE 2: Intraoperative picture. There were multiple small nodules on serosal surface of upper stomach.

GIST. There were no alterations in either the c-kit gene (exons 8, 9, 11, 13, and 17) or PDGFRA gene (exons 12, 14, and 18). The patient's normal gastric mucosal tissue also showed no mutations in the c-kit gene (exons 8, 9, 11, 13, and 17) or PDGFRA gene (exons 12, 14, and 18), confirming that this was

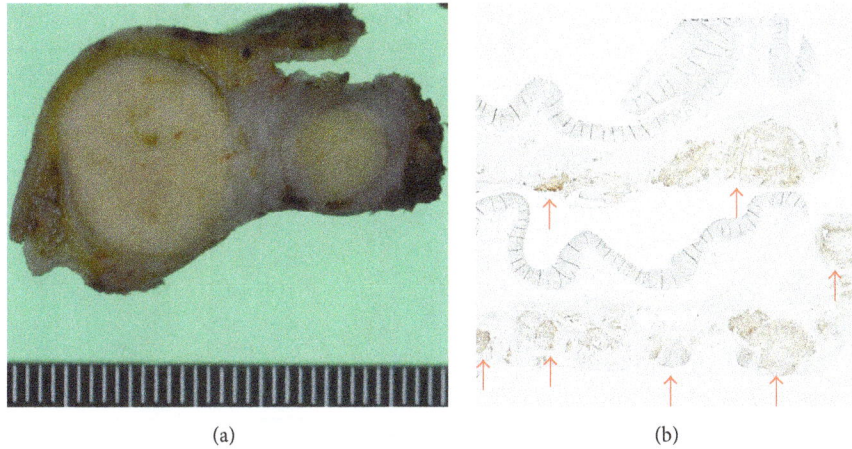

(a)

(b)

FIGURE 3: (a) SMT of the middle gastric wall contained two intramural lesions (1.4 × 1.2 cm and 0.8 × 0.6 cm). There were no findings indicating tumor rupture in these two lesions. (b) Multiple nodules located in subserosa of upper stomach. These nodules were positive for KIT (CD117).

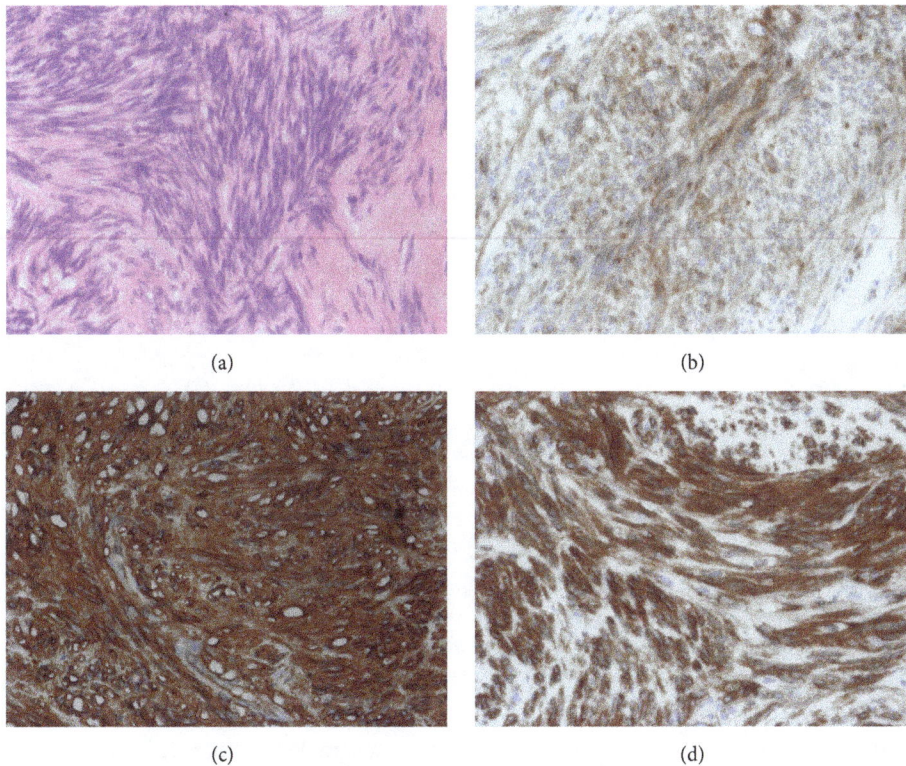

(a)

(b)

(c)

(d)

FIGURE 4: Histopathological analysis. (a) The tumors consisted of spindle cells. (b) Positive for KIT (CD117). (c) Positive for CD34. (d) Positive for DOG-1.

not a case of familial GISTs with a germline mutation in the c-*kit* or *PDGFRA* gene.

The patient is being followed up without the administration of a tyrosine kinase inhibitor.

3. Discussion

GIST is the most common mesenchymal tumor in the digestive tract, originating from the interstitial cell of Cajal [4]. Sporadic GISTs are most commonly located in the stomach (60–70% of cases), followed by the small intestine (20–25%) and other locations [5]. In sporadic GISTs, 85–90% of cases have mutations in the c-*kit* gene. In addition, 35–62.5% of cases without c-*kit* gene mutations have mutations in the *PDGFRA* gene [6].

On the other hand, GISTs in NF 1 patients differ from sporadic GISTs in several aspects. A PubMed search of the literature revealed 126 case reports concerning GISTs associated with NF 1 (keywords: "Gastrointestinal stromal tumor" and "Neurofibromatosis 1"; language: English). Only

TABLE 1: Cases of gastric GISTs in patients with NF 1.

Case number	Age	Sex	Total number of GISTs	Site	Number of GISTs	Size (cm)	Genetic analysis		Reference number
							c-kit	PDGFRA	
1	32	F	4	Stomach	ND	2–10	NE	NE	[7]
				Jejunum	ND				
2	82	F	Numerous	Stomach	ND	0.5–2.5	WT	WT	[7]
				Small intestine	ND				
				Colon	ND				
3	77	M	5	Stomach	ND	0.3–2.0	WT	WT	[7]
				Esophagus	ND				
				Jejunum	ND				
				Ileum	ND				
4	64	M	>100	Stomach	ND	0.1–3.5	WT	WT	[7]
				Small intestine	ND				
				Colon	ND				
5	58	M	5	Stomach	2	0.3, 3.0	WT	WT	[8]
				ND	3	ND			
6	64	F	Multiple	Stomach	1	11	WT	WT	[9]
				Small intestine	Multiple	Maximum 3.5			
7	40	F	1	Stomach	1	2.5	WT	WT	[10]
8	67	M	1	Stomach	1	Voluminous	NE	NE	[11]
9	71	M	1	Stomach	1	3.6	NE	NE	[3]
10	38	F	1	Stomach	1	8	NE	NE	[12]
11	59	F	4	Stomach	2	0.2, 0.5	WT	WT	[1]
				Jejunum	2	0.8, 3.0			

ND: not described, NE: not examined, and WT: wild type.

11 (8.7%) patients had gastric GISTs (Table 1) [1, 3, 7–12], of whom seven had multiple GISTs in the stomach and four had only one gastric GIST. Six patients also had GISTs in the small intestine. One patient had GISTs on another site, but with no description of the site involved. In contrast, 120 (95.2%) patients had GISTs in the small intestine, including the duodenum. In addition, there were two or more GISTs in 82 (65.1%) patients. Mutations in the c-kit gene were detected in only 2 of 51 patients (3.9%), and those in the PDGFRA gene were not detected (0/47). Thus, typical GISTs associated with NF 1 are located in the small intestine, show multiplicity, and have a mutation in neither the c-kit nor PDGFRA gene. Our NF 1 case with more than 90 GISTs on the serosal surface of the stomach is extremely unusual. To the best of our knowledge, there are no similar case reports.

GISTs associated with NF 1 are generally of low grade [3]. Our NF 1 case was also of low grade, with a maximum GIST size of 1.4 cm and with 3/50 HPF mitotic figures. In addition, GISTs without a mutation in the c-kit/PDGFRA gene appear to respond less well to a tyrosine kinase inhibitor than GISTs with this mutation. Therefore, a tyrosine kinase inhibitor may show no effect on GISTs associated with NF 1 [13]. In our case, left lesions or recurrences on the residual stomach were the major concerns. Nevertheless, we did not perform adjuvant chemotherapy with a tyrosine kinase inhibitor because the resected GISTs were low risk and a response to a tyrosine kinase inhibitor could not be guaranteed. For GISTs with NF 1, the importance of a routine follow-up is unknown. Our plan of follow-up for our patient is CT every 6 months for 5 years. When recurrences are detected, we will observe them unless they cause some symptoms such as obstruction or bleeding because multiple and metachronal recurrences are anticipated.

Familial and multiple GISTs caused by germline mutations in the c-kit or PDGFRA gene have been reported [14]. In such situations, multiple GISTs develop in both the stomach and the small intestine. All multiple GISTs have the same mutation in the c-kit or PDGFRA gene. Moreover, patients display the same mutation, even in the normal tissue. In the current case report, there was no mutation in the c-kit or PDGFRA gene not only in the GIST tissue but also in the normal gastric mucosa. This indicates that this is not a case of familial GISTs caused by germline mutations in the c-kit or PDGFRA gene.

In summary, we encountered an extremely rare case of multiple gastric GISTs associated with NF 1.

Competing Interests

The authors declare that there are no competing interests regarding the publication of this paper.

References

[1] M. Vlenterie, U. Flucke, L. C. Hofbauer et al., "Pheochromocytoma and gastrointestinal stromal tumors in patients with neurofibromatosis type I," *The American Journal of Medicine*, vol. 126, no. 2, pp. 174–180, 2013.

[2] A. Gorgel, D. D. Cetinkaya, F. Salgur et al., "Coexistence of gastrointestinal stromal tumors (GISTs) and pheochromocytoma in three cases of neurofibromatosis type 1 (NF1) with a review of the literature," *Internal Medicine*, vol. 53, no. 16, pp. 1783–1789, 2014.

[3] P. F. Salvi, L. Lorenzon, S. Caterino, L. Antolino, M. S. Antonelli, and G. Balducci, "Gastrointestinal stromal tumors associated with neurofibromatosis 1: a single centre experience and systematic review of the literature including 252 cases," *International Journal of Surgical Oncology*, vol. 2013, Article ID 398570, 8 pages, 2013.

[4] S. Hirota, K. Isozaki, Y. Moriyama et al., "Gain-of-function mutations of c-kit in human gastrointestinal stromal tumors," *Science*, vol. 279, no. 5350, pp. 577–580, 1998.

[5] M. Miettinen and J. Lasota, "Gastrointestinal stromal tumors—definition, clinical, histological, immunohistochemical, and molecular genetic features and differential diagnosis," *Virchows Archiv*, vol. 438, no. 1, pp. 1–12, 2001.

[6] K. Isozaki and S. Hirota, "Gain-of-function mutations of receptor tyrosine kinases in gastrointestinal stromal tumors," *Current Genomics*, vol. 7, no. 8, pp. 469–475, 2006.

[7] J. Andersson, H. Sihto, J. M. Meis-Kindblom, H. Joensuu, N. Nupponen, and L.-G. Kindblom, "NF1-associated gastrointestinal stromal tumors have unique clinical, phenotypic, and genotypic characteristics," *The American Journal of Surgical Pathology*, vol. 29, no. 9, pp. 1170–1176, 2005.

[8] Y. Takazawa, S. Sakurai, Y. Sakuma et al., "Gastrointestinal stromal tumors of neurofibromatosis type I (von Recklinghausen's disease)," *The American Journal of Surgical Pathology*, vol. 29, no. 6, pp. 755–763, 2005.

[9] M. Miettinen, J. F. Fetsch, L. H. Sobin, and J. Lasota, "Gastrointestinal stromal tumors in patients with neurofibromatosis 1: a clinicopathologic and molecular genetic study of 45 cases," *The American Journal of Surgical Pathology*, vol. 30, no. 1, pp. 90–96, 2006.

[10] B. Liegl, J. L. Hornick, C. L. Corless, and C. D. M. Fletcher, "Monoclonal antibody DOG1.1 Shows higher sensitivity than KIT in the diagnosis of gastrointestinal stromal tumors, including unusual subtypes," *American Journal of Surgical Pathology*, vol. 33, no. 3, pp. 437–446, 2009.

[11] G. Cavallaro, U. Basile, A. Polistena et al., "Surgical management of abdominal manifestations of type 1 neurofibromatosis: experience of a single center," *American Surgeon*, vol. 76, no. 4, pp. 389–396, 2010.

[12] S. K. Swain, R. Smile, T. Arul, and D. David, "Unusual presentation of gastrointestinal stromal tumor of stomach in neurofibromatosis type 1: a case report," *Indian Journal of Surgery*, vol. 75, no. 1, pp. 398–400, 2013.

[13] K. Kinoshita, S. Hirota, K. Isozaki et al., "Absence of c-kit gene mutations in gastrointestinal stromal tumours from neurofibromatosis type 1 patients," *The Journal of Pathology*, vol. 202, no. 1, pp. 80–85, 2004.

[14] K. Yamanoi, K. Higuchi, H. Kishimoto et al., "Multiple gastrointestinal stromal tumors with novel germline c-kit gene mutation, K642T, at exon 13," *Human Pathology*, vol. 45, no. 4, pp. 884–888, 2014.

38

Minimally Invasive Treatment of Sporadic Burkitt's Lymphoma Causing Ileocaecal Invagination

Paolo Panaccio [ID],[1] Michele Fiordaliso,[1] Domenica Testa,[1] Lorenzo Mazzola,[2] Mariangela Battilana,[1] Roberto Cotellese,[1] and Federico Selvaggi[2]

[1]*Department of Medical and Oral Sciences and Biotechnologies, "G. d'Annunzio" University, Chieti, Italy*
[2]*General Surgery Unit, Renzetti Hospital, Lanciano, Italy*

Correspondence should be addressed to Paolo Panaccio; paolo.panaccio@gmail.com

Academic Editor: Robert Stein

Introduction. Primary NHL (non-Hodgkin lymphoma) of the colon represents only 0.2% to 1.2% of all colonic malignancies. Burkitt's lymphoma (BL) is usually a disease reported in children and young people, most of them associated with EBV or HIV infection. We describe a rare case of intestinal obstruction due to sporadic Burkitt's lymphoma causing ileocaecal invagination explaining our experience *Methods.* A 31-year-old man presented with diffuse colic pain and weight loss. Clinical examination revealed an abdominal distension with pain in the right iliac fossa. Colonoscopy documented a caecal large lesion with ulcerated mucosa. Computed tomography (CT) have shown a 60×50 mm right colic parietal lesion with signs of ileocolic intussusception. *Results.* Laparoscopic right hemicolectomy was performed. Postoperative period was uneventful. CD20+ high-grade B-cell Burkitt's lymphoma was confirmed by immunohistochemistry (CD20+, CD79+, and CD10+) and FISH test (t (8;14) (q24; q32). The patient was subsequently treated with adjuvant combination chemotherapy (Hyper-CVAD) and is alive and disease-free at 8 months follow-up. *Discussion.* Adult sporadic Burkitt's lymphoma (BL) causing intestinal obstruction due to ileocaecal intussusception is an extremely rare occurrence and a diagnostic dilemma. Despite the surgical approach is selected based on patient's conditions and surgeon's expertise, minimally invasive method could be preferred.

1. Introduction

Burkitt's lymphoma (BL) is usually viewed in children and young adults and rarely in middle-aged adults. BL is caused by chromosomal translocation and deregulation of the c-MYC oncogene; in nonendemic BL regions, it manifests highly aggressive and fast-growing B-cell malignancy. BL cause 5% of all bowel intussusception and 1% of all bowel obstruction. The localization of BL in the ileocaecal region is rare, especially in adults [1]. Intussusception in adults is often associated with organic pathology. We describe a case of BL-related ileocaecal intussusception in a young man successfully managed by laparoscopic-assisted surgery.

2. Case Report

A 31-year-old man without previous medical history, except for a posttraumatic pneumothorax, presented to our emergency department with a 2-week history of diffuse colic pain and weight loss. Physical examination showed abdominal distension, a localized pain, and a palpable mass in the right lower quadrant. Laboratory studies were normal (WBC $4.99 \times 10^3/\mu L$; HGB 9.9 g/dL; HIV-EBV tests were negative; CEA and CA 19–9 were negative). A computed tomography (CT) of the abdomen showed a three-layered structure giving the characteristic target-shaped appearance in the ascending colon. Moreover, the CT showed a hyperdense 60×50 mm right colic parietal lesion, signs of ileocolic intussusception with adjacent lymphadenopathy measuring 20 mm (Figure 1). Flexible colonoscopy documented a caecal large submucosal lesion with ulcerated mucosa (Figure 2).

Laparoscopic exploration was performed: the 5-port method is generally used. A 10 mm trocar is inserted 1 cm below the umbilicus as an observation port. Another 12 mm trocar is introduced in the left flank 3 cm above the upper iliac crest as a major hand port. A 5 mm trocar is then

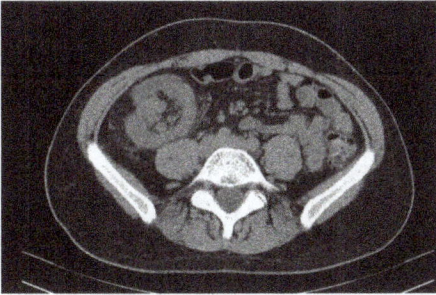

FIGURE 1: CT showed a hyperdense 60×50 mm right colic parietal lesion, signs of ileocolic intussusception with adjacent lymphadenopathy.

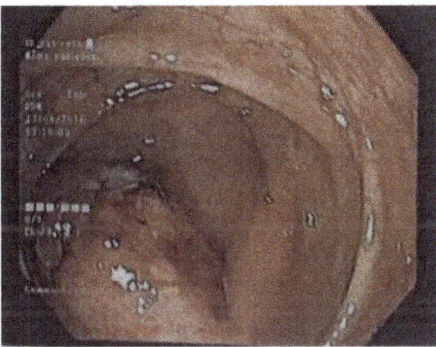

FIGURE 2: Flexible colonoscopy documented a caecal large submucosal lesion with ulcerated mucosa.

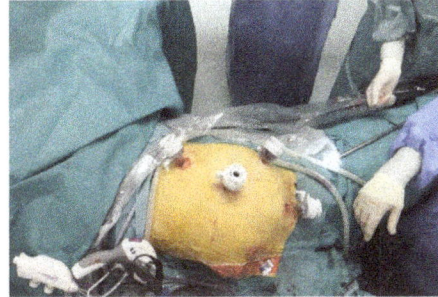

FIGURE 3: Trocar's disposition. Laparoscopic right hemicolectomy.

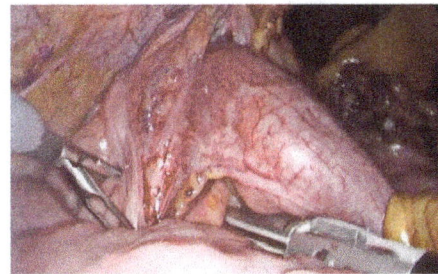

FIGURE 4: Intraoperative view of ileocolic intussusception.

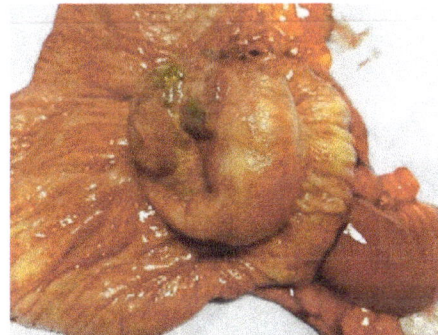

FIGURE 5: Surgical specimen after opening of the colon with appearance of tumor at the ileocaecal valve.

inserted in the epigastrium (1 cm below xiphoid process). Two accessory trocars (5 mm and 10 mm) were positioned, respectively, in the right iliac fossa and suprapubic region. The surgical table is declined about 10–15° into the Trendelenburg position with a slight rotation on the left flank. The surgeon was between the patient's legs, and the camera operator/assistant was on the left side (Figure 3). Ileocolic intussusception causing occlusive status with multiple lymphadenopathies along the ileocaecal artery was observed intraoperatively (Figure 4). Laparoscopic right hemicolectomy was performed following strictly oncologic principles with ileocolic, right colic, and right branch of middle colic artery ligation. Previous reduction of the invaginated segments was not attempted. The specimen was exteriorized through periumbilical midline incision, and primary extracorporeal anastomosis was performed using double-layer manual sutures. Gross examination of the specimen revealed a tumor mass of the ileocaecal valve measuring 50×45 mm which seemed infiltrate muscular layer (Figure 5).

Microscopy examination showed ileocaecal valve section presenting dense proliferation of large-sized atypical lymphoid cells with eosinophilic cytoplasm and one or various irregular nucleoli next to the basal membrane. Histopathology of 25 regional and omental lymph nodes revealed focal lymphomatous involvement. Immunophenotypic profile was CD20+, CD79 alfa+, CD10+, BCL2−−+, BCL6−−+, CD5−++, Ciclina D1−, CD3−, CD30−, and ALK−. Proliferation index was high (Ki67/MIB-1 > 95%) (Figure 6).

Fluorescent in situ hybridization (FISH) showed typical Burkitt's disease chromosomal translocation: t(8;14)(q24;q32).

Postoperative course was uneventful, and patient was discharged 4 days after surgery. Six weeks after surgery, the patient underwent bone marrow biopsy and full-body CT scan for a further evaluation of the disease. Bone marrow biopsy demonstrated normal proliferation and maturation of all cell lines; CT scan did not show other disease localizations. The patient received a hyper-CVAD combined chemotherapy (cyclophosphamide, doxorubicin, vincristine, and prednisone). At 8-month follow-up before this report, patient is still alive and free of disease.

3. Discussion

BL is a B-cell lymphoma with a short doubling time and usually developing an enormous tumoral mass (bulky disease) [2]. BL is characterized by a chromosomal translocation that

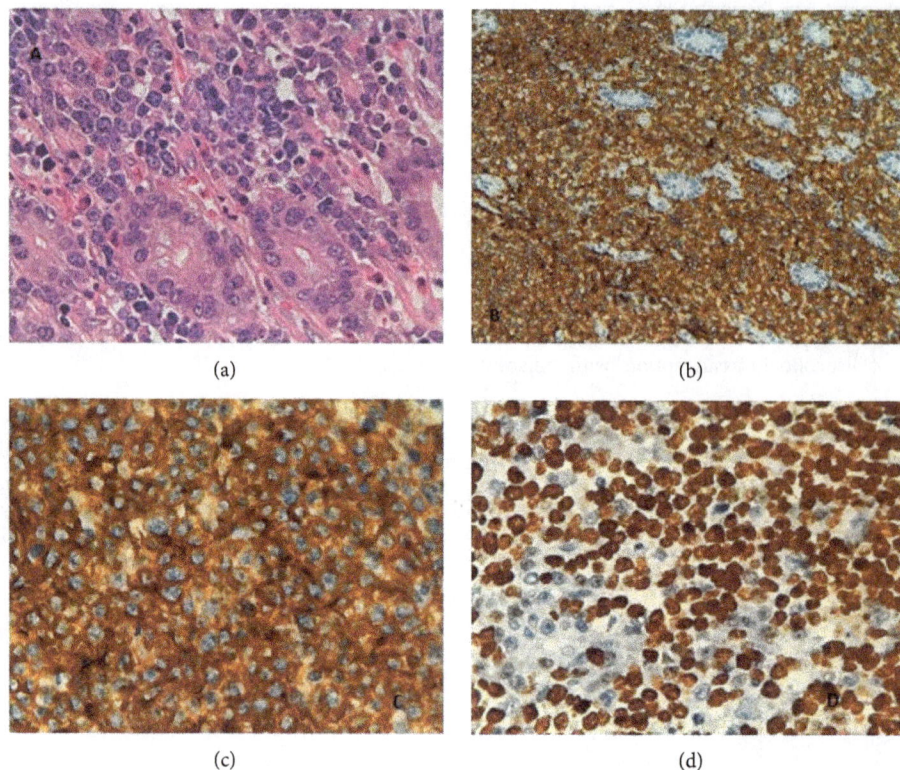

FIGURE 6: Histological and immunohistological examination of the specimens showing diffuse large B-cell non-Hodgkin's lymphoma. (a) Magnification ×400, HE staining, polymorphic large B-cells with irregular nuclei. (b) Magnification ×400, CD20(+). (c) Magnification ×400, CD79(+). (d) Magnification ×400, Ki67/Mib1 > 95% (high-grade B-cell lymphoma).

results in deregulation of the c-MYC oncogene. Burkitt's lymphoma (BL) is a disease usually affecting children and young adults, rarely adults. The first case of Burkitt's lymphoma (BL) was observed in African children by Burkitt in 1958 [3].

Burkitt's lymphoma is more frequent in males rather than females with a ratio of 2:1 [4, 5]. In reviews including a considerable number of adult patients with abdominal Burkitt's lymphoma, a percentage from 33% to 50% were more than 20 years old [4, 5].

In endemic areas, BL usually involves the facial bones, particularly the jaw, maxilla, and orbit, especially in young children, associated with Epstein-Barr virus (EBV) infection [6, 7]. Bone marrow involvement is observed in progressive disease [8].

In nonendemic BL, the presence of an abdominal mass is a common finding at the first medical examination. Burkitt's and MALT lymphoma are the most common lymphomas of the small bowel and represent the 42.5% of all lymphomas. American Burkitt's differs from the African type described by Burkitt in 1958 because of the increased propensity for widespread involvement within the abdominal cavity [9].

Intussusception was first described by Barbette of Amsterdam in 1674 [10]. Intussusception in leukemia patients is found almost exclusively in the pediatric population, rarely in adults [11, 12]. In the literature, we found 4 clinical cases of intussusception in adult leukemia patients [11, 13]. In most cases, the leukemic infiltration of the bowel acted like a lead point for the development of the

intussusception, even if it is described as a case in which imaging and histological studies have not revealed any leukemic infiltration of the organ [13].

In contrast with children intussusception, a demonstrable etiology is found in 70–95% of cases of adult intussusception and primitive or secondary neoplasms are responsible/the cause of 40% of this condition. Malignancies represent 30% of all small bowel intussusceptions and from 63% up to 68% of large bowel ones [14, 15].

A previous history of chemotherapy and radiotherapy could be potential risk factors for secondary ileocaecal BL [16].

While intussusception in children has a well-known/well-defined clinical presentation for its frequency, intussusception in adults may present with nonspecific symptoms. In Begos et al.' series, 75% of patients presented with obstruction symptoms, 5% with acute abdomen. At physical examination, a palpable abdominal mass was found in a third of cases [17]. The most frequent symptoms are abdominal pain of various character and intensity, vomit, weight loss, permanent fatigue, night perspiration, and sporadic gastrointestinal bleeding. Rarely, complications like acute peritonitis, in case of small bowel perforation, or small bowel obstruction may occur [18].

Laboratory findings are nonspecific in adult intussusception. Transabdominal sonographic study of the bowel intussusception demonstrated an elevated diagnostic accuracy [19], and it is considered a first level diagnostic technique, used directly in the patient's rooms [20]. Sonographically, intussusception appears as a superficial oval formation in longitudinal section with a target shape in transversal section, often with intraperitoneal free fluid [21]. TC scan is a gold standard in ileocolic intussusception diagnosis.

Surgery, chemotherapy, radiotherapy, and radioimmunotherapy are different weapons to fight with GI lymphoma [22].

The role of surgery in GI Burkitt's lymphoma remains controversial. Burkitt's lymphoma responds dramatically to chemotherapies inducing rapid tumor regression and often long-term remission [23]. The surgical treatment in Burkitt's lymphoma intussusception due to localized disease consists in resection and anastomosis of the pathological tract [24]. On the other hand, Magrath et al., considering a study in Burkitt's lymphoma patients in Uganda, suggest that an aggressive operative debulking, with a tumor removal of 90%, performed before the chemotherapy may increase survival [25].

In the emergency settings, there are no evidence-based guidelines leading to which surgical techniques (laparoscopic or laparotomic) to prefer. This choice should be made based on clinical judgment and surgeon's experience. Laparoscopic approach was useful because it allowed us to diagnose the cause of occlusion and resolve it in oncological way considering the risk of an underlying malignancy. Outcomes following laparoscopic colectomy in this setting resulted in reduced length of stay, lower complication rates, and lower costs. Increased adoption of laparoscopy in the nonelective settings should be considered [26]. The laparoscopic approach to acute abdomen, when performed by experienced surgeon, is a feasible alternative to open surgery [27]. Nevertheless, some authors prefer the open technique in colic intussusception, because of the high probability of associated malignant lesions [28].

Thanks to the better understanding of the biology of the disease, for there has been an improvement in chemotherapeutic drugs [29]. The current 5-year survival for advanced Burkitt's lymphoma in children and young adults has increased of 2-3 times in the last 3 decades, from 85% to 90% with less than 6 months of intensive chemotherapy [30].

4. Conclusions

Burkitt's lymphoma determining ileocaecal intussusception, although rare in adults, must be considered in intestinal obstruction differential diagnosis, especially when a palpable mass in the right iliac region is present. Imaging studies, particularly abdominal CT, may consent a correct preoperative diagnosis. Definitive treatment and management of intussusception should be individualized according to the patient's age and tumour localization. The surgical approach in GI Burkitt's lymphoma has not yet been coded. In our case, considering intestinal obstruction, early surgical intervention and total tumor removal may be mandatory.

Surgery is always indicated in case of organic obstruction causing the intussusception. Several studies showed that laparoscopic-assisted right colectomy results in less blood loss, a shorter length of hospital stay, and lower postoperative short-term morbidity compared with open resections, also in emergency settings. Minimally invasive surgery should be preferred for abdominal emergencies, like ileocaecal intussusception.

Disclosure

A previous version of this work was presented as an abstract at the 7th National Congress of the Italian Society of Colorectal Surgery, Rome, September 30 to October 3, 2017, published on Tech Coloproctol (2017) 21: 823 (https://doi.org/10.1007/s10151-017-1674-0).

References

[1] L. Zhai, Y. Zhao, L. Lin et al., "Non-Hodgkin's lymphoma involving the ileocecal region: a single-institution analysis of 46 cases in a chinese population," *Journal of Clinical Gastroenterology*, vol. 46, no. 6, pp. 509–514, 2012.

[2] S. J. Jang, D. H. Yoon, S. Kim et al., "A unique pattern of extranodal involvement in Korean adults with sporadic Burkitt lymphoma: a single center experience," *Annals of Hematology*, vol. 91, no. 12, pp. 1917–1922, 2012.

[3] D. Burkitt, "A sarcoma involving the jaws in African children," *British Journal of Surgery*, vol. 46, no. 197, pp. 218–223, 1958.

[4] M. Khan, A. Agrawal, and P. Strauss, "Ileocolic intussusception - a rare cause of acute intestinal obstruction in adults; case report and literature review," *World Journal of Emergency Surgery*, vol. 3, no. 1, p. 26, 2008.

[5] M. M. Kemeny, I. T. Magrath, and M. F. Brennan, "The role of surgery in the management of American Burkitt's lymphoma and its treatment," *Annals of Surgery*, vol. 196, no. 1, pp. 82–86, 1982.

[6] R. J. Q. Mcnally and L. Parker, "Environmental factors and childhood acute leukemias and lymphomas," *Leukemia & Lymphoma*, vol. 47, no. 4, pp. 583–598, 2006.

[7] D. Kiresi, L. G. Karabekmez, Y. Koksal, and D. Emlik, "A case of Burkitt lymphoma re-presenting as periportal hepatic and multiple organ infiltration," *Clinical Lymphoma and Myeloma*, vol. 8, no. 1, pp. 59–61, 2008.

[8] J. T. Yustein and C. V. Dang, "Biology and treatment of Burkitt's lymphoma," *Current Opinion in Hematology*, vol. 14, no. 4, pp. 375–381, 2007.

[9] M. A. Rathore, S. I. Andrabi, and M. Mansha, "Adult intussusception—a surgical dilemma," *Journal of Ayub Medical College, Abbottabad*, vol. 18, no. 3, pp. 3–6, 2006.

[10] A. S. Krasniqi, A. R. Hamza, L. M. Salihu et al., "Compound double ileoileal and ileocecocolic intussusception caused by lipoma of the ileum in an adult patient: a case report," *Journal of Medical Case Reports*, vol. 5, no. 1, p. 452, 2011.

[11] M. F. Law, C. K. Wong, C. Y. Pang et al., "Rare case of intussusception in an adult with acute myeloid leukemia," *World Journal of Gastroenterology*, vol. 21, no. 2, pp. 688–693, 2015.

[12] M. V. Manglani, J. Rosenthal, N. F. Rosenthal, P. Kidd, and L. J. Ettinger, "Intussusception in an infant with acute lymphoblastic leukemia: a case report and review of the literature," *Journal of Pediatric Hematology/Oncology*, vol. 20, no. 5, pp. 467-468, 1998.

[13] F. T. Hoxha, S. I. Hashani, A. S. Krasniqi et al., "Intussusceptions as acute abdomen caused by Burkitt lymphoma: a case report," *Cases Journal*, vol. 2, no. 1, article 9322, 2009.

[14] S. Y. Pan and H. Morrison, "Epidemiology of cancer of the small intestine," *World Journal of Gastrointestinal Oncology*, vol. 3, no. 3, pp. 33–42, 2011.

[15] S. S. Gill, D. M. Heuman, and A. A. Mihas, "Small intestinal neoplasms," *Journal of Clinical Gastroenterology*, vol. 33, no. 4, pp. 267–282, 2001.

[16] F. Parente, A. Anderloni, S. Greco, P. Zerbi, and G. B. Porro, "Image of the month," *Gastroenterology*, vol. 127, no. 1, pp. 8–368, 2004.

[17] D. G. Begos, A. Sandor, and I. M. Modlin, "The diagnosis and management of adult intussusception," *The American Journal of Surgery*, vol. 173, no. 2, pp. 88–94, 1997.

[18] P. D. McLaughlin and M. M. Maher, "Primary malignant diseases of the small intestine," *American Journal of Roentgenology*, vol. 201, no. 1, pp. W9–14, 2013.

[19] J. P. Pracros, V. A. Tran-Minh, C. H. Morin de Finfe, P. Deffrenne-Pracros, D. Louis, and T. Basset, "Acute intestinal intussusception in children. Contribution of ultrasonography (145 cases)," *Annales de Radiologie*, vol. 30, no. 7, pp. 525–530, 1987.

[20] K. E. Applegate, "Intussusception in children: evidence-based diagnosis and treatment," *Pediatric Radiology*, vol. 39, Supplement 2, pp. 140–S143, 2009.

[21] H. Williams, "Imaging and intussusception," *Archives of Disease in Childhood - Education and Practice*, vol. 93, no. 1, pp. 30–36, 2008.

[22] P. Ghimire, G. Y. Wu, and L. Zhu, "Primary gastrointestinal lymphoma," *World Journal of Gastroenterology*, vol. 17, no. 6, pp. 697–707, 2011.

[23] J. L. Ziegler, "Burkitt's lymphoma," *New England Journal of Medicine*, vol. 305, no. 13, pp. 735–745, 1981.

[24] H. Gupta, A. M. Davidoff, C. H. Pui, S. J. Shochat, and J. T. Sandlund, "Clinical implications and surgical management of intussusception in pediatric patients with Burkitt lymphoma," *Journal of Pediatric Surgery*, vol. 42, no. 6, pp. 998–1001, 2007.

[25] I. T. Magrath, C. Janus, B. K. Edwards et al., "An effective therapy for both undifferentiated (including Burkitt's) lymphomas and lymphoblastic lymphomas in children and young adults," *Blood*, vol. 63, no. 5, pp. 1102–1111, 1984.

[26] D. S. Keller, R. Pedraza, J. R. Flores-Gonzalez, J. P. LeFave, A. Mahmood, and E. M. Haas, "The current status of emergent laparoscopic colectomy: a population-based study of clinical and financial outcomes," *Surgical Endoscopy*, vol. 30, no. 8, pp. 3321–3326, 2016.

[27] M. E. Franklin Jr, J. J. Gonzalez Jr, D. B. Miter, J. L. Glass, and D. Paulson, "Laparoscopic diagnosis and treatment of intestinal obstruction," *Surgical Endoscopy*, vol. 18, no. 1, pp. 26–30, 2004.

[28] L. K. Eisen, J. D. Cunningham, and A. H. Aufses Jr, "Intussusception in adults: institutional review," *Journal of the American College of Surgeons*, vol. 188, no. 4, pp. 390–395, 1999.

[29] I. T. Aldoss, D. D. Weisenburger, K. Fu et al., "Adult Burkitt lymphoma: advances in diagnosis and treatment," *Oncology (Williston Park)*, vol. 22, no. 13, pp. 1508–1517, 2008.

[30] L. de Leval and R. P. Hasserjian, "Diffuse large B-cell lymphomas and Burkitt lymphoma," *Hematology/Oncology Clinics of North America*, vol. 23, no. 4, pp. 791–827, 2009.

39

Giant Adrenal Myelolipoma in a Patient without Endocrine Disorder: A Case Report and a Review of the Literature

Yoshifumi Nakayama ⓘ,[1,2] Nobutaka Matayoshi,[1] Masaki Akiyama,[1,2]
Yusuke Sawatsubashi,[1,2] Jun Nagata,[1,2] Masanori Hisaoka,[3] and Keiji Hirata[1]

[1]Department of Surgery 1, University of Occupational and Environmental Health, 1-1 Iseigaoka, Yahata-nishi-ku, Kitakyushu 807-8555, Japan
[2]Department of Gastroenterological and General Surgery, Wakamatsu Hospital of University of Occupational and Environmental Health, 1-17-1 Hamamachi, Wakamatsu-ku, Kitakyushu 808-0024, Japan
[3]Department of Pathology and Oncology, School of Medicine, University of Occupational and Environmental Health, 1-1 Iseigaoka, Yahata-nishi-ku, Kitakyushu 807-8555, Japan

Correspondence should be addressed to Yoshifumi Nakayama; nakayama@med.uoeh-u.ac.jp

Academic Editor: Baran Tokar

We herein present a surgically treated case of huge adrenal myelolipoma. A 62-year-old woman presented to our surgical outpatient clinic with a retroperitoneal tumor. A clinical examination revealed an elastic soft, smooth-surfaced, painless, child-head-sized tumor with poor mobility, which was located in the left upper abdomen. Computed tomography (CT) and magnetic resonance imaging (MRI) of the abdomen revealed an uneven tumor surrounding the stomach, spleen, pancreas, and left kidney, which was $20 \times 18 \times 10$ cm in size. The retroperitoneal tumor was resected. The tumor was attached to the surrounding organs, including the pancreas, spleen, and left kidney, but had not directly invaded these organs. The tumor was yellow and elastic soft and covered with a thin film. The origin of the tumor was suggested to be the left adrenal gland. The weight of the excised tumor was 1500 g. The histopathological diagnosis was adrenal myelolipoma. The patient had an uneventful recovery and was discharged from the hospital on the thirteenth day after the operation. She has been followed up in our outpatient clinic.

1. Introduction

Adrenal myelolipoma (AML) is a relatively rare benign tumor composed of mature adipose tissues and a variable amount of hematopoietic elements. The male-to-female ratio is 1 : 1. The incidence of AML is reported to be 0.08–0.4% at autopsy [1]. AMLs are nonfunctional tumors that are usually asymptomatic; however, they have been known to coexist with other endocrine disorders, such as Cushing's syndrome, congenital adrenal hyperplasia (CAH), Conn's syndrome, and pheochromocytoma [2–4]. Recently, AMLs have been reported in patients with CAH with increasing frequency. One study indicated that myelolipoma was detected in 4% of patients with CAH [5].

The largest AML (size, $31 \times 24.5 \times 11.5$ cm; weight, 6000 g) in a patient without endocrine disorder was described by Akamatsu et al. [6], while the largest AML in a patient with CAH (size, $34 \times 24 \times 10.5$ cm; weight, 5900 g) was described by Boudreaux et al. [7].

We herein report a relatively rare case of a giant AML of 1500 g in weight in a patient without endocrine disorder and discuss our analysis of the literature.

2. Case Report

A 62-year-old Japanese female patient presented with a left abdominal mass. She was referred to our surgical outpatient clinic to undergo a detailed examination and treatment for the left abdominal mass. A clinical examination revealed an elastic soft, smooth-surfaced, painless, child-head-sized tumor with poor mobility, which was located in the left upper abdomen. Abdominal computed tomography (CT)

(a)   (b)

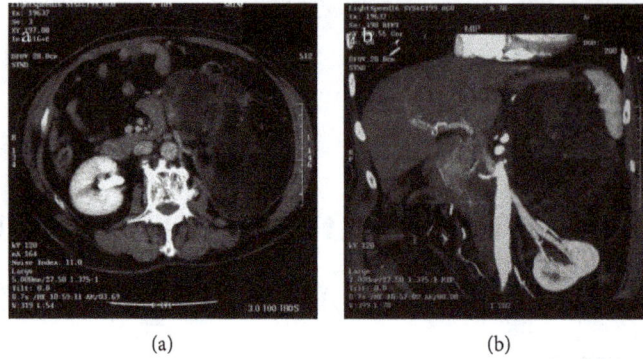

FIGURE 1: Abdominal computed tomography (CT) demonstrated a child-head-sized mass with heterogeneous contrast located in the left upper abdomen around the stomach, spleen, pancreas, and left kidney on the horizontal (a) and coronal (b) images.

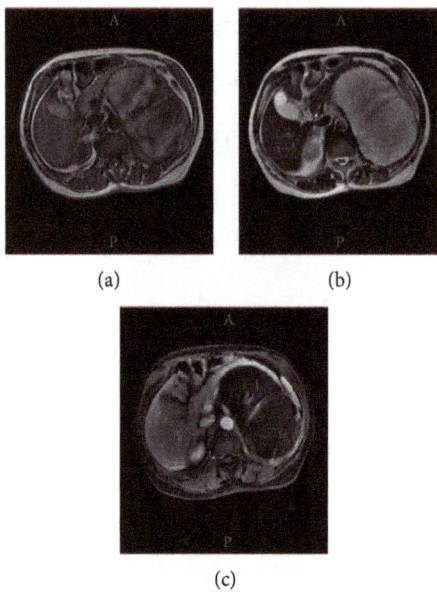

(a)   (b)

(c)

FIGURE 2: Magnetic resonance imaging (MRI) revealed a heterogeneously hyperintense mass on T1-weighted imaging (a), a relatively uniform and hyperintense mass on T2-weighted imaging (b), and a hypointense mass with an enhanced border on Gd-enhanced imaging (c).

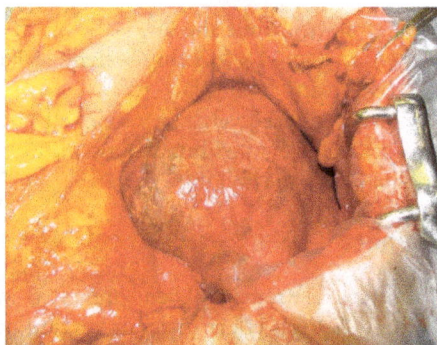

FIGURE 4: An examination of the cut surface of this tumor revealed a multilobular yellow mass with bleeding in places.

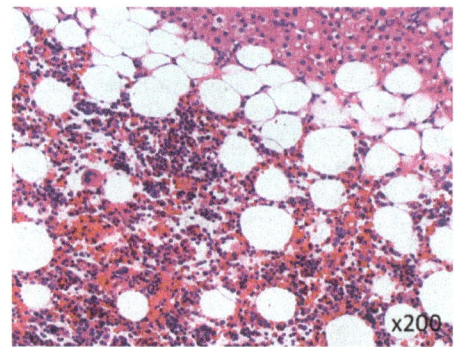

FIGURE 5: A histopathological examination (×200) with hematoxylin and eosin staining revealed that tumor was composed of a proliferation of mature and variable-sized adipocytes admixed with aggregates of hematopoietic elements.

FIGURE 3: The operative findings revealed a yellow mass covered with a thin layer that was located at the left side of the stomach, posteriorly to the transverse mesocolon and pancreas, on the cranial side of the left kidney.

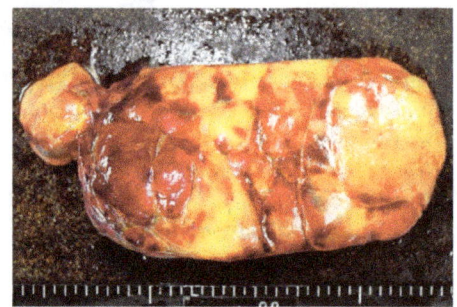

demonstrated a child-head-sized mass with heterogeneous contrast at the left upper abdomen around the stomach, spleen, pancreas, and left kidney on a horizontal image (Figure 1(a)) and coronal image (Figure 1(b)).

Magnetic resonance imaging (MRI) revealed a heterogeneously hyperintense mass on T1-weighted imaging (Figure 2(a)), a relatively uniform and hyperintense mass on T2-weighted imaging (Figure 2(b)), and a hypointense mass with an enhanced border on gadolinium- (Gd-) enhanced imaging (Figure 2(c)). A retroperitoneal tumor was diagnosed. Her laboratory data were white blood cell count, 4600/mm^3; hemoglobin, 12.8 g/dl; hematocrit, 36.5%;

TABLE 1: Giant myelolipoma more than 1500 g without endocrine disorder.

Number	Author	Year	Gender	Age	Site	Size (cm)	Weight (g)	Symptoms	Ref. number
1	Akamatsu	2004	Male	51	Right	$31 \times 24.5 \times 11.5$	6000	Abd. mass, abd. pain	[6]
2	Wilhelmus	1981	Female	70	Left	$30 \times 22 \times 16$	5500	Abd. mass, abd. pain	[21]
3	Mukherjee	2010	Male	56	Right	$28 \times 26 \times 17$	5500	Abd. mass, weight loss	[22]
4	Kumar	2015	Male	40	Right	$38 \times 20 \times 16$	5200	Abd. pain, dyspnea, dizziness	[23]
5	Brogna	2011	Male	52	Left	$25 \times 20 \times 20$	4400	No	[24]
6	O'Daniel-Pierce	1996	Male	67	Right	$30 \times 20 \times 11$	4370	Abd. pain, abd. mass	[25]
7	Reshi	2007	Male	45	Right	$25 \times 14 \times 11$	>4000	Abd. mass	[26]
8	Gautam	2013	Male	52	Right	$28 \times 18 \times 12$	3850	Abd. pain, headache	[27]
9	Tanaka	1998	Male	50	Right	$30 \times 25 \times 23$	3500	Abd. mass	[28]
10	Dell'Avanzato	2009	Male	43	Right	$22 \times 18 \times 9$	3500	ND	[29]
11	Saha	2015	Female	59	Left	$23 \times 16 \times 9$	3300	Abd. distension, dragging sensation	[30]
12	Kumaresan	2011	Female	24	Right	$30 \times 20 \times 18$	3000	Abd. pain, abd. mass	[31]
13	Gerson	2015	Female	62	Right	$21 \times 18 \times 9$	2468	Abd. pain, nausea	[32]
14	Takahashi	2005	Male	48	Right	$20 \times 18 \times 16$	2400	Abd. distension, fever, diarrhea	[33]
15	Fernandes	2010	Male	48	Right	$28 \times 20 \times 15$	2200	Abd. pain, abd. mass	[34]
16	Chand	2017	Male	35	Right	$24 \times 15 \times 12$	2000	Pain in the right thigh	[35]
17	Répássy	2001	Female	50	Right	20×14	1650	Abd. pain, abd. discomfort	[36]
18	Andersom	2010	Man	35	Right	$23.8 \times 11.6 \times 7.5$	1575	Right-sided abd. discomfort	[37]
19	Goldman	1996	Male	42	Right	$20.5 \times 15 \times 8.5$	1550	Right frank pain, dizziness, vomiting	[38]
20	Ersoy	2006	Male	67	Right	12×10	1500	Abd. pain, fever	[39]
21	Chakrabarti	2012	Female	40	Right	$15 \times 10 \times 8$	1500	Abd. pain	[40]
22	Our case	2018	Female	62	Left	$20 \times 18 \times 10$	1500	Abd. mass	

ND: not described in abstract.

and platelet count, $182,000/mm^3$, with normal electrolytes, as well as normal blood urea nitrogen levels, but slight liver dysfunction. Her serum levels of corticosteroid and/or androgen were 13.3 ng/ml (10.4–35.0 in female) and 173 pg/dl (35.7–240.0), respectively, which are within the normal ranges; however, her serum level of ACTH was elevated at 138.70 pg/ml (7.2–63.3).

The retroperitoneal tumor was resected (Figure 3). The tumor was located at the left side of the stomach, posteriorly to the transverse mesocolon and pancreas, on the cranial side of the left kidney (Figures 1 and 2), but has not invaded the surrounding organs (Figures 1 and 2). The right adrenal gland was normal in size. The resected tumor was $20 \times 18 \times 10$ cm in diameter and weighted 1500 g. An examination of the cut surface of the tumor revealed a multilobular yellow mass with bleeding in places (Figure 4).

A histopathological examination with hematoxylin and eosin staining revealed that the tumor was composed of a proliferation of mature and variable-sized adipocytes admixed with aggregates of hematopoietic elements, associated with adrenal gland tissue in the peripheral region within the tumor (Figure 5). These findings were compatible with AML.

The patient had an uneventful recovery and was discharged from the hospital on the 6th day after the operation. She has been followed up in our outpatient clinic without recurrence for approximately 12 years since undergoing the operation.

3. Discussion

The etiology of AML remains unclear. Some of the hypothesized etiologies include extramedullary hematopoiesis due to the autonomous proliferation of bone marrow cells transferred during embryogenesis, degeneration of epithelial tissues of the adrenal cortex, and adrenocortical cell metaplasia of the reticuloendothelial cells of the blood capillaries in response to stimuli such as necrosis, infection, or stress [1, 8–10]. The most widely accepted theory is that myelolipomas arise due to metaplasia of the reticuloendothelial cells of the blood capillaries in the adrenal gland in response to stimuli such as chronic stress, infection, necrosis, or inflammation [11, 12].

Although the diameter of AMLs ranges from less than 1 cm to more than 30 cm, they are usually less than 5 cm in diameter [13, 14]. AML is often asymptomatic, sometimes leading to very large adrenal masses (≥10 cm in diameter). These are often called "giant AML" [15]. Lawler et al. proposed a definition of the often quoted term "giant" AML [16]. We propose that giant AMLs of ≥1, 500 g should be called "real giant AMLs." According to this criterion, we found the 21 cases involving giant AMLs in patients without endocrine disorders (Table 1) and the 6 cases involving giant AMLs in patients with CAH (Table 2).

Ultrasonography (US), computed tomography (CT), and magnetic resonance imaging (MRI) are effective for diagnosing AML in ≥90% of cases [4, 17]. Recently, with the

TABLE 2: Giant adrenal myelolipoma more than 1500 g with CAH.

Number	Author	Year	Gender	Age	Site	Size (cm)	Weight (g)	Symptoms	Ref. number
1	Boudreaux	1979	Male	56		34 × 24 × 10.5	5900	Dyspnea, low thoracic pain	[7]
2	McGeoch	2012	Male	34	Left	23 × 19 × 11	5800	Adb. mass	[41]
3	Kale	2015	Male	51	Left	34 × 20 × 13	4700	Back pain	[42]
4	Alvarez	2014	Female	44	Left	26 × 24 × 9.5	5090	Abd. pain, nausea, bilious emesis	[43]
5	Al-Bahri	2014	Male	39	Left, right	30 × 25 × 20 25 × 20 × 13	4100, 2700	Abd. distension, fatigue	[44]
6	German-Mena	2011	Male	45	Left	24.4 × 19.0 × 9.5	2557	Abd. distension, abd. pain	[45]

CAH: congenital adrenal hyperplasia.

widespread use of imaging studies such as US, CT, and MRI, the incidental detection of AML has been more common, and they now represent up to 10–15% of incidentally detected adrenal masses [18]. US shows myelolipoma as a well-defined tumor with varying degrees of hyperechoic (fatty tissue) and hypoechoic (myeloid tissue) components. CT shows myelolipoma as a well-delineated mass with heterogeneous attenuation and low-density fat tissue with more dense areas of myeloid tissue. MRI demonstrates myelolipoma as an area of high signal intensity on T1-weighted and T2-weighted sequences with reduced signal intensity on fat suppression and opposite phase imaging [18, 19].

Management of AML should be individualized. Small lesions, which are asymptomatic and measure less than 5 cm, should be monitored over a period of 1-2 years with imaging controls [20]. On the other hand, surgery is indicated when the patient is symptomatic, when the lesion is more than 5 cm in size due to rupture—which is a rare event—or when malignancy is suspected [20]. The most recognized complication of AML is spontaneous retroperitoneal hemorrhage [14, 16]. Daneshmand et al. suggested that symptomatic tumors or myelolipomas of ≧7 cm in size should be removed because they are associated with an increased risk of spontaneous rupture with retroperitoneal hemorrhage [4].

4. Conclusion

We reported a relatively rare case of a real giant AML that weighted 1500 g in a patient without an endocrine disorder. It is very important to provide suitable management on an individual basis.

Authors' Contributions

Yoshifumi Nakayama contributed to drafting and editing of the paper. Masaki Akiyama and Yusuke Sawatsubashi contributed to obtaining the clinical details. Jun Nagata contributed to literature search. Nobutaka Matayoshi helped in

drafting the paper. Masanori Hisaoka and Keiji Hirata helped in editing the paper.

References

[1] C. A. Olsson, R. J. Krane, R. C. Klugo, and S. M. Selikowitz, "Adrenal myelolipoma," Surgery, vol. 73, no. 5, pp. 665–670, 1973.

[2] H. Wagnerová, I. Lazúrová, J. Bober, L. Sokol, and M. Zachar, "Adrenal myelolipoma. 6 cases and a review of the literature," Neoplasma, vol. 51, no. 4, pp. 300–305, 2004.

[3] L. Yildiz, I. Akpolat, K. Erzurumlu, O. Aydin, and B. Kandemir, "Giant adrenal myelolipoma: case report and review of the literature," Pathology International, vol. 50, no. 6, pp. 502–504, 2000.

[4] S. Daneshmand and M. L. Quek, "Adrenal myelolipoma: diagnosis and management," Urology Journal, vol. 3, no. 2, pp. 71–74, 2006.

[5] I. Nermoen, J. Rørvik, S. H. Holmedal et al., "High frequency of adrenal myelolipomas and testicular adrenal rest tumours in adult Norwegian patients with classical congenital adrenal hyperplasia because of 21-hydroxylase deficiency," Clinical Endocrinology, vol. 75, no. 6, pp. 753–759, 2011.

[6] H. Akamatsu, M. Koseki, H. Nakaba et al., "Giant adrenal myelolipoma: report of a case," Surgery Today, vol. 34, no. 3, pp. 283–285, 2004.

[7] D. Boudreaux, J. Waisman, D. G. Skinner, and R. Low, "Giant adrenal myelolipoma and testicular interstitial cell tumor in a man with congenital 21-hydroxylase deficiency," The American Journal of Surgical Pathology, vol. 3, no. 2, pp. 109–123, 1979.

[8] D. C. Collins, "Formation of bone marrow in the suprarenal gland," The American Journal of Pathology, vol. 8, no. 1, pp. 97–106.1, 1932.

[9] A. Plaut, "Myelolipoma in the adrenal cortex; myeloadipose structures," The American Journal of Pathology, vol. 34, no. 3, pp. 487–515, 1958.

[10] H. B. Rubin, F. Hirose, and J. R. Benfield, "Myelolipoma of the adrenal gland: angiographic findings and review of the literature," The American Journal of Surgery, vol. 130, no. 3, pp. 354–358, 1975.

[11] K. Y. Lam and C. Y. Lo, "Adrenal lipomatous tumours: a 30 year clinicopathological experience at a single institution," Journal of Clinical Pathology, vol. 54, no. 9, pp. 707–712, 2001.

[12] A. Meyer and M. Behrend, "Presentation and therapy of mye-lolipoma," *International Journal of Urology*, vol. 12, no. 3, pp. 239–243, 2005.

[13] F. M. Enzinger and W. W. Sharen, "Benign lipomatous tumors," in *Soft Tissue Tumors*, F. M. Enzinger and W. W. Sharen, Eds., pp. 409-410, Mosby, St Louis, 3rd edition, 1995.

[14] J. P. Meaglia and J. D. Schmidt, "Natural history of an adrenal myelolipoma," *The Journal of Urology*, vol. 147, no. 4, pp. 1089-1090, 1992.

[15] B. Iorio, G. Gravante, D. Pietrasanta et al., "Description of a case of giant adrenal myelolipoma and survey of the litera-ture," *Minerva Chirurgica*, vol. 58, no. 4, pp. 595–600, 2003.

[16] L. P. Lawler and P. J. Pickhardt, "Giant adrenal myelolipoma presenting with spontaneous hemorrhage. CT, MR and pathology correlation," *Irish Medical Journal*, vol. 94, no. 8, pp. 231–233, 2001.

[17] P. J. Kenney, B. J. Wagner, P. Rao, and C. S. Heffess, "Myeloli-poma: CT and pathologic features," *Radiology*, vol. 208, no. 1, pp. 87–95, 1998.

[18] N. A. Wani, T. Kosar, I. A. Rawa, and A. Qayum, "Giant adre-nal myelolipoma: incidentaloma with a rare incidental associ-ation," *Urology Annals*, vol. 2, no. 3, pp. 130–133, 2010.

[19] K. M. Cyran, P. J. Kenney, D. S. Memel, and I. Yacoub, "Adre-nal myelolipoma," *AJR. American Journal of Roentgenology*, vol. 166, no. 2, pp. 395–400, 1996.

[20] S. I. Tyritzis, I. Adamakis, V. Migdalis, D. Vlachodimitropoulos, and C. A. Constantinides, "Giant adrenal myelolipoma, a rare urological issue with increasing incidence: a case report," *Cases Journal*, vol. 2, no. 1, p. 8863, 2009.

[21] J. L. Wilhelmus, G. R. Schrodt, M. T. Alberhasky, and M. O. Alcorn, "Giant adrenal myelolipoma: case report and review of the literature," *Archives of Pathology & Laboratory Medi-cine*, vol. 105, no. 10, pp. 532–535, 1981.

[22] S. Mukherjee, S. Pericleous, R. R. Hutchins, and P. S. Freed-man, "Asymptomatic giant adrenal myelolipoma," *Urology Journal*, vol. 7, no. 1, pp. 66–68, 2010.

[23] S. Kumar, K. Jayant, S. Prasad et al., "Rare adrenal gland emer-gencies: a case series of giant myelolipoma presenting with massive hemorrhage and abscess," *Nephro-Urology Monthly*, vol. 7, no. 1, article e22671, 2015.

[24] A. Brogna, G. Scalisi, R. Ferrara, and A. M. Bucceri, "Giant secreting adrenal myelolipoma in a man: a case report," *Jour-nal of Medical Case Reports*, vol. 5, no. 1, article 298, 2011.

[25] M. E. O'Daniel-Pierce, J. A. Weeks, and P. C. Mcgrath, "Giant adrenal myelolipoma," *Southern Medical Journal*, vol. 89, no. 11, pp. 1116–1118, 1996.

[26] R. Reshi, M. L. Bhat, S. M. Kadri et al., "Giant myelolipoma of the adrenal gland with adenocarcinoma of the colon: a rare surgico-pathological presentation," *Laboratory Medicine*, vol. 38, no. 8, pp. 491-492, 2007.

[27] S. C. Gautam, H. Raafat, S. Sriganesh et al., "Giant adrenal myelolipoma," *Qatar Medical Journal*, vol. 2013, no. 1, pp. 2–11, 2013.

[28] D. Tanaka, T. Oyama, H. Niwatsukino, and M. Nakajo, "A case of asymptomatic giant myelolipoma of the adrenal gland," *Radiation Medicine*, vol. 16, no. 3, pp. 213–216, 1998.

[29] R. Dell'Avanzato, F. Castaldi, C. Giovannini, E. Mercadante, P. Cianciulli, and M. Carlini, "Giant symptomatic myeloli-poma of the right adrenal gland: a case report," *Chirurgia Italiana*, vol. 61, no. 2, pp. 231–236, 2009.

[30] M. Saha, S. Dasgupta, S. Chakrabarti, and J. Chakraborty, "Giant myelolipoma of left adrenal gland simulating a retro-peritoneal sarcoma," *International Journal of Advanced Medi-cal and Health Research*, vol. 2, no. 2, p. 122, 2015.

[31] K. Gupta, N. Kalra, R. Das, and K. Kumaresan, "A rare associ-ation of giant adrenal myelolipoma in a young female double heterozygous for HbD Punjab and β-thalassemia trait," *Indian Journal of Pathology and Microbiology*, vol. 54, no. 3, p. 635, 2011.

[32] G. Gerson, M. P. F. G. Bêco, C. G. Hirth et al., "Giant retroper-itoneal myelolipoma: case report and literature review," *Jornal Brasileiro de Patologia e Medicina Laboratorial*, vol. 51, no. 1, 2015.

[33] H. Takahashi, T. Yamaguchi, R. Takeda, S. Sakata, and M. Yamamoto, "A case of giant adrenal myelolipoma," *Nihon Rinsho Geka Gakkai Zasshi (Journal of Japan Surgical Associa-tion)*, vol. 66, no. 1, pp. 197–201, 2005.

[34] G. C. Fernandes, R. K. Gupta, and B. M. Kandalkar, "Giant adrenal myelolipoma," *Indian Journal of Pathology & Microbi-ology*, vol. 53, no. 2, pp. 325-326, 2010.

[35] G. Chand, "Giant adrenal myelolipoma presenting as an inci-dentaloma: a case report and review of literature," *Journal of Investigative Genomics*, vol. 4, no. 2, 2017.

[36] D. L. Répássy, S. Csata, G. Sterlik, and A. Iványi, "Giant adre-nal myelolipoma," *Pathology Oncology Research*, vol. 7, no. 1, pp. 72-73, 2001.

[37] B. B. Anderson, L. J. Hampton, C. M. Johnson, and G. E. Gur-uli, "Symptomatic giant adrenal myelolipoma," *World Journal of Endocrine Surgery*, vol. 2, no. 3, pp. 143-144, 2010.

[38] H. B. Goldman, R. C. Howard, and A. L. Patterson, "Spontane-ous retroperitoneal hemorrhage from a giant adrenal myeloli-poma," *The Journal of Urology*, vol. 155, no. 2, p. 639, 1996.

[39] E. Ersoy, M. Ozdoğan, A. Demirağ et al., "Giant adrenal mye-lolipoma associated with small bowel leiomyosarcoma: a case report," *The Turkish Journal of Gastroenterology*, vol. 17, no. 2, pp. 126–129, 2006.

[40] I. Chakrabarti, N. Ghosh, and V. Das, "Giant adrenal myeloli-poma with hemorrhage masquerading as retroperitoneal sar-coma," *Journal of Mid-life Health*, vol. 3, no. 1, pp. 42–44, 2012.

[41] S. C. McGeoch, S. Olson, Z. H. Krukowski, and J. S. Bevan, "Giant bilateral myelolipomas in a man with congenital adre-nal hyperplasia," *The Journal of Clinical Endocrinology & Metabolism*, vol. 97, no. 2, pp. 343-344, 2012.

[42] G. Kale, E. M. Pelley, and D. B. Davis, "Giant myelolipomas and inadvertent bilateral adrenalectomy in classic congenital adrenal hyperplasia," *Endocrinology, Diabetes & Metabolism Case Reports*, vol. 2015, article 150079, 2015.

[43] J. F. Alvarez, L. Goldstein, N. Samreen et al., "Giant adrenal myelolipoma," *Journal of Gastrointestinal Surgery*, vol. 18, no. 9, pp. 1716–1718, 2014.

[44] S. al-Bahri, A. Tariq, B. Lowentritt, and D. V. Nasrallah, "Giant bilateral adrenal myelolipoma with congenital adrenal hyper-plasia," *Case Reports in Surgery*, vol. 2014, Article ID 728198, 5 pages, 2014.

[45] E. German-Mena, G. B. Zibari, and S. N. Levine, "Adrenal myelolipomas in patients with congenital adrenal hyperplasia: review of the literature and a case report," *Endocrine Practice*, vol. 17, no. 3, pp. 441–447, 2011.

40

Sapovirus Gastroenteritis in Young Children Presenting as Distal Small Bowel Obstruction: A Report of 2 Cases and Literature Review

Lynn Model and Cathy Anne Burnweit

Nicklaus Children's Hospital, Miami, FL, USA

Correspondence should be addressed to Lynn Model; lynnsmodel@gmail.com

Academic Editor: Baran Tokar

Abdominal pain and distention in children are commonly encountered problems in the pediatric emergency room. The majority of complaints are found to be due to benign entities such as gastroenteritis and constipation. What confounds these diagnoses is that young children often deliver a challenging and unreliable exam. Thus, it often becomes exceedingly problematic to differentiate these benign conditions from surgical conditions requiring prompt attention including small or large bowel obstruction, volvulus, and appendicitis. The cases highlight *Sapovirus* as a cause of severe abdominal distention and vomiting in children and this report is the first to describe and demonstrate the impressive radiologic findings that may be associated with this infection. Surgeons should heed this information and hesitate to emergently operate on similar children.

1. Introduction

Severe abdominal distention in young children, with symptoms and X-rays consistent with bowel obstruction, causes significant concern for physicians and families. An English language literature review revealed that *Sapovirus* as a cause of this clinical picture has not been described. In this report, we outline the courses of 2 children presenting with what appeared to be small bowel obstruction but who, after *Sapovirus* infectious gastroenteritis was diagnosed, went on to resolve their illnesses spontaneously.

2. Case 1

A 2-year-old male with no significant past medical history and normal stooling history presented to the emergency room (ER) with nonbilious vomiting and severe abdominal distention for one week. He was initially seen at an urgent care center where he was given ondansetron intramuscularly and discharged home. He had slight improvement and then subsequent worsening of the vomiting. During the 2 days prior to presentation in the ER, the patient had been irritable, fussy, and less active than normal. He was also reported to have anorexia and diarrhea containing "red flakes." The patient's mother denied urinary symptoms, upper respiratory symptoms, or recent travel in the boy but noted a sibling with gastroenteritis approximately 3 weeks prior.

Exam revealed a markedly distended, tympanic abdomen without significant tenderness (Figure 1). Plain films demonstrated markedly dilated loops of bowel with air-fluid levels (Figure 2); distal bowel obstruction was suspected. Ultrasound was negative for intussusception. Laboratory studies revealed a slight leukocytosis at 11,500/mL with a monocytosis of 17.8% and low neutrophils at 19.7%. Electrolytes and liver functions were all within normal ranges. Stool for culture and polymerase chain reaction (PCR) was sent. Fecal hemoccult test was negative.

The patient was admitted for hydration and control of nausea with ondansetron. A nasogastric tube was placed but was promptly removed by the patient repeatedly. Abdominal distention resolved over the next 24 hours; the patient was fed a regular diet and discharged home. Stool PCR returned positive for *Sapovirus*, and neither PCR nor culture revealed other pathogens.

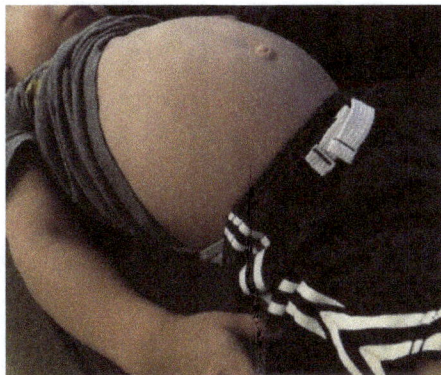

FIGURE 1: Photograph of severe abdominal distention in the 2-year-old male presented in Case 1.

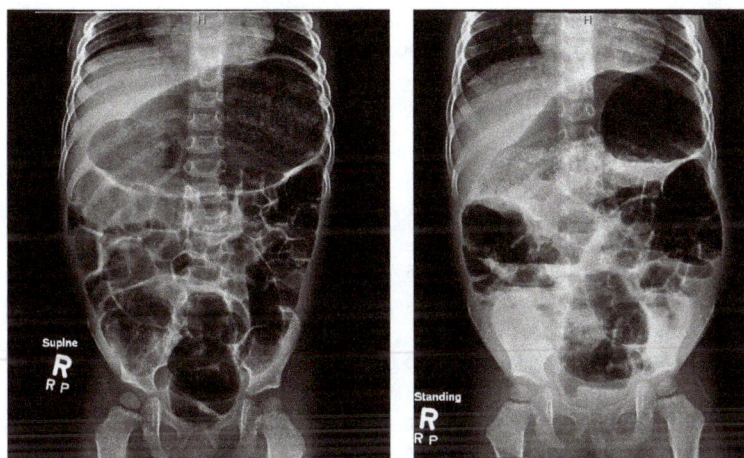

FIGURE 2: Supine and upright plain X-rays of the patient presented in Case 1. Moderate dilatation of the bowel is seen with significant gaseous distention of the stomach being seen. Multiple air-fluid levels are seen. No free intra-abdominal air is identified.

3. Case 2

A 2-year-old male with a history of mild prematurity (35 weeks of gestational age), laryngomalacia, and vocal cord paralysis with tracheostomy presented to the ER with severe abdominal distention and pain. The boy's mother described one week of nonbloody diarrhea and then no bowel movement in the prior 3 days and prior to that no problems with stooling. The patient had a history of gastrostomy and fundoplication as an infant but had been maintaining nutrition by oral feeding for the past 7 months. He was not vomiting but was brought in due to the concern for his massive abdominal girth.

Exam revealed a distended, nontender, tympanitic abdomen and no other abnormalities. X-ray showed markedly dilated loops of bowel with air-fluid levels (Figure 3), and small bowel obstruction was the lead diagnosis, given his surgical history. Laboratory exams revealed normal electrolytes, liver function tests, and white cell count (9,100/mL with normal differentiation).

The patient was admitted for observation, with hydration and withholding of oral intake. Shortly after admission, he began passing profuse amounts of flatus. His distention

significantly improved. On hospital day 2, he had a stool, and feeding was begun. The fecal PCR returned positive for *Sapovirus* and no other pathogens. The patient recovered quickly and was discharged home.

4. Discussion

The differential diagnosis of suspected bowel obstruction in young children is vast. It includes such entities as postoperative adhesions, intussusception, Meckel's diverticulum, appendicitis, and foreign body ingestion, all of which may require prompt surgical intervention. Other nonsurgical etiologies are gastroenteritis, constipation, medication-related side effects, and enteric neuropathies, such as Hirschsprung's disease or pseudoobstruction syndromes [1, 2]. To complicate matters, young children often deliver a difficult and unreliable exam.

Sapovirus is a member of the Caliciviridae family that worldwide is responsible for 2.2–12.7% of gastroenteritis and has been reported in more than 35 countries [3–5]. Incubation period is from 1 to 4 days, and there is a median of 6 days of symptoms. Major symptoms include diarrhea and vomiting, as well as other common viral symptoms such as

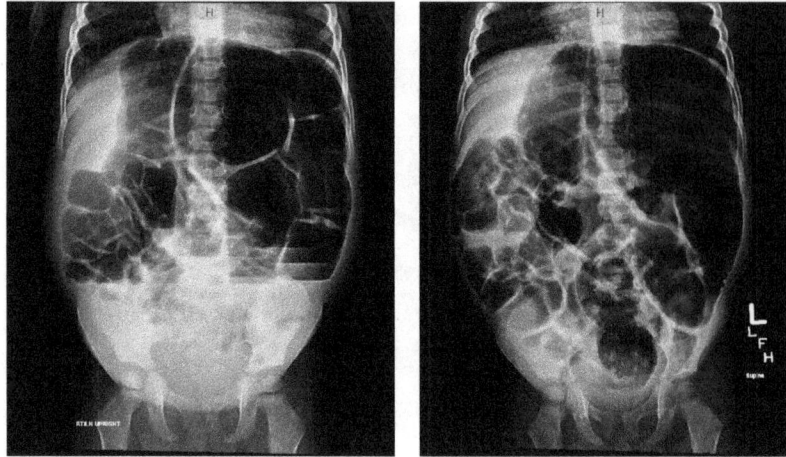

FIGURE 3: Supine and upright plain X-rays of the patient presented in Case 2. The stomach is markedly distended and filled with air. There is moderate and severe distention of several bowel loops, with air-fluid levels.

nausea, abdominal pain, headaches, myalgia, and malaise. Fever is rare, and the symptoms are usually self-limited [5]. This entity more commonly affects children under 5 years of age than in older children and adults, though outbreaks in hospitalized adult populations have been described [6]. Asymptomatic viral shedding has been reported as well. *Sapovirus* has been studied significantly less than other more common Caliciviridae like norovirus. The clinical presentation of nonbloody diarrhea and vomiting is generally milder than seen with rotavirus or norovirus, but hospitalizations and deaths have been reported [5], particularly in rural areas without running water and in immunocompromised children [3]. PCR assays are the best current method for detection of viral strains [7]. *Sapovirus* is often detected concomitantly with other viruses such as *norovirus, rotavirus, adenovirus,* and human *astrovirus* in children with gastroenteritis [8].

The pathophysiology of *Sapovirus* is not well-studied but it is believed to act similar to *rotavirus* and other Caliciviridae such as *norovirus*. For example, *rotavirus* causes infectious diarrhea through production of enterotoxins that alter the epithelial cell function and permeability and through activation of the enteric nervous system. *Norovirus* similarly damages the villi of the small bowel and causes diminished activity of intestinal disaccharidases leading to malabsorption [9]. Effects on the enteric nervous system along with increased luminal contents from malabsorption may thus explain the bowel dilation seen in the presented cases.

We have presented a report of 2 children with exams and imaging greatly concerning for bowel obstruction but who were found to have gastroenteritis with *Sapovirus* as the causative organism. Thus, the approach to a child with abdominal distention, even those with significant air-fluid levels on X-ray and profuse vomiting, should be to consider a wide differential diagnosis. Surgical consultation should be called when there is concern for mechanical obstruction. Clinicians should recognize that even when patients have worrisome symptoms and X-rays, if they lack findings of an acute abdomen, it may be prudent to postpone invasive testing or surgical intervention for a period of observation, while stool cultures and PCR results are evaluated.

Competing Interests

The authors declare that there is no conflict of interests regarding the publication of this paper.

References

[1] L. Ambartsumyan and L. Rodriguez, "Gastrointestinal motility disorders in children," *Gastroenterology & Hepatology*, vol. 10, no. 1, pp. 16–26, 2014.

[2] S. Gfroerer and U. Rolle, "Pediatric intestinal motility disorders," *World Journal of Gastroenterology*, vol. 21, no. 33, pp. 9683–9687, 2015.

[3] N. Page, M. J. Groome, T. Murray et al., "Sapovirus prevalence in children less than five years of age hospitalised for diarrhoeal disease in South Africa, 2009–2013," *Journal of Clinical Virology*, vol. 78, pp. 82–88, 2016.

[4] X. Liu, D. Yamamoto, M. Saito et al., "Molecular detection and characterization of sapovirus in hospitalized children with acute gastroenteritis in the Philippines," *Journal of Clinical Virology*, vol. 68, pp. 83–88, 2015.

[5] T. Oka, Q. Wang, K. Katayama, and L. J. Saif, "Comprehensive review of human sapoviruses," *Clinical Microbiology Reviews*, vol. 28, no. 1, pp. 32–53, 2015.

[6] S. Svraka, H. Vennema, B. van Der Veer et al., "Epidemiology and genotype analysis of emerging sapovirus-associated infections across Europe," *Journal of Clinical Microbiology*, vol. 48, no. 6, pp. 2191–2198, 2010.

[7] C. M. Osborne, A. C. Montano, C. C. Robinson, S. Schultz-Cherry, and S. R. Dominguez, "Viral gastroenteritis in children in Colorado 2006–2009," *Journal of Medical Virology*, vol. 87, no. 6, pp. 931–939, 2015.

[8] A. Thongprachum, P. Khamrin, N. Maneekarn, S. Hayakawa, and H. Ushijima, "Epidemiology of gastroenteritis viruses in Japan: prevalence, seasonality, and outbreak," *Journal of Medical Virology*, vol. 88, no. 4, pp. 551–570, 2016.

41

Isolated Superior Mesenteric Vein Tumor Thrombus in a Patient with Gastric Cancer

Barış Özcan ⓘ,[1] Metin Çevener,[2] Ayşegül Kargı,[3] Mustafa Özdoğan,[3] and Alihan Gürkan[1]

[1]Department of General Surgery, Medstar Antalya Hospital, Antalya, Turkey
[2]Department of Radiology, Medstar Antalya Hospital, Antalya, Turkey
[3]Department of Medical Oncology, Medstar Antalya Hospital, Antalya, Turkey

Correspondence should be addressed to Barış Ozcan; barisozcan2004@yahoo.com

Academic Editor: Alexander R. Novotny

Tumor thrombus in the portal vein can rarely originate from gastric cancer via hematogenous spread, with only few case reports published in the literature. Isolated superior mesenteric vein tumor thrombus in gastric cancer has not been previously reported. A 61-year-old male patient who had undergone distal gastrectomy and gastroenterostomy for gastric ulcer 20 years ago was diagnosed with an obstructive tumor originating from the gastroenterostomy anastomosis site on upper gastrointestinal endoscopy that was performed for complaints of fatigue, oral feeding problems, and anemia. The PET-CT imaging revealed a hypermetabolic mass in the gastroenterostomy region along with hypermetabolic suspected tumor thrombus in the superior mesenteric vein (SMV). A suspected tumor thrombus with contrast enhancement that completely obstructed the SMV was detected on triphasic abdominal computed tomography. Decision for surgery was made due to gastric tumor obstruction. Firstly, lesions suspected with tumor thrombus were extirpated from the SMV and sent to frozen section. Then, it was completely recanalized. A locally advanced tumor originating from the gastroenterostomy anastomosis site that totally obliterated the lumen was observed on surgical exploration. After proving tumor thrombus by frozen, near-total gastrectomy was performed for palliative purposes. Histopathologic examination of the specimen showed gastric invasive adenocarcinoma and tumor thrombi in the SMV (T4N2M1). The patient received adjuvant chemotherapy, and he is at his 22nd-month follow-up with extensive hepatic metastases and intra-abdominal disease. It should be kept in mind that gastric cancer may lead to portal vein tumor thrombus or that it may rarely be associated with an isolated SMV tumor thrombus, both of which are associated with poor prognosis.

1. Introduction

Gastric cancer mainly spreads via lymphatic and hematogenous routes. In gastric cancer, tumor cells enter into the portal system by hematogenous route and lead to hepatic metastases. Nevertheless, tumor thrombi in the portal vein itself can rarely be detected in patients with gastric cancer [1]. Only few cases have been reported in the literature regarding portal vascular tumor thrombosis due to gastric cancer, which is considered as a poor prognostic factor, and the survival rate is reported to be quite low in these patients [2, 3].

In the literature, it has been shown that portal vein tumor thrombus in patients with gastric cancer may be associated with splenic vein, right and/or left gastric vein, or superior mesenteric vein (SMV) tumor thrombi [4]. Tumor thrombus development in these locations is attributed to gastric venous drainage pathways, while gastric cancer associated with isolated superior mesenteric vein tumor thrombus has not been previously reported in the literature.

In this case report, we aimed at presenting the diagnostic and therapeutic stages of an obstructive gastric cancer, which was diagnosed in a patient who had undergone partial gastrectomy for benign causes who then presented with gastric cancer in the gastrojejunostomy site along with isolated superior mesenteric vein tumor thrombus.

2. Case Report

A 61-year-old male patient who had undergone distal gastrectomy and gastroenterostomy due to gastric ulcer 20 years ago presented with new onset fatigue, oral feeding problems, and anemia. The upper gastrointestinal system endoscopy

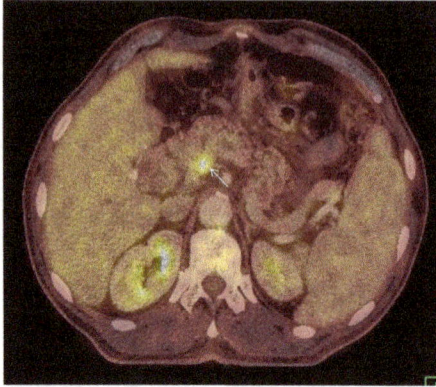

FIGURE 1: Fused axial image of 18-FDG-PET/CT scan shows 18-FDG uptake of thrombus in the superior mesenteric vein. This finding was considered as hypermetabolic tumor thrombus.

revealed an obstructing tumor at the gastroenterostomy site. Histopathologic examination of the endoscopic biopsy showed moderately differentiated adenocarcinoma. The PET-CT revealed a hypermetabolic mass in the gastric anastomosis site along with hypermetabolic activity in the superior mesenteric vein (SMV) suspected with tumor thrombus (Figure 1). A contrast-enhanced thrombus misgiving for tumor was detected within a 4 cm segment of the SMV proximal to the splenic confluence that completely obstructed the lumen on triphasic computed tomography (Figure 2). Mesenteric venous drainage was maintained through collateral veins that drained into the portal vein. Portal vein tumor involvement was not detected, and the portal vein was fully patent.

Decision for surgery was made due to tumor obstruction. On surgical exploration, a tumor that originated from the gastroenterostomy anastomosis site with near-complete obstruction, infiltrating the surrounding tissues was observed. Firstly, to ensure that thrombus was tumor, the SMV was dissected and opened vertically near the splenic confluence under vascular control (Figure 3). The SMV was completely occluded with no blood flow. The thrombus was extirpated within the SMV by direct removal and by using a Fogarty catheter (Figure 4). Following recanalization of the SMV, reflow was allowed and the vein was closed with primary repair. The thrombus was sent to frozen section, and the result revealed tumor. Therefore, the patient was considered to be in the metastatic stage, but palliative surgery for gastric cancer was decided due to luminal obstruction. Gastric tumor tissue was completely dissected from the surrounding tissues followed by near-total gastrectomy and Roux-en-Y gastroenterostomy. The patient was discharged with low-molecular-weight heparin treatment without any problems in the intraoperative and postoperative period.

Histopathologic examination of the surgical specimen revealed gastric invasive adenocarcinoma. Infiltrated surrounding serosal fat planes by gastric tumor was detected (T4). Six surrounding lymph nodes from specimens were resulted as metastatic (N2). Lesions removed from the SMV have been reported to be tumor thrombi (T4N2M1) (Figure 5).

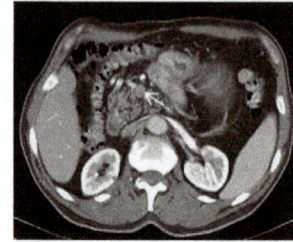

(a)

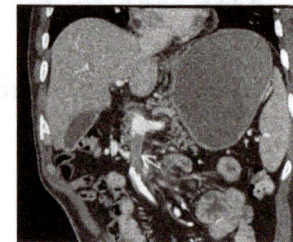

(b)

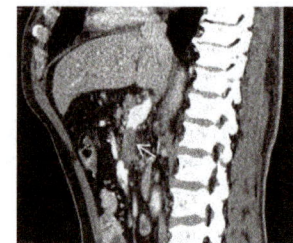

(c)

FIGURE 2: Axial (a), coronal (b), and sagittal (c) slices of abdominal CT show contrast media defect due to tumor thrombus (arrows) in the superior mesenteric vein.

Postoperative abdominal computed tomography showed no evidence of thrombus in the SMV, but the SMV was obliterated and the drainage was still provided by collateral veins. The patient received 5 cycles of systemic paxlitaxel and carboplatin adjuvant chemotherapy. He is at his 22nd-month follow-up with extensive liver, peritoneal, and omental metastases.

3. Discussion

Gastric cancer spreads via lymphatic, hematogenous, and peritoneal routes and local invasion. Perigastric and para-aaortic lymph nodes are involved first through lymphatic spread, whereas liver metastases develop via the portal venous system by hematogenous spread [5]. Although rare, portal vein tumor thrombi can also be detected in case of hematogenous dissemination [6–11].

Although gastric veins usually drain directly into the portal vein, they can also drain first into the superior mesenteric vein (SMV) and then the portal vein via the right and left gastroepiploic veins. Therefore, tumor cells may spread into the portal system in patients with gastric cancer to cause a tumor thrombus there or, rarely, to create a tumor thrombus within the SMV [1, 4].

Furui et al. reviewed published patients with gastric cancer in whom portal vein thrombosis was detected in the

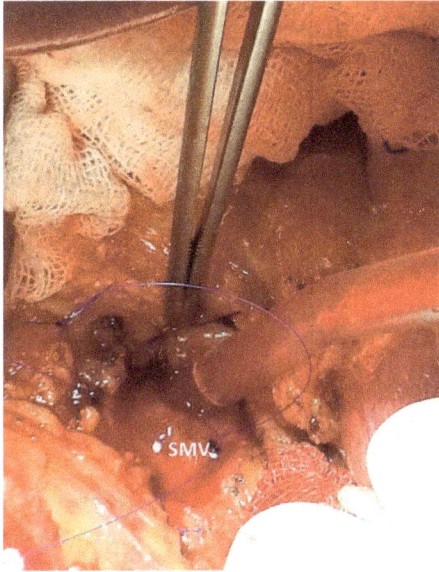

FIGURE 3: The SMV dissection near the splenic confluence.

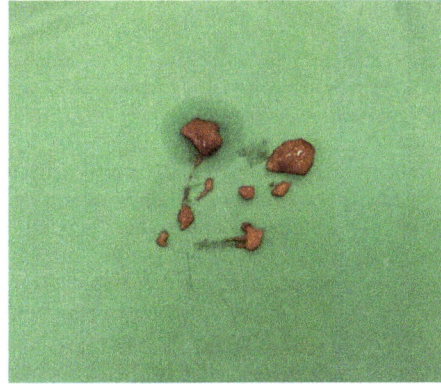

FIGURE 4: Extirpated tumor thrombus within the SMV.

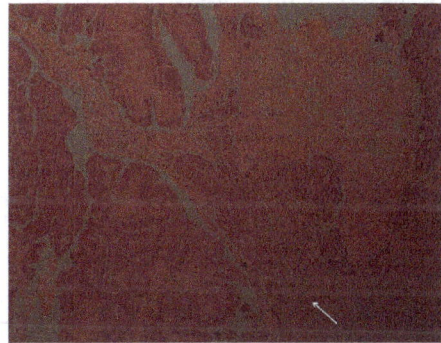

FIGURE 5: H&E (×100) shows tumor cells (arrow) in bloody background.

literature along with their own series in 1996 [4]. Isolated SMV tumor thrombus was not detected in any of the 15 patients presented in that review. It was reported that tumor thrombus in the SMV was usually accompanied by concurrent portal vein or right gastroepiploic vein tumor thrombus.

In our case, we thought that the gastric venous drainage route into the SMV was altered due to the previous distal gastrectomy, especially because of absence of the right gastroepiploic venous drainage. Since a tumor originating from the gastrojejunostomy site was detected in our case, it was concluded that venous drainage was obtained by jejunal mesenteric veins instead of gastric drainage routes, thus resulting in an isolated tumor thrombosis within the SMV. Similar to our case, Ishigami et al. [7] reported a patient who had received distal gastrectomy and gastroenterostomy due to peptic ulcer about 40 years ago who then presented with remnant gastric cancer along with a tumor thrombus in the splenic vein extending into the portal vein. However, to the best of our knowledge, there are no previous reports in the literature of a patient with tumor thrombus in the SMV via direct jejunal venous drainage.

Portal venous tumor thrombus in patients with gastric cancer, with or without liver metastasis, is a poor prognostic factor, and the survival of these patients is dismal [2, 3, 7, 11]. The overall survival is reported to be no longer than 6 months in such cases [2]. Although not based on literature data, it is thought that isolated tumor thrombus in the SMV might also be associated with poor prognosis. As a matter of fact, our case developed multiple liver metastases and peritoneal involvement within 22 months of follow-up.

Eom et al. retrospectively evaluated 51 gastric cancer patients with portal tumor thrombosis and reported that this patient group had a very poor prognosis with an average survival of 5.4 months [2]. In 2016, Sato et al. reviewed 71 cases of gastric cancer with portal vein thrombosis who received 2 to 4 cycles of S-1 and cisplatin therapy in Japan [3]. They reported 10 patients with a survival over 36 months in their study. Because splenic vein and SMV both drain into the portal system, the presence of a tumor thrombus in these vascular structures is also accepted as a poor prognostic factor and the life expectancy is very short in these patients.

4. Conclusion

It should be kept in mind that gastric cancer may lead to portal vein tumor thrombus or that it may rarely be associated with an isolated SMV tumor thrombus. The presence of SMV tumor thrombus indicates a poor prognosis. Tumor thrombosis in the SMV might be expected in patients with gastric cancer who had previously undergone partial gastrectomy, due to alterations in venous drainage routes.

Disclosure

This study was first presented at the 20th National Congress of Surgery, April 2016, Antalya, Turkey.

References

[1] A. Tanaka, R. Takeda, S. Mukaihara et al., "Tumor thrombi in the portal vein system originating from gastrointestinal tract cancer," *Journal of Gastroenterology*, vol. 37, no. 3, pp. 220–228, 2002.

[2] B. W. Eom, J. H. Lee, J. S. Lee et al., "Survival analysis of gastric cancer patients with tumor thrombus in the portal vein," *Journal of Surgical Oncology*, vol. 105, no. 3, pp. 310–315, 2012.

[3] S. Sato, E. Nagai, Y. Taki et al., "A long-surviving case of gastric cancer with main portal vein tumor thrombus after surgical resection and postoperative S-1 therapy," *Clinical Journal of Gastroenterology*, vol. 9, no. 4, pp. 233–237, 2016.

[4] J. Furui, A. Enjyoji, S. Okudaira, K. Takayama, and T. Kanematsu, "Successful surgical treatment of gastric cancer with a tumor thrombus in the portal and splenic veins: report of a case," *Surgery Today*, vol. 28, no. 10, pp. 1046–1050, 1998.

[5] E. Viadana, I. D. Bross, and J. W. Pickren, "The metastatic spread of cancers of the digestive system in man," *Oncology*, vol. 35, no. 3, pp. 114–126, 1978.

[6] Y. Sugawara, T. Konishi, M. Hiraishi et al., "Portal tumor thrombi due to gastric cancer," *Hepatogastroenterology*, vol. 43, pp. 1000–1005, 1996.

[7] S. Ishigami, T. Arigami, K. Okubo et al., "Successful treatment of advanced gastric adenocarcinoma with portal tumor thrombosis by total gastrectomy following CDDP and S-1 therapy," *Clinical Journal of Gastroenterology*, vol. 5, no. 3, pp. 230–233, 2012.

[8] K. Morishima, Y. Hosoya, K. Kurashina et al., "A case of gastric cancer with portal tumor thrombus successfully treated by surgical resection," *Journal of Japan Surgical Association*, vol. 71, no. 5, pp. 1170–1174, 2010.

[9] T. Araki, K. Suda, T. Sekikawa, Y. Ishii, T. Hihara, and K. Kachi, "Portal venous thrombosis associated with gastric adenocarcinoma," *Radiology*, vol. 174, no. 3, pp. 811–814, 1990.

[10] M. Ishikawa, S. Koyama, T. Ikegami, H. Fukutomi, and T. Gohongi, "Venous tumor thrombosis and cavernous transformation of the portal vein in a patient with gastric carcinoma," *Journal of Gastroenterology*, vol. 30, no. 4, pp. 529–533, 1995.

[11] S. Nakao, B. Nakata, M. Tendo et al., "Salvage surgery after chemotherapy with S-1 plus cisplatin for a-fetoprotein-producing gastric cancer with a portal vein tumor thrombus: a case report," *BMC Surgery*, vol. 15, no. 1, 2015.

42

Adult Intussusception due to Gastrointestinal Stromal Tumor: A Rare Case Report, Comprehensive Literature Review, and Diagnostic Challenges in Low-Resource Countries

Paddy Ssentongo (ID),[1] **Mark Egan,**[2] **Temitope E. Arkorful,**[3] **Theodore Dorvlo,**[3] **Oneka Scott,**[4] **John S. Oh** (ID),[5] **and Forster Amponsah-Manu**[3]

[1]*Center for Neural Engineering, Department of Engineering, Science and Mechanics, Pennsylvania State University, University Park, PA, USA*
[2]*Department of Pathology, Eastern Regional Hospital, P.O. Box 201, Koforidua, Ghana*
[3]*Department of Surgery, Eastern Regional Hospital, P.O. Box 201, Koforidua, Ghana*
[4]*Ministry of Public Health, 1 Brickdam, Georgetown, Guyana*
[5]*Department of Surgery, Penn State Hershey College of Medicine and Milton S. Hershey Medical Center, Hershey, PA, USA*

Correspondence should be addressed to Paddy Ssentongo; pssentongo@pennstatehealth.psu.edu

Academic Editor: Beth A. Schrope

We present a rare case of gastrogastric intussusception due to gastrointestinal stromal tumor (GIST) and the largest comprehensive literature review of published case reports on gastrointestinal (GI) intussusception due to GIST in the past three decades. We found that the common presenting symptoms were features of gastrointestinal obstruction and melena. We highlight the diagnostic challenges faced in low-resource countries. Our findings emphasize the importance of early clinical diagnosis in low-resource settings in order to guide timely management. In addition, histological analysis of the tumor for macroscopic and microscopic characteristics including mitotic index and c-Kit/CD117 status should be obtained to guide adjuvant therapy with imatinib mesylate. Periodic follow-up to access tumor recurrence is fundamental and should be the standard of care.

1. Introduction

Intussusception is the telescoping or invagination of the proximal part of the gastrointestinal tract (intussusceptum) into an adjacent section (intussuscipiens). Intussusception mostly occurs in childhood and is rare in adults with the incidence of approximately 2-3 per 1,000,000 per year, causing only 1% of all bowel obstruction in adults [1, 2]. Unlike the presentation of pediatric intussusception, in adults, the presentation is variable. Symptoms may be acute or chronic [3–5].

Furthermore, unlike intussusception in children where approximately 90% of cases are idiopathic, approximately 70%–90% of cases of adult intussusception are secondary to an underlying pathology, with 65% being due to benign or malignant neoplasms including GIST [1, 4, 6].

GISTs are mesenchymal tumors found in the GI tract possessing a range of malignant potential. They originate from neoplastic transformation of the interstitial cells of Cajal [7–10]. Although they can be found at any location along the GI tract, they frequently arise from the stomach or small intestines [10]. Their dynamic of growth being exophytic, they have a potential to invade the adjacent organs, and in some cases cause perforation into the peritoneal cavity [7]. With such pattern of growth, they rarely cause intussusception or obstruction. Here, we present a rare case of gastrogastric intussusception due to GIST in an 85-year-old woman and discuss diagnostic challenges and management in the low-resource environment. We also review 18 published cases of intussusception caused by GIST.

2. Methods

We present a rare case of gastrogastric intussusception due to GIST and a literature review of published studies on GI intussusception due to GIST. Searches were performed in the PubMed Central and Google Scholar databases. Keywords used were gastrointestinal stromal tumor, adult intussusception and intussusception caused by gastrointestinal stromal tumor, and GIST presenting as intussusception. The citations received via Google Scholar and PubMed Central were each further examined to determine if they satisfy the inclusion criteria. The database search included all articles from 1983 to February 2018. We extracted the following clinical characteristics: publication year, country of origin, patient age, sex, clinical history, duration of complaint, presence of palpable mass, imaging tools, surgical approach, tumor location, tumor size (largest dimension), CD117 expression, tumor mitotic index, length of follow-up after surgery, and recurrence status. If pertinent information was missing, corresponding authors were contacted with a list of variables to provide. We excluded articles of adult intussusception due to GIST that failed to report immunohistochemical staining of CD117 to confirm GIST.

3. Case Report

An 85-year-old Ghanaian female patient presented to our emergency department referred from a district hospital in Ghana with a 1-day history of melena associated with epigastric pain following food ingestion, dyspepsia, dizziness, and palpitations. The patient denied any history of hematemesis associated with this pain. The reason for referral from the district hospital was for a blood transfusion due to severe anemia. Prior to this, she also had a 14-day history of postprandial nausea and nonbloody vomiting. Physical examination revealed severe conjunctival pallor and melenic stool on digital rectal examination with a blood pressure = 110/70 mmHg, heart rate = 114 beats per minute, and afebrile temperature = 36.1°C. There was no abdominal tenderness or distention and no palpable abdominal mass on physical exam. Laboratory investigations showed macrocytic anemia (hemoglobin, 4.4 g/dL (normal: 12.3–18 g/dL), a hematocrit of 12% (normal: 40–54%), mean cell volume of 104.8 fL (normal: 80–100 fL), mean cell hemoglobin 53.5 pg (normal: 27–33 pg), and red blood cell distribution width 17.2% (normal: 11.0–16.0%)). Blood cell counts revealed a leukocytosis of 19,350/μL (normal: 2600–8500/μL), a neutrophilia of 14,570/μL (normal: 2500–7500/μL), and a platelet count of 392,000/μL (normal: 150,000–400,000/μL). The patient was resuscitated with 4 units of whole blood, normal saline, and ringers lactate. The differential diagnosis was upper GI bleeding secondary to peptic ulcer disease. The patient was started empirically on esomeprazole and had a nasogastric tube inserted. The patient continued to pass melenic stools and sustained severe anemia requiring continued

blood transfusion. Due to the lack of resources including endoscopy, a functional computed tomography (CT) imaging unit, and inability to refer the patient 2 hours away to obtain imaging diagnostics, a clinical diagnosis of upper gastrointestinal bleeding was made based on the presence of melena and severe anemia, contrary to lower GI bleeding which usually presents with hematochezia. A decision for an emergent explorative laparotomy was done. Because this is a low-resource setting, there was no availability of endoscopy for laparoscopic surgery.

Under general anesthesia, the abdominal cavity was entered through an upper midline incision. A gastrogastric intussusception was found. The gastric fundus was intussuscepting into the body of the stomach (Figure 1(a)). A tumor measuring 2.5 cm × 2.5 cm was found at the anterior fundal area (Figure 1(b)). The portion of the stomach at the level of the tumor was devascularized. The intussusception was reduced by gently applying pressure on the body of the stomach to reduce the intussusception. Wedge resection was performed at the fundus followed by primary anastomosis. The resected segment of the stomach measured 10 cm × 4 cm and weighed 0.2 kg. Macroscopic examination showed a cream to dark brown soft tissue mass. The tumor was completely resected with at least 0.2 cm clearance (Figure 1(c)). The hematoxylin and eosin staining (H&E) showed spindle cell in the muscularis of the stomach (Figure 2(a)). On immunohistochemical analysis, the spindle cells were positive for both c-Kit protein (CD117) and CD34 but negative for smooth muscle actin and desmin (Figure 2(b)). There were less than 5 mitoses per 50 high-power fields. A diagnosis of a low-risk gastrointestinal stromal tumor of the stomach was made. The patient recovered without complications, discharged 10 days later, and has remained well and symptom-free 2 years after discharge. She was not started on imatinib mesylate due to the small size and low mitotic index of the tumor.

3.1. Literature Review. We identified 28 reports concerning 28 cases of intussusception due to GIST. We excluded 10 reports because they failed to report immunohistochemical (IHC) staining for CD117 or failed to report the results of the analysis discovered on GIST-1 (DOG-1) or platelet-derived growth factor receptor alpha (PDGFRA) markers for the CD117-negative tumors. Therefore, we only included 18 reports concerning 18 cases of intussusception due to GIST in the literature review. The patients were aged 34 to 95 years (mean, 60 ± 15.8 years); 72% (n = 13) were women. 56% (n = 10) of GISTs were located in the stomach, 22% (n = 4) in the jejunum, 17% (n = 3) in the ileum, and 6% (n = 1) in the duodenum. 94% (n = 17) were CD117-positive, and 6% (n = 1) were CD117-negative. In 73% of the patients, there was no palpable mass on abdominal examination. The tumor dimensions ranged from 2.2 to 15 cm (mean, 6.2 ± 3.7 cm), and the median follow-up period was 12 months (range 3–33 months). There were no tumor recurrences reported. Regarding the types of intussusception, 56% (n = 10) of the cases were gastroduodenal, 17% (n = 3) were jejunojejunal, and 17% (n = 3) were ileoileal. Ileojejunal and duodenal-jejunal each contributed 6% (n = 1). None was

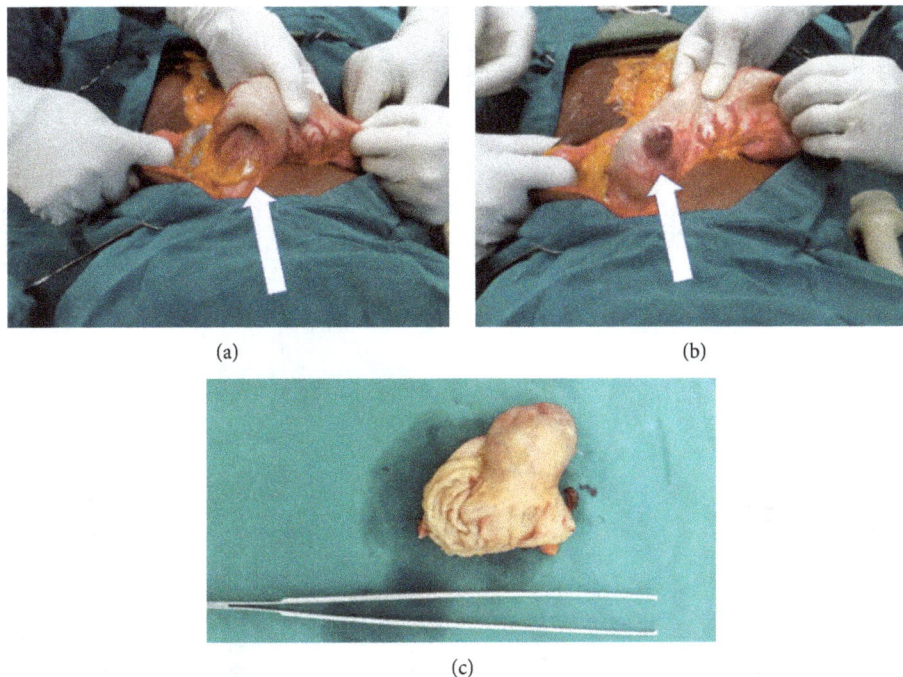

(a)   (b)

(c)

FIGURE 1: Intraoperative photograph of gastrogastric intussusception. (a) The fundus intussuscepting into the body of the stomach (white arrow). (b) GIST after reduction of the intussusception. The GIST is extending exophytically (white arrow). (c) A 2.5 cm × 2.5 cm excised GIST.

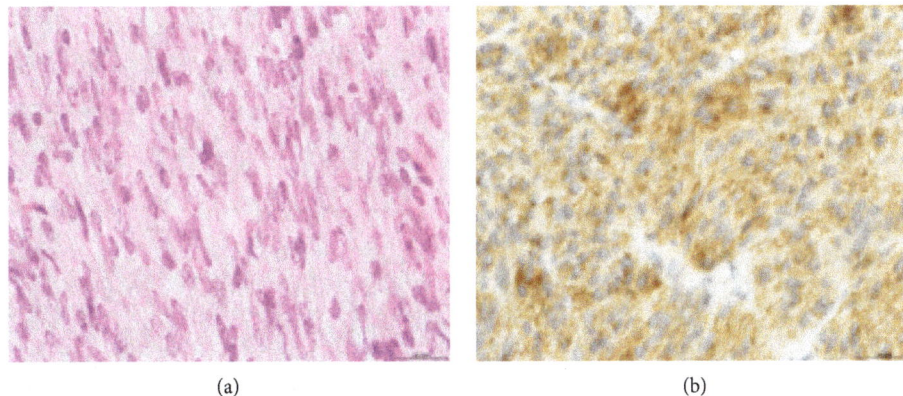

(a)   (b)

FIGURE 2: GIST histology. (a) H&E staining demonstrating spindle cells ×400. (b) IHC staining showing CD117 positive cells ×400.

gastrogastric. The clinicopathological characteristics of the 18 patients are summarized in Table 1.

4. Discussion

GISTs may occur anywhere along the GI tract with 60–70% of tumors occurring in the stomach and 20–25% in the small bowel [11]. This is in agreement with our findings in the literature analysis. In 1983, Mazur and Clark proposed the name stromal tumor to differentiate it from other smooth muscle gastrointestinal tumors [12]. The proposed cellular origin of GISTs are the interstitial cells of Cajal, intestinal pacemaker cells that regulate autonomous contraction of the GI tract [13]. Publications by two different groups in 1998 showed that GISTs commonly express CD117 and CD34 that are morphologically and immunophenotypically similar to the interstitial cells of Cajal [14, 15].

GISTs are one of the most common sarcomatous tumors of the gastrointestinal tract, with an incidence rate of 6 to 14 cases per million people in the United States of America and Europe [16] and approximately 16 to 22 cases per million people in Asia [17]. The incidence in Africa is unknown. The incidence rose as a result of the introduction of anti-CD117 antibody for immunohistochemical staining in 2001. This was due to the change in diagnostic methods and to the reclassification of many mesenchymal gastrointestinal tumors previously diagnosed as smooth muscle tumors such as leiomyosarcomas [18].

A review of 18 cases of intussusception secondary to GIST found that approximately 56% of GISTs were located

TABLE 1: General characteristics of 18 cases of intussusception due to gastrointestinal stromal tumor reported between 1983 and 2018.

Reference	Country	Age (year)	Gender	Presentation	Duration of complaints	Palpable mass	Imaging tool	Surgical approach	Tumor location	Tumor size largest dimension (cm)	Expression for c-Kit/CD117, mitotic index	Follow-up/ recurrence
[32]	Greece	79	F	Lower right abdominal colicky pain, abdominal distention, N + V	5 days	No	Plain X-ray, contrast CT	Laparotomy, end-to-end ileoileal anastomosis	Ileum	2.2	Positive, 7-8 mitoses/ 50 HPF	11 months, no recurrence
[33]	Brunei	62	F	Epigastric pain, melena	3 days	No	Endoscopy, CT	Billroth II, partial gastrectomy	Distal body of the stomach	5.2	Positive, 6 mitoses/ 50 HPF	Taking imatinib mesylate, no recurrence
[34]	China	34	F	Epigastric pain, vomiting	1 month	No	CT, endoscopy	Laparoscopic, wedge resection	Fundus	6.5	Positive, 2 mitoses/ 50 HPF	No recurrence, on follow-up
[35]	USA	52	F	Epigastric pain, vomiting	1 day	No	CT, endoscopy	Laparoscopic, wedge resection	Fundus	5.0	Positive, 4 mitoses/ 50 HPF	5 months, no recurrence, taking imatinib mesylate
[36]	Japan	95	F	Vomiting and loss of appetite, melena	1 week	NR	CT, endoscopy	Endoscopic submucosal dissection	Posterior wall of distal body	4.2	Positive, 4 mitoses/ 50 HPF	No recurrence, patient died of old age 55 months later
[37]	Japan	51	M	N + V, melena, and severe anemia	4 days	No	CT, endoscopy		Antrum	5.5	Positive/NR	No recurrence
[38]	India	65	F	Upper abdominal pain, intermittent vomiting 30 minutes after meals	6 months	Yes	CT, endoscopy	Laparotomy, wedge resection	Pylorus	6.0	Positive, 0-1 mitosis/ 50 HPF	1 year, no recurrence
[39]	Ireland	78	F	Upper abdominal discomfort, vomiting, and anorexia	1 week	NR	CT	Endoscopic reduction, laparoscopic, wedge resection	Body and antrum	4.5	Positive, NR	No recurrence on follow-up
[40]	Ghana	59	F	Intermittent vomiting	1 week	Yes	US	Laparotomy, wedge resection	Anterior wall stomach	NR	Positive, <1 mitosis/ 50 HPF	12 months, no recurrence
[41]	India	60	F	Intermittent vomiting 30 minutes after meals, loss of appetite and weight	NR	NR	CT, endoscopy	Laparoscopic, Billroth II, partial gastrectomy	Antrum	8.0	Positive, 2 mitoses/ 50 HPF	14 months, no recurrence

TABLE 1: Continued.

Reference	Country	Age (year)	Gender	Presentation	Duration of complaints	Palpable mass	Imaging tool	Surgical approach	Tumor location	Tumor size largest dimension (cm)	Expression for c-Kit/CD117, mitotic index	Follow-up/ recurrence
[42]	China	69	F	Acute abdominal pain, N + V	6 hours	No	Endoscopy	Laparoscopic wedge resection	Antrum	4.5	Negative, but DOG-1 and CD34-positive, no PDGFRA mutation, <5 mitoses/ 50 HPF	33 months, no recurrence
[43]	UK	68	M	Abdominal pain and distension, vomiting, constipation, melena	NR	NR	CT	Laparotomy	Jejunum	4.0	Positive, 0-1 mitosis/ 50 HPF	NR, no recurrence
[44]	UK	70	M	Abdominal pain, nausea, bilious vomiting, constipation	1 week	NR	Abdominal X-ray, CT	Laparotomy, primary anastomosis	Jejunum	4.0	Positive/NR	3 months, no recurrence, taking imatinib mesylate
[45]	Morocco	59	F	Abdominal distension, pain, constipation, vomiting	6 months	No	CT	Laparotomy, primary ileoileal anastomosis	Ileum	NR	Positive/NR	NR
[46]	India	46	F	Abdominal pain, abdominal distension, anorexia, vomiting, constipation	36 hours	Yes	Endoscopy, US, CT	Laparotomy, primary jejunojejunal anastomosis	Jejunum	4.0	Positive, 6 mitoses/ 50 HPF	2 years, no recurrence, taking imatinib mesylate
[47]	India	38	M	Abdominal pain	2 months	Yes	US, CT enteroclysis	Laparotomy, tumor resection	Jejunum	15.0	Positive, 6 mitoses/ 50 HPF	Six months, no recurrence, taking imatinib mesylate
[48]	India	59	M	Abdominal pain, distension, bilious vomiting, constipation	3 days	No	Plain X-ray abdomen, US	Laparotomy, primary ileoileal anastomosis	Ileum	NR	Positive/NR	NR

TABLE 1: Continued.

Reference	Country	Age (year)	Gender	Presentation	Duration of complaints	Palpable mass	Imaging tool	Surgical approach	Tumor location	Tumor size largest dimension (cm)	Expression for c-Kit/CD117, mitotic index	Follow-up/ recurrence
[49]	UK	36	F	Collapse, melena, hypotension (82/46 mmHg), tachycardia (150 bpm)	NR	No	CT	Laparotomy, pancreaticoduodenectomy	Duodenum	15.0	Positive/NR	No recurrence

F: female; M: male; NR: not reported; US: ultrasonography; CT: computed tomography; N + V: nausea and vomiting; HPF: high-power field; USA: United States of America; UK: United Kingdom; bpm: beats per minute; DOG-1: discovered on GIST-1; PDGFRA: platelet-derived growth factor receptor alpha.

in the stomach followed by a quarter of tumors arising from the jejunum. We also found that over half of the types of intussusception were gastroduodenal. Mucosal ulceration or fistulation occurs in about 15–50% of these tumors. The associated bleeding in our patient likely contributed to her anemia. Pathohistologically, GISTs are defined by positive immunostaining for c-Kit protooncogene-CD117 (overexpressed in 95%) and CD34 (positive in 60% to 70%) [19].

GISTs most commonly present with dyspepsia and GI bleeding presenting as melena caused by pressure necrosis and ulceration of the overlying mucosa [20]. Rarely, they may present with bowel obstruction or tumor rupture with hemoperitoneum. In our study, 28% of patients presented with melena and 83% presented with vomiting. The classic triad of intussusception, abdominal tenderness, palpable abdominal mass, and hemoglobin-positive stools, is rarely found in adults [21]. Therefore, an accurate diagnosis is based on a combination of accurate medical history, thorough physical examination, and imaging modalities.

Abdominal X-ray is the first diagnostic tool used due to the obstructive symptoms that dominate the clinical picture in most cases. However, due to its high sensitivity (98–100%), specificity (88%), and a lower cost, abdominal ultrasound scan (US) is the diagnostic tool of choice [22]. The typical imaging features of abdominal US consist of the doughnut or target sign in the transverse view and the pseudokidney or sandwich sign in the longitudinal view. Barium studies in upper GI series show stacked coin or coiled spring sign due to edematous mucosal folds and a cup-shaped filling defect in barium enemas when evaluating colocolic or ileocolic intussusception [23]. However, due to the higher sensitivity of abdominal computed tomography (CT) scans [24] and the characteristic "target sign," it has been reported to be the most useful and accurate imaging modality for diagnosis of intestinal intussusception and may be superior to the abovementioned studies.

In low-resource countries where access to imaging modalities like CT scan and endoscopy is a challenge [25], a timely diagnosis should be made based on a clinical history and physical examination. The clinical presentation includes abdominal pain, nausea and vomiting, and melena. The definitive diagnosis of intussusception is made intraoperatively due to the paucity of preoperative imaging. In light of the patient's massive bleeding, with no endoscopic capability and limited blood products, the decision to perform an exploratory laparotomy for hemorrhage control was made. If the laparotomy was not done urgently, the patient would have died due to severe anemia. In our case, we performed a laparotomy on the grounds of clinical findings and in the absence of access to imaging means such as an abdominal US and CT scan or a plain X-ray. In this environment, any delay in surgery resulting in necrotic bowel complicates management and may necessitate an otherwise avoidable bowel resection. The resulting complications may include the need for an ostomy, anastomotic leak, and reoperation. All of these complications further burden the healthcare system in an economically overstressed system.

Treatment of adult intussusception is always surgical [26]. However, optimal management remains controversial. The surgical approach is either primary *en* block resection or initial reduction of the intussusception followed by a limited resection [27]. However, suspicion of malignancy is a contraindication to reduction to avoid the likelihood of intraluminal seeding, venous embolization in regions of ulcerated mucosa, and anastomotic leak [28]. Laparoscopy as a minimally invasive procedure for both diagnosis and treatment of adult intussusceptions has recently gained popularity [29]. For surgical resection of a gastric GIST, a laparoscopic approach is associated with low morbidity, mortality, and short length of stay, and therefore, if available, is the preferred resection technique in the majority of patients having small- and medium-sized gastric GISTs [30]. In addition to surgical management of GIST, imatinib mesylate is used if the tumor is aggressive. This drug was approved by the FDA in 2001 for the treatment of gastrointestinal stromal tumors. Its mechanism of action is to selectively inhibit the KIT signal-transduction pathway (the mutated exon 11 of the KIT receptor) [31]. Patient age, tumor size, mitotic index, tumor ulceration, and necrosis significantly influence tumor recurrence. However, the presence of 10 or more mitotic figures per 50 high-power fields is an independent and a significant predictor of disease progression [30]. The 2-year survival of patients with advanced disease has risen to 75–80% following treatment with imatinib mesylate. In our literature review, we found that approximately 28% of the patients were started on imatinib mesylate after surgery. There was no tumor recurrence reported in the median 12 months of follow-up.

5. Conclusion

Although gastric GIST is not uncommon, presentation in the form of gastrogastric intussusception is very rare. This diagnosis should be entertained in a patient with acute gastric outlet obstruction and melena. In low-resource countries with limited access to imaging modalities, clinical history and physical exams should be the basis of early diagnosis and surgical management. Surgical management is the best treatment modality. After reduction of the intussusception, GIST requires surgical resection and should be histologically analyzed to quantify its aggressiveness.

Additional Points

SCARE Checklist (2013) Statement. The authors have read the CARE Checklist (2013), and the manuscript was prepared according to the CARE Checklist (2013).

Authors' Contributions

Paddy Ssentongo, John S. Oh, and Forster Amponsah-Manu designed the research. Mark Egan performed the pathological analysis. All authors performed the research. Paddy Ssentongo performed the literature search, data analysis, and drafted the manuscript. All authors reviewed and agreed on the final version of the manuscript.

Acknowledgments

This study was supported by the Global Surgery Program, Penn State Hershey College of Medicine, Hershey, PA, United States.

References

[1] N. Wang, X.-Y. Cui, Y. Liu et al., "Adult intussusception: a retrospective review of 41 cases," *World Journal of Gastroenterology: WJG*, vol. 15, no. 26, pp. 3303–3308, 2009.

[2] S. M. H. Kashfi, F. Behboudi Farahbakhsh, M. Golmohammadi et al., "Jejunojejunal intussusception caused by a jejunal villous adenoma polyp in an adult," *Annals of Colorectal Research*, vol. 2, no. 4, 2014.

[3] F. P. Agha, "Intussusception in adults," *American Journal of Roentgenology*, vol. 146, no. 3, pp. 527–531, 1986.

[4] D. Brayton and W. J. Norris, "Intussusception in adults," *The American Journal of Surgery*, vol. 88, no. 1, pp. 32–43, 1954.

[5] A. M. Cotlar and I. Cohn Jr., "Intussusception in adults," *The American Journal of Surgery*, vol. 101, no. 1, pp. 114–120, 1961.

[6] S. Akbulut, M. M. Sevinc, B. Cakabay, S. Bakir, and A. Senol, "Giant inflammatory fibroid polyp of ileum causing intussusception: a case report," *Cases Journal*, vol. 2, no. 1, p. 8616, 2009.

[7] M. Miettinen and J. Lasota, "Gastrointestinal stromal tumors: review on morphology, molecular pathology, prognosis, and differential diagnosis," *Archives of pathology & laboratory medicine*, vol. 130, no. 10, pp. 1466–1478, 2006.

[8] T. L. Robinson, K. Sircar, B. R. Hewlett, K. Chorneyko, R. H. Riddell, and J. D. Huizinga, "Gastrointestinal stromal tumors may originate from a subset of CD34-positive interstitial cells of Cajal," *The American Journal of Pathology*, vol. 156, no. 4, pp. 1157–1163, 2000.

[9] C. Sturgeon, G. Chejfec, and N. J. Espat, "Gastrointestinal stromal tumors: a spectrum of disease," *Surgical Oncology*, vol. 12, no. 1, pp. 21–26, 2003.

[10] M. Miettinen and J. Lasota, "Gastrointestinal stromal tumors: pathology and prognosis at different sites," *Seminars in Diagnostic Pathology*, vol. 23, no. 2, pp. 70–83, 2006.

[11] M. A. Sorour, M. I. Kassem, A. E. H. A. Ghazal, M. T. el-Riwini, and A. Abu Nasr, "Gastrointestinal stromal tumors (GIST) related emergencies," *International Journal of Surgery*, vol. 12, no. 4, pp. 269–280, 2014.

[12] M. T. Mazur and H. B. Clark, "Gastric stromal tumors. Reappraisal of histogenesis," *American Journal of Surgical Pathology*, vol. 7, no. 6, pp. 507–520, 1983.

[13] K. M. Sanders, S. D. Koh, and S. M. Ward, "Interstitial cells of Cajal as pacemakers in the gastrointestinal tract," *Annual Review of Physiology*, vol. 68, no. 1, pp. 307–343, 2006.

[14] L.-G. Kindblom, H. E. Remotti, F. Aldenborg, and J. M. Meis-Kindblom, "Gastrointestinal pacemaker cell tumor (GIPACT): gastrointestinal stromal tumors show phenotypic characteristics of the interstitial cells of Cajal," *The American Journal of Pathology*, vol. 152, no. 5, pp. 1259–1269, 1998.

[15] S. Hirota, K. Isozaki, Y. Moriyama et al., "Gain-of-function mutations of c-kit in human gastrointestinal stromal tumors," *Science*, vol. 279, no. 5350, pp. 577–580, 1998.

[16] B. Nilsson, P. Bümming, J. M. Meis-Kindblom et al., "Gastrointestinal stromal tumors: the incidence, prevalence, clinical course, and prognostication in the preimatinib mesylate era," *Cancer*, vol. 103, no. 4, pp. 821–829, 2005.

[17] M.-Y. Cho, J. H. Sohn, J. M. Kim et al., "Current trends in the epidemiological and pathological characteristics of gastrointestinal stromal tumors in Korea, 2003-2004," *Journal of Korean Medical Science*, vol. 25, no. 6, pp. 853–862, 2010.

[18] E. A. Perez, A. S. Livingstone, D. Franceschi et al., "Current incidence and outcomes of gastrointestinal mesenchymal tumors including gastrointestinal stromal tumors," *Journal of the American College of Surgeons*, vol. 202, no. 4, pp. 623–629, 2006.

[19] P. A. R. Bucher, P. Villiger, J. F. Egger, L. H. Buhler, and P. Morel, "Management of gastrointestinal stromal tumors: from diagnosis to treatment," *Swiss Medical Weekly*, vol. 134, no. 11-12, pp. 145–153, 2004.

[20] H. C. Kang, C. O. Menias, A. H. Gaballah et al., "Beyond the GIST: mesenchymal tumors of the stomach," *Radiographics*, vol. 33, no. 6, pp. 1673–1690, 2013.

[21] G. Lianos, N. Xeropotamos, C. Bali, G. Baltoggiannis, and E. Ignatiadou, "Adult bowel intussusception: presentation, location, etiology, diagnosis and treatment," *Il Giornale di chirurgia*, vol. 34, no. 9-10, pp. 280–283, 2013.

[22] G. Del-Pozo, J. C. Albillos, D. Tejedor et al., "Intussusception in children: current concepts in diagnosis and enema reduction," *Radiographics*, vol. 19, no. 2, pp. 299–319, 1999.

[23] P. A. Ongom and S. C. Kijjambu, "Adult intussusception: a continuously unveiling clinical complex illustrating both acute (emergency) and chronic disease management," *OA Emergency Medicine*, vol. 1, no. 1, p. 3, 2013.

[24] A. Marinis, A. Yiallourou, L. Samanides et al., "Intussusception of the bowel in adults: a review," *World journal of gastroenterology: WJG*, vol. 15, no. 4, pp. 407–411, 2009.

[25] P. Ssentongo, X. Candela, A. K. Sakyi Amoah et al., "Jejunal atresia causing failure to thrive: the role of camera mobile phones in aiding diagnosis in limited resource settings," *Journal of Pediatric Surgery Case Reports*, vol. 36, pp. 67–69, 2018.

[26] D. G. Begos, A. Sandor, and I. M. Modlin, "The diagnosis and management of adult intussusception," *The American Journal of Surgery*, vol. 173, no. 2, pp. 88–94, 1997.

[27] M. Rathore, S. Andrabi, and M. Mansha, "Adult intussusception-a surgical dilemma," *Journal of Ayub Medical College, Abbottabad*, vol. 18, no. 3, pp. 3–6, 2006.

[28] L. K. Eisen, J. D. Cunningham, and A. H. Aufses Jr., "Intussusception in adults: institutional review1," *Journal of the American College of Surgeons*, vol. 188, no. 4, pp. 390–395, 1999.

[29] C. Palanivelu, M. Rangarajan, R. Senthilkumar, and M. V. Madankumar, "Minimal access surgery for adult intussusception with subacute intestinal obstruction: a single center's decade-long experience," *Surgical Laparoscopy, Endoscopy & Percutaneous Techniques*, vol. 17, no. 6, pp. 487–491, 2007.

[30] Y. W. Novitsky, K. W. Kercher, R. F. Sing, and B. T. Heniford, "Long-term outcomes of laparoscopic resection of gastric gastrointestinal stromal tumors," *Annals of Surgery*, vol. 243, no. 6, pp. 738–747, 2006.

[31] G. D. Demetri, M. von Mehren, C. D. Blanke et al., "Efficacy and safety of imatinib mesylate in advanced gastrointestinal stromal tumors," *New England Journal of Medicine*, vol. 347, no. 7, pp. 472–480, 2002.

[32] K. Vasiliadis, E. Kogopoulos, M. Katsamakas et al., "Ileoileal intussusception induced by a gastrointestinal stromal tumor," *World Journal of Surgical Oncology*, vol. 6, no. 1, p. 133, 2008.

[33] B. S. Begawan and B. Darussalam, "Gastroduodenal intussusception as a first manifestation of gastric gastrointestinal stromal tumor," *The Turkish Journal of Gastroenterology*, vol. 23, no. 2, pp. 185–197, 2012.

[34] C. T. Y. Chan, S. K. H. Wong, Y. Ping Tai, and M. K. W. Li, "Endo-laparoscopic reduction and resection of gastroduodenal intussuction of gastrointestinal stromal tumor (GIST): a synchronous endoscopic and laparoscopic treatment," *Surgical Laparoscopy, Endoscopy & Percutaneous Techniques*, vol. 19, no. 3, pp. e100–e103, 2009.

[35] D. W. Rittenhouse, P. W. Lim, L. A. Shirley, and K. A. Chojnacki, "Gastroduodenal intussusception of a gastrointestinal stromal tumor (GIST): case report and review of the literature," *Surgical Laparoscopy, Endoscopy & Percutaneous Techniques*, vol. 23, no. 2, pp. e70–e73, 2013.

[36] K. Yamauchi, M. Iwamuro, E. Ishii, M. Narita, N. Hirata, and H. Okada, "Gastroduodenal intussusception with a gastric gastrointestinal stromal tumor treated by endoscopic submucosal dissection," *Internal Medicine*, vol. 56, no. 12, pp. 1515–1519, 2017.

[37] H. S. Seok, C. I. Shon, H. I. Seo, Y. G. Choi, W. G. Chung, and H. S. Won, "Gastroduodenal intussusception due to pedunculated polypoid gastrointestinal stromal tumor," *The Korean Journal of Gastroenterology*, vol. 59, no. 5, pp. 372–376, 2012.

[38] A. R. A. Jameel, D. Segamalai, G. Murugaiyan, R. Shanmugasundaram, and N. B. Obla, "Gastroduodenal intussusception due to gastrointestinal stromal tumour (GIST)," *Journal of Clinical and Diagnostic Research*, vol. 11, no. 8, 2017.

[39] M. H. Wilson, F. Ayoub, P. McGreal, and C. Collins, "Gastrointestinal stromal tumour presenting as gastroduodenal intussusception," *BMJ Case Reports*, vol. 2012, 2012.

[40] A. Gyedu, S. Reich, and P. Hoyte-Williams, "Gastrointestinal stromal tumour presenting acutely as gastroduodenal intussusception," *Acta Chirurgica Belgica*, vol. 111, no. 5, pp. 327–328, 2011.

[41] C. Palanivelu, M. Rangarajan, and S. Annapoorni, "Laparoscopic distal gastrectomy for gastroduodenal intussusception due to a benign gastric tumour," *Hellenic Journal of Surgery*, vol. 88, no. 2, pp. 135–138, 2016.

[42] Y. Zhou, X. D. Wu, Q. Shi, C. H. Xu, and J. Jia, "Gastroduodenal intussusception and pylorus obstruction induced by a c-KIT-negative gastric gastrointestinal stromal tumor: case report and review of the literature," *Zeitschrift für Gastroenterologie*, vol. 56, no. 4, pp. 374–379, 2018.

[43] P. Sadeghi and S. Lanzon-Miller, "A jejunal GIST presenting with obscure gastrointestinal bleeding and small bowel obstruction secondary to intussusception," *BMJ Case Reports*, vol. 2015, 2015.

[44] R. E. Sankey, M. Maatouk, A. Mahmood, and M. Raja, "Case report: jejunal gastrointestinal stromal tumour, a rare tumour, with a challenging diagnosis and a successful treatment," *Journal of Surgical Case Reports*, vol. 2015, no. 5, 2015.

[45] K. Rabbani, Y. Narjis, B. Finech, and A. Elidrissi, "Unusual malignant cause of adult intussusception: stromal tumor of the small bowel," *Journal of Emergencies, Trauma, and Shock*, vol. 3, no. 3, p. 306, 2010.

[46] A. Basu, M. K. Dutta, U. De, and S. Biswas, "Jejunojejunal intussusception caused by a jejunal gastrointestinal stromal tumour (GIST)," *Hellenic Journal of Surgery*, vol. 86, no. 1, pp. 37–41, 2014.

[47] A. K. Dhull, V. Kaushal, R. Dhankhar, R. Atri, H. Singh, and N. Marwah, "The inside mystery of jejunal gastrointestinal stromal tumor: a rare case report and review of the literature," *Case Reports in Oncological Medicine*, vol. 2011, Article ID 985242, 4 pages, 2011.

[48] A. Gupta, S. Gupta, A. Tandon, M. Kotru, and S. Kumar, "Gastrointestinal stromal tumor causing ileo-ileal intussusception in an adult patient a rare presentation with review of literature," *Pan African Medical Journal*, vol. 8, no. 1, 2011.

[49] M. L. Wall, M. A. Ghallab, M. Farmer, and D. J. Durkin, "Gastrointestinal stromal tumour presenting with duodenal-jejunal intussusception: a case report," *The Annals of The Royal College of Surgeons of England*, vol. 92, no. 7, pp. e32–e34, 2010.

43

Primary Leiomyosarcoma of the Colon: A Report of Two Cases, Review of the Literature, and Association with Immunosuppression for IBD and Rheumatoid Arthritis

Jessica S. Crystal,[1] Kristin Korderas,[2] David Schwartzberg ⓘ,[2] Steven C. Tizio,[3] Min Zheng,[3] and Glenn Parker ⓘ[3]

[1]Rutgers Robert Wood Johnson Medical School, New Brunswick, NJ, USA
[2]Monmouth Medical Center, Long Branch, NJ, USA
[3]Jersey Shore University Medical Center, Neptune, NJ, USA

Correspondence should be addressed to Glenn Parker; eginvest7@aol.com

Academic Editor: Marcus L. Quek

Primary leiomyosarcomas (LMS) of the colon are rare and aggressive neoplasms and have been infrequently reported in the literature. These tumors are more aggressive and have poorer prognoses than adenocarcinoma of the colon and are often mistaken as such on initial evaluation. While the former has a clear association with inflammatory bowel disease (IBD), this correlation is not known to exist with LMS and IBD. Nor is there a known link between LMS and the immunosuppression for IBD, despite the known association between malignancy and immunosuppression for other diseases. Due to the low prevalence of this disease entity, there is limited knowledge and literature on the approach to diagnosing and treating these neoplasms, especially in the setting of the aforementioned comorbidities. Here, we describe two cases of this rare entity, presenting in two different circumstances: one in the setting of immunosuppression for IBD and arthritis, with a synchronous urothelial carcinoma, and the second appearing as the source of an acute abdomen. Both diagnoses were established following pathologic analysis.

1. Introduction

Primary mesenchymal sarcomas of the gastrointestinal tract are rare and constitute only 0.1–3% of all gastrointestinal tumors [1]. Leiomyosarcoma (LMS) is the most common variant of these tumors and represents only 0.12% of all colon malignancies [2]. Amongst the variety of soft tissue sarcomas, leiomyosarcomas represent 10–20% of these malignancies. LMS most commonly originates in the uterus, GI tract, and retroperitoneum. Within the GI tract, the stomach is the most common site followed by the small intestine, colon, and rectum [3]. LMS of the colon has such a low prevalence that there is a paucity of data describing the true demographic, clinical, or gross features of the disease. We herein report 2 cases of primary LMS of the colon, each of which presented in unusual settings and review the literature to highlight the diagnosis, treatment, association with other diseases, and prognosis of these uncommon malignancies.

2. Case Presentations

2.1. Case 1. A 57-year-old female with a past medical history significant for Crohn's disease and arthritis, currently being treated with Humira (adalimumab, AbbVie Inc., North Chicago, IL) and Lialda (mesalamine, Shire US Inc., Lexington, MA), presented for a screening colonoscopy and was found to have a friable mass 40 cm proximal to the anal verge. Initial pathology was consistent with a spindle cell tumor. Further imaging showed extension of the mass towards the bladder. At the time, the patient denied any symptoms of abdominal pain or change in bowel habits. On physical exam, she had a benign abdomen and no other significant findings. Pre-op lab values were within normal limits. The patient then underwent an elective, rectosigmoid colon resection with primary anastomosis, cystoscopy, and transurethral resection of the bladder tumor. Immunosuppression was held for the procedure. Final pathology showed

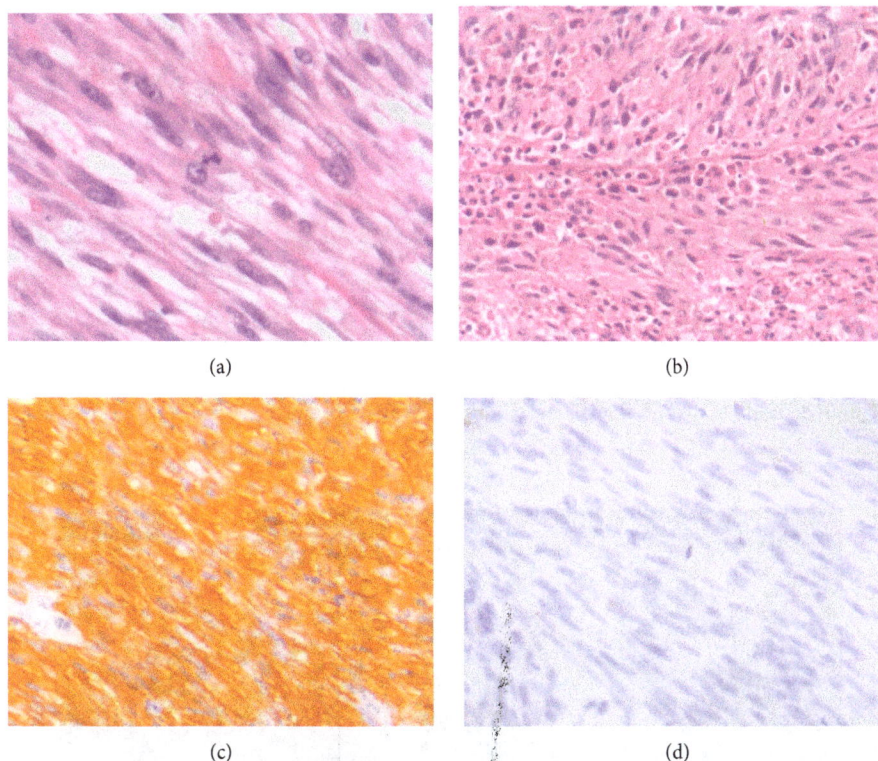

(a)   (b)

(c)   (d)

FIGURE 1: Leiomyosarcoma of the colon. (a) Fascicular tumor cell growth with high mitotic rate (H&E stain, original magnification ×630). (b) Tumor cell necrosis (H&E stain, original magnification ×400). (c) SMA staining positive (×400). (d) c-kit/CD117 staining negative (×400).

a well circumscribed, pedunculated, firm rectosigmoid colon mass with slightly friable/ulcerated surface. The mass was found to be of high grade (mitotic count up to 40 per 50 high power fields) and showed high Ki67/MIB1 labeling index of up to 70% and stained positive for smooth muscle actin (SMA). The tumor cells were negative for c-KIT/CD117, DOG-1, pankeratin, CD34, and S100 stains (Figure 1). The bladder mass was a tan, pale-pink lesion found to be a high-grade papillary, urothelial carcinoma without invasion into the muscularis propria and no lymphovascular invasion (Figure 2). The patient's postoperative course was complicated by an intra-abdominal abscess which was percutaneously drained and resolved shortly thereafter. She then was discharged home to follow-up for systemic therapy.

2.2. Case 2. An 88-year-old male presented to the emergency room with complaints of abdominal pain, fever, and chills. He had an extensive past medical history including atrial fibrillation, obesity, hypertension, chronic kidney disease, hyperlipidemia, left ventricular hypertrophy, benign prostatic hyperplasia, and aortic and mitral valve disease. Abdominal/pelvic computed tomography (CT) revealed an 8.3 × 9.5 × 8 cm cecal mass with thickening of the ascending colon and pericolonic fat stranding. There was no evidence of pneumoperitoneum. There were also several masses in the liver suggestive of metastatic disease, the largest of which measured 12.7 × 11.7 cm (Figure 3). The patient was febrile to 101.5°F and in rapid atrial fibrillation. On physical exam,

a tender palpable mass was appreciated in the right lower quadrant along with peritoneal signs. Laboratory work revealed leukocytosis of 20,800 cells/mL and anemia with a hemoglobin value of 10.8 g/dL. The patient underwent an emergent exploratory laparotomy in the setting of his acute peritonitis. Upon entering the peritoneal cavity, foul-smelling fluid was encountered without feculent contamination. A large, dusky cecal tumor was seen covered in fibrinous exudate without any overt focal perforation. A right hemicolectomy was performed. Gross pathologic analysis showed a 6.5 × 5.5 × 5.5 cm firm, partially circumferential cecal tumor with a lobulated, white-gray surface invading into the terminal ileal wall involving the ileal mucosa and mesenteric adipose tissue. Microscopic evaluation of the tumor revealed high-grade leiomyosarcoma. Immunohistochemistry stains revealed CD117 negativity and smooth muscle actin (SMA) positivity confirming leiomyosarcoma. Final pathology revealed a high-grade (grade 3) T2bN0 leiomyosarcoma with abscess and perforation; 12 lymph nodes were negative for malignancy. The patient had a difficult postoperative course with ventilator-dependent respiratory failure and a prolonged stay in the intensive care unit. Eventually, he was transferred to hospice for palliative care and expired within a few months postoperatively.

3. Discussion

Leiomyosarcoma is a rare entity to arise primarily from the colon. It originates from the muscularis propria layer of the

(a)   (b)

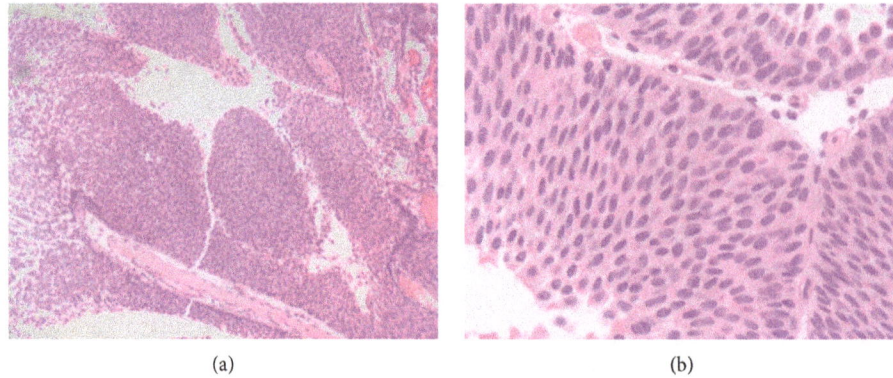

FIGURE 2: High-grade noninvasive urothelial carcinoma. H&E stain, original magnification: (a) ×100 and (b) ×400.

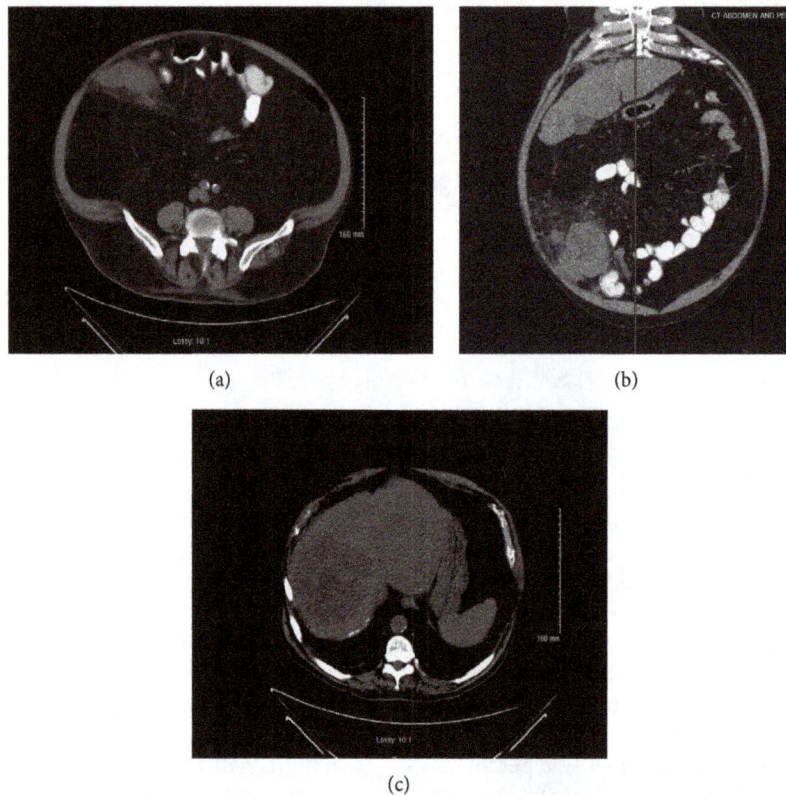

(a)   (b)

(c)

FIGURE 3: CT scan of the abdomen and pelvis. (a) Axial view of the large tumor in the cecum. (b) Coronal view of the tumor with surrounding inflammatory changes. (c) Large lesion in the right lobe of the liver also seen on CT scan suggestive of metastatic disease.

bowel. While it has been found throughout the colon, it most commonly originates primarily from the sigmoid and transverse colon [4, 5]. It is important to distinguish the diagnosis of LMS from other GI mesenchymal tumors, particularly GIST, as the two diseases have different treatments and prognoses [3]. The introduction of targeted therapies for GISTs contributed to the establishment of further criteria for describing leiomyosarcomas as a separate condition from GIST. Prior to identification of GIST, mesenchymal tumors had been labeled as leiomyosarcomas but were later found to be GISTs [4]. The hallmark histochemical stain that differentiates LMS from GIST is KIT,

which is uniformly positive in GIST but are generally negative in LMS. In addition, LMS will stain positive for smooth muscle actin and desmin and will have negative CD117, CD34, and DOG1.1 stains which are positive in GIST [2]. In general, the pathologic analysis of LMS has shown that, like other sarcomas, increased size, mitotic activity, and presence of necrosis confer a poorer prognosis; however, according to case reports, primary colonic LMSs are highly aggressive regardless of size or mitotic activity [1, 6].

The typical presentation of leiomyosarcoma of the gastrointestinal tract is in middle-aged patients with a mean age of diagnosis of 50 years of age [1]. Initial symptoms include abdominal pain, rectal bleeding, intra-abdominal bleeding, weight loss, constipation, diarrhea, bowel obstruction, tenesmus, or fever, which are nonspecific, generally reflect the tumor size and location, and can mimic those symptoms of colonic adenocarcinoma or other gastrointestinal diseases [1, 2]. LMS of the colon was found to be more aggressive compared to other colonic tumors and has a high local recurrence rate and significant hematogenous spread, and rarely lymph node involvement [1, 5]. These tumors are most commonly diagnosed on biopsy obtained during colonoscopy. There has not been any established correlation with any specific tumor markers [2]. When present, metastases most commonly occur in the lungs and peritoneum but can occur in the liver as well. The most common cause of death in these patients is secondary to spread of disease to the lung and liver [5].

Due to the paucity of data, the prognostic factors have been poorly defined and vary by studies. Amongst those identified, poor prognostic factors include age greater than 45 years, necrotic areas within the tumor, dissemination of disease, and tumor size [1, 7]. Accurately predicting patient outcome is difficult due to the rarity of the disease and the short survival once diagnosis has been established. In a recent review of 11 patients with colonic leiomyosarcoma by Aggarwal et al. in 2012, only 2 of the 11 patients survived 5 years, with an average survival of twenty months [6]. Yamamoto et al. reported an estimated 5-year tumor-specific overall survival rate of 51.6% [7].

While the more commonly prevalent colon malignancies, particularly adenocarcinoma, have an increased incidence in patients with inflammatory bowel disease (IBD), sarcomas arising in this setting are quite rare. To our knowledge and by review of PubMed literature, only eight cases of associated sarcoma and IBD have been reported, including three cases of LMS in ulcerative colitis and five cases of sarcomas found in the setting of Crohn's disease [3, 8]. There is however a relationship between malignancy and immunosuppressed patients. Commonly, these patients develop lymphomas or skin cancer; however, recently, there have been a few reports of leiomyosarcoma and other Epstein–Barr virus (EBV) associated smooth muscle tumors arising in younger patients with human immunodeficiency virus (HIV) and those that have been immunosuppressed after receiving transplanted organs [6, 9]. However, this association has not been shown for the immunosuppression that is given to patients with IBD [9, 10]. It is believed that these neoplasms arise in this setting following the complex interaction of several factors. These include the presence of impaired immune surveillance, the role immunosuppressive drugs play in malignancies, a persistently activated lymphoreticular system in response to foreign allograft antigens, and the vulnerability of immunosuppressed patients to viral infections, including ones with malignant potential, such as EBV. It is possible that the poor prognosis of these immunosuppressed patients with tumors may be related to delays in diagnosis in these patients and to the exceptionally aggressive behavior of smooth muscle tumors in the setting of their damaged immune systems [11]. In addition, few cases of urothelial carcinoma of the bladder have been reported in the setting of synchronous leiomyosarcoma of the same organ or presenting simultaneously in 2 different organs [12]. Similarly as rare is the existence of urothelial carcinoma in the setting of IBD [13].

Currently, the best treatment for leiomyosarcoma of the colon is surgical resection. This is true for both those LMS cases that arise independently and those that occur in the setting of immunosuppression and/or IBD [3, 5]. However, since these malignancies are often not detected until late, outcomes are poor, and there is only a 50–60% success rate. Adjuvant chemotherapy is also used, is typically anthracycline or docetaxel based, and does not significantly improve survival [6]. Radiotherapy has not been shown to be as effective [1].

4. Conclusion

In conclusion, leiomyosarcoma of the colon is a rare and aggressive neoplasm with poor prognosis. It can mimic other tumors and GI diseases but should be distinguished as a separate entity as the prognosis and treatment vary. While rare, it should be included on the differential diagnoses when a patient presents with a abdominal pain.

Disclosure

This study was presented at the Society of American Gastrointestinal and Endoscopic Surgeons (SAGES), March 17-18, 2016, Boston, Massachusetts. It was also presented at New York Colorectal Society Residents' Night, March 26, 2015.

References

[1] A. Yaren, S. Değirmencioğlu, N. Callı Demirkan, A. Gökçen Demiray, B. Taşköylü, and G. G. Doğu, "Primary mesenchymal tumors of the colon: a report of three cases," Turkish Journal of Gastroenterology, vol. 25, pp. 314–318, 2014.

[2] K. Iwasa, K. Taniguchi, M. Noguchi, H. Yamashita, and M. Kitagawa, "Leiomyosarcoma of the colon presenting as acute suppurative peritonitis," Surgery Today, vol. 27, no. 4, pp. 337–344, 1997.

[3] P. Singh, B. Bello, C. Weber, and K. Umanskiy, "Rectal leiomyosarcoma in association with ulcerative colitis: a rare condition with an unusual presentation," International Journal of Colorectal Disease, vol. 29, no. 7, pp. 887-888, 2014.

[4] M. Kono, N. Tsuji, N. Ozaki et al., "Primary leiomyosarcoma of the colon," Clinical Journal of Gastroenterology, vol. 8, no. 4, pp. 217–222, 2015.

[5] W. Faraj, J. El-Kehdy, G. E. Nounou et al., "Liver resection for metastatic colorectal leiomyosarcoma: a single center experience," Journal of Gastrointestinal Oncology, vol. 6, no. 5, pp. E70–E76, 2015.

[6] G. Aggarwal, S. Sharma, M. Zheng et al., "Primary leiomyosarcoma of the gastrointestinal tract in the post-gastrointestinal stromal tumor era," Annals of Diagnostic Pathology, vol. 16, no. 6, pp. 532–540, 2012.

[7] H. Yamamoto, M. Handa, T. Tobo et al., "Clinicopathological features of primary leiomyosarcoma of the gastrointestinal

tract following recognition of gastrointestinal stromal tumours," *Histopathology*, vol. 63, pp. 194–207, 2013.

[8] D. Akutsu, Y. Mizokami, H. Suzuki et al., "A rare case of colonic leiomyosarcoma in association with ulcerative colitis," *Internal Medicine*, vol. 55, no. 19, pp. 2799–2803, 2016.

[9] H. Chelimilla, K. Badipatla, A. Ihimoyan, and M. Niazi, "A rare occurrence of primary hepatic leiomyosarcoma associated with Epstein Barr virus infection in an AIDS patient," *Case Reports in Gastrointestinal Medicine*, vol. 2013, Article ID 691862, 5 pages, 2013.

[10] R. G. Armstrong, J. West, and T. R. Card, "Risk of cancer in inflammatory bowel disease treated with azathioprine: a UK population-based case–control study," *American Journal of Gastroenterology*, vol. 105, no. 7, pp. 1604–1609, 2010.

[11] H. Fujita, M. Kiriyama, T. Kawamura et al., "Primary hepatic leiomyosarcoma in a woman after renal transplantation: report of a case," *Surgery Today*, vol. 32, no. 5, pp. 446–449, 2002.

[12] S. Bakaris, S. Resim, A. I. Tasci, and G. Demirpolat, "A rare case of synchronous leiomyosarcoma and urothelial cancer of the bladder," *Canadian Journal of Urology*, vol. 15, no. 1, pp. 3920–3923, 2008.

[13] Y. Fujimura, T. Kihara, J. Uchida et al., "Transitional cell carcinoma of the bladder associated with Crohn's disease: case report and review of the literature," *British Journal of Radiology*, vol. 65, no. 779, pp. 1040–1042, 1992.

44

An Unusual Cause of Intestinal Obstruction in a Young Adult Patient: Inflammatory Fibroid Polyp

Meryem Rais,[1] **Hafsa Chahdi,**[1] **Mohammed Elfahssi,**[2]
Abderrahmane Albouzidi,[1] **and Mohamed Oukabli**[1]

[1]*Department of Pathology, Faculty of Medicine and Pharmacy and Mohammed V Military Hospital,
Mohammed V University, Rabat, Morocco*
[2]*Department of Digestive Surgery, Faculty of Medicine and Pharmacy and Mohammed V Military Hospital,
Mohammed V University, Rabat, Morocco*

Correspondence should be addressed to Meryem Rais; meryemmrais@gmail.com

Academic Editor: Paola De Nardi

Inflammatory fibroid polyps are uncommon benign lesions that originate in the submucosa of the gastrointestinal tract. The stomach and the ileum are the most commonly affected sites. Although inflammatory fibroid polyp is one of the rare conditions leading to intestinal obstruction in adults, it should be considered as a possible diagnosis in obstructive tumors of the small bowel causing intussusceptions. We present one case of inflammatory fibroid polyp as a rare cause of intussusception in a young adult patient.

1. Introduction

Inflammatory fibroid polyps (IFPs) are rare, benign lesions arising from the submucosa of the gastrointestinal tract. The average age of presentation is the 6th to 7th decade of life. Most cases occur in the stomach, followed by the small bowel, and, more rarely, the large bowel, duodenum, gallbladder, and oesophagus [1, 2]. The clinical symptoms vary depending on the location of the lesion. In the small bowel, IFPs rarely cause intussusceptions [3]. We report an unusual case of ileoileal intussusception caused by an IFP, whose diagnosis was confirmed by immunohistochemistry.

2. Case Report

A 22-year-old man presented to our hospital with acute abdominal pain, vomiting, and nausea. He had a history of intermittent constipation and weight loss in the previous year. He had no previous surgical intervention. Physical examination found abdominal distention. Abdominal X-ray showed dilated small bowel segments with marked small bowel air-fluid levels. Computerized tomography of the abdomen demonstrated a thickening of small bowel loops with a pseudokidney pattern, suggestive of intussusception (Figure 1). Exploratory laparotomy showed an ileoileal intussusception completely obstructing the ileal lumen. Segmental resection of the obstructed ileal segment and end-to-end anastomosis were performed. Macroscopic examination of the resected ileal segment found a 3 × 3 × 3 cm firm pedunculated polyp projecting into the bowel lumen (Figure 2). Microscopic examination revealed a mucosal and submucosal proliferation of loose spindle cells arranged in short fascicles or whorled structures, often in an "onion-skin" disposition around the abundant blood vessels (Figure 3). There was an associated abundant inflammatory infiltrate comprising mainly eosinophils (Figure 4). On immunohistochemical studies, the spindle cells were diffusely positive for CD34 (Figure 5) and negative for CD117. The morphological features were typical of IFP and the immunoprofile was consistent with this diagnosis.

A diagnosis of IFP of the ileum was made. The patient was discharged following an uneventful postoperative recovery.

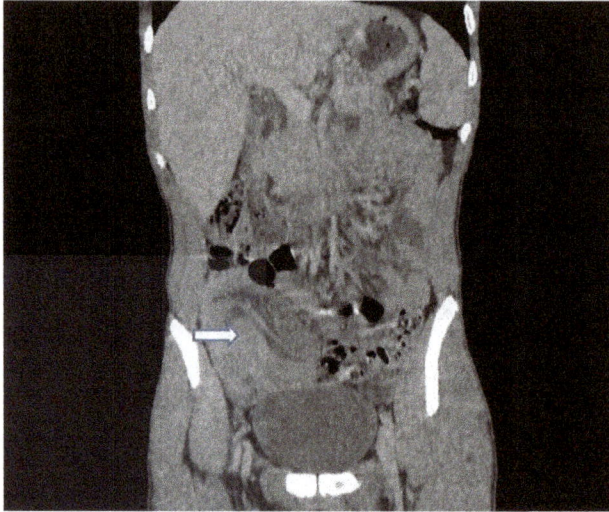

FIGURE 1: Coronal CT scan of the abdomen and pelvis showing a pseudokidney mass (arrow).

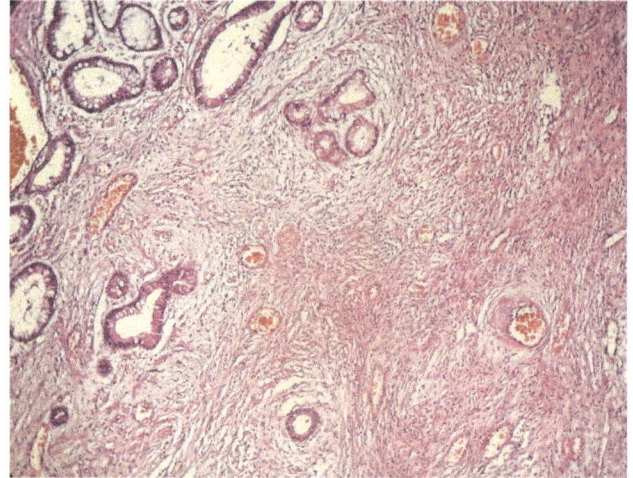

FIGURE 2: Macroscopic appearance of the resected specimen, showing a 3 cm pedunculated polyp.

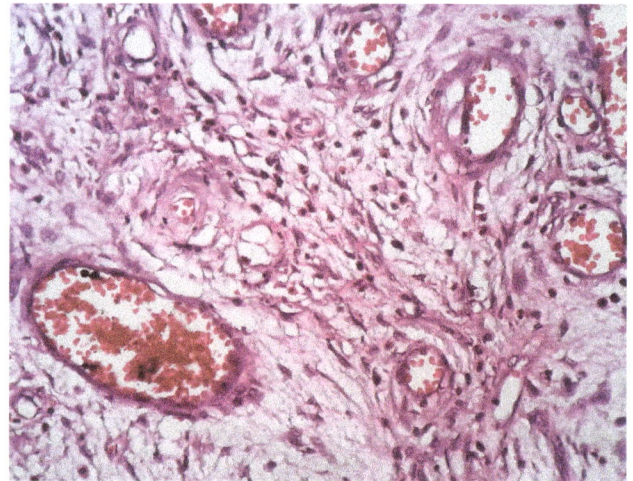

FIGURE 3: Hematoxylin and eosin (H&E) stain demonstrating a mucosal and submucosal spindle cell proliferation showing an "onion-skin" disposition around the abundant blood vessels.

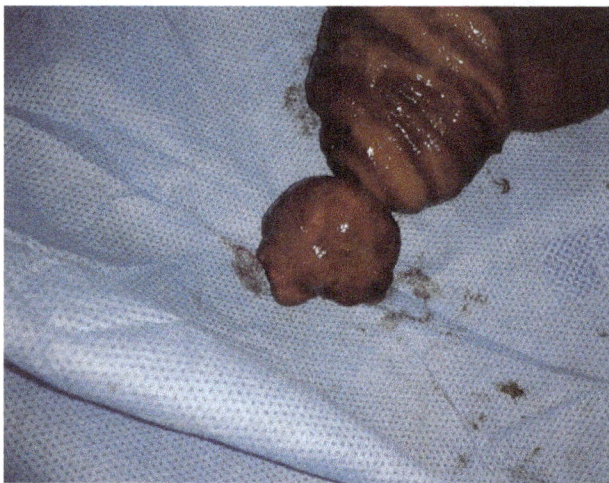

FIGURE 4: H&E stain demonstrating an associated abundant inflammatory infiltrate dominated by eosinophils.

3. Discussion

Inflammatory fibroid polyp (IFP) is an uncommon benign lesion of the gastrointestinal tract [4]. It was first described by Vanek in 1949 as an eosinophilic submucosal granuloma [5]. The term inflammatory fibroid polyp was later introduced by Helwig and Ranier [6], suggesting an inflammatory nature of the lesion. However, recent studies have discovered that IFPs harbor mutations of PDGFRA gene, this being in favor of a neoplastic origin of IFPs [7–9].

These tumors can be found throughout the gastrointestinal tract, but the most common site is the gastric antrum, followed by the small bowel, colorectal region, gallbladder, esophagus, duodenum, and appendix [1]. They can affect any age group, but peak incidence is between the sixth and seventh decades, and there is a slight predominance in men [1]. Presenting symptoms depend on the size of the tumor

and its localization in the gastrointestinal tract. In the small bowel, IFPs can cause chronic episodes of abdominal pain, lower gastrointestinal bleeding, anemia, and, more rarely, intestinal obstruction due to intestinal intussusception [10]. These clinical characteristics are similar to those of our patient, except for the age which is 22 years.

Intussusception is an invagination of a proximal part of bowel along with its mesentery into an immediately adjacent segment [1]. This condition is uncommon in adults, accounting for only 1%–5% of all cases of intestinal obstruction [11]. Preoperative diagnosis of intussusceptions, as in this patient, is challenging. Clinically, an abdominal mass can be found. Ultrasonography is the imaging exam of choice; classical features of intussusceptions comprise a target sign in transverse view and a pseudokidney sign in longitudinal view [12]. On computed tomography, a bowel-within-bowel configuration, with fat and vessels compressed between the walls of the small

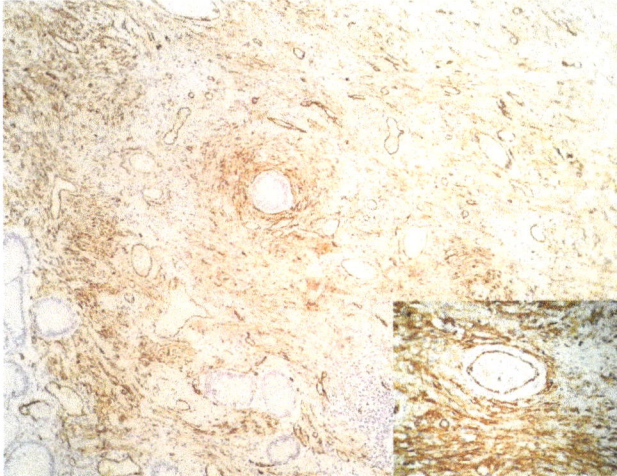

FIGURE 5: CD34 immunostaining showing diffuse positivity in the spindle cells.

bowel, is pathognomonic of intussusceptions [11]. Seventy to ninety percent of all adult intussusceptions happen as a result of a malignant or benign lesion usually appearing at the head of the invagination [13]. Benign lesions that can induce intussusception in the small bowel include lipomas, hamartomatous and inflammatory polyps, and adenomas. Malignant tumors include lymphomas, gastrointestinal stromal tumors (GISTs), and adenocarcinomas [13]. Although imaging examinations are required to identify the intussusceptions as the cause of obstruction, pathological confirmation is needed for the definitive diagnosis of IFPs. Macroscopically, they present as pedunculated or sessile polyps, measuring between 2 and 5 cm in most cases (extremes 0,2–20 cm), and they are usually submucosal and protrude into the bowel lumen [1]. Microscopically, IFPs are made of bland spindled stromal cells admixed to an inflammatory infiltrate consisting mainly of eosinophils, with numerous small blood vessels in an edematous background. The spindle cells are often arranged concentrically around blood vessels, and this is referred to as "onion skinning" [14, 15]. The lesions are usually centered on the submucosa, and they rarely extend to the muscularis propria and exceptionally reach the serosa [16]. On immunohistochemistry, these tumors show positive staining with CD34 and vimentin and variable staining with smooth muscle actin. They are negative for CD117, S100, and ALK1 [14, 17, 18]. IFPs should be differentiated from other spindle cell tumors of the gastrointestinal tract, which include GISTs, schwannomas, and inflammatory myofibroblastic tumors (IMTs) [8, 18]. This distinction is more challenging in the absence of the characteristic microscopic features of IFPs and requires immunohistochemistry. Gastrointestinal stromal tumors are positive with CD117 while IFPs are not [1]. IMTs have an inflammatory infiltrate with more lymphoid cells and less eosinophils than IFPs, and they express ALK1 while IFTs do not [18]. Schwannomas are positive for S100, which differentiates them from IFTs [8].

The optimal surgical management of intussusceptions in adult patients depends on the presence of a malignancy or

manifestations of ischemia of the involved bowel. Intussusceptions in the small intestine result from malignant lesions in 1% to 47% of cases, and the majority of these lesions are metastatic. Consequently, recent reports have recommended initial reduction of externally viable small bowel prior to resection. The incidence of malignancy as the cause of ileocolic and colocolic intussusceptions ranges from 43% to 100%, most of these lesions appear as primary lesions, and a resection without reduction is therefore recommended on those cases [1].

Disclosure

This case was presented as a poster in the International Academy of Pathology-Arab Division 26th Annual Meeting, Sousse, Tunisia.

References

[1] S. Akbulut, "Intussusception due to inflammatory fibroid polyp: a case report and comprehensive literature review," World Journal of Gastroenterology, vol. 18, no. 40, pp. 5745–5752, 2012.

[2] A. P. Wysocki, G. Taylor, and J. A. Windsor, "Inflammatory fibroid polyps of the duodenum: a review of the literature," Digestive Surgery, vol. 24, no. 3, pp. 162–168, 2007.

[3] D. Stewart, M. Hughes, and W. W. Hope, "Laparoscopic-assisted small bowel resection for treatment of adult small bowel intussusception: a case report," Cases Journal, vol. 1, no. 1, p. 432, 2008.

[4] S. Rehman, Z. Gamie, T. R. Wilson, A. Coup, and G. Kaur, "Inflammatory fibroid polyp (Vanek's tumour), an unusual large polyp of the jejunum: a case report," Cases Journal, vol. 2, no. 5, article 7152, 2009.

[5] J. Vanek, "Gastric submucosal granuloma with eosinophilic infiltration," The American Journal of Pathology, vol. 25, no. 3, pp. 397–411, 1949.

[6] J. M. Johnstone and B. C. Morson, "Inflammatory fibroid polyp of the gastrointesthal tract," Histopathology, vol. 2, no. 5, pp. 349–361, 1978.

[7] K. M. Joyce, P. S. Waters, R. M. Waldron et al., "Recurrent adult jejuno-jejunal intussusception due to inflammatory fibroid polyp—Vanek's tumour: a case report," Diagnostic Pathology, vol. 9, no. 1, article 127, 2014.

[8] H.-U. Schildhaus, T. Caviar, E. Binot, R. Büttner, E. Wardelmann, and S. Merkelbach-Bruse, "Inflammatory fibroid polyps harbour mutations in the platelet-derived growth factor receptor alpha (PDGFRA) gene," The Journal of Pathology, vol. 216, no. 2, pp. 176–182, 2008.

[9] J. Lasota, Z.-F. Wang, L. H. Sobin, and M. Miettinen, "Gain-of-function PDGFRA mutations, earlier reported in gastrointestinal stromal tumors, are common in small intestinal inflammatory fibroid polyps. A study of 60 cases," Modern Pathology, vol. 22, no. 8, pp. 1049–1056, 2009.

[10] R. Nonose, J. S. Valenciano, C. M. G. Da Silva, C. A. F. De Souza, and C. A. R. Martinez, "Ileal intussusception caused by Vanek's tumor: a case report," Case Reports in Gastroenterology, vol. 5, no. 1, pp. 110–116, 2011.

[11] A. Marinis, A. Yiallourou, L. Samanides et al., "Intussusception of the bowel in adults: a review," *World Journal of Gastroenterology*, vol. 15, no. 4, pp. 407–411, 2009.

[12] S. Yakan, C. Caliskan, O. Makay, A. G. Denecli, and M. A. Korkut, "Intussusception in adults: clinical characteristics, diagnosis and operative strategies," *World Journal of Gastroenterology*, vol. 15, no. 16, pp. 1985–1989, 2009.

[13] J. Y.-M. Chiang and Y.-S. Lin, "Tumor spectrum of adult intussusception," *Journal of Surgical Oncology*, vol. 98, no. 6, pp. 444–447, 2008.

[14] T.-C. Liu, M.-T. Lin, E. A. Montgomery, and A. D. Singhi, "Inflammatory fibroid polyps of the gastrointestinal tract: spectrum of clinical, morphologic, and immunohistochemistry features," *American Journal of Surgical Pathology*, vol. 37, no. 4, pp. 586–592, 2013.

[15] Y. I. Kim and W. H. Kim, "Inflammatory fibroid polyps of gastrointestinal tract. Evolution of histologic patterns," *American Journal of Clinical Pathology*, vol. 89, no. 6, pp. 721–727, 1988.

[16] S. Tajima and K. Koda, "Locally infiltrative inflammatory fibroid polyp of the ileum: report of a case showing transmural proliferation," *Gastroenterology Report*, pp. 1–5, 2016.

[17] O. Daum, J. Hatlova, V. Mandys et al., "Comparison of morphological, immunohistochemical, and molecular genetic features of inflammatory fibroid polyps (Vanek's tumors)," *Virchows Archiv*, vol. 456, no. 5, pp. 491–497, 2010.

[18] C. Forasté-Enríquez, R. Mata-Hernández, A. Hernández-Villaseñor, G. Alderete-Vázquez, and P. Grube-Pagola, "Intestinal obstruction in adults due to ileal intussusception secondary to inflammatory fibroid polyp: a case report," *Revista de Gastroenterología de México (English Edition)*, 2016 (English).

45

Endolumenal Vacuum Therapy and Fistulojejunostomy in the Management of Sleeve Gastrectomy Staple Line Leaks

Kyle Szymanski [ID],[1] Estrellita Ontiveros [ID],[1] James S. Burdick,[2] Daniel Davis,[1,3] and Steven G. Leeds [ID][1]

[1]Division of Minimally Invasive Surgery, Baylor University Medical Center at Dallas, Dallas, TX 75246, USA
[2]Department of Gastroenterology, Baylor University Medical Center at Dallas, Dallas, TX 75246, USA
[3]Division of Bariatric Surgery, Baylor University Medical Center at Dallas, Dallas, TX 75246, USA

Correspondence should be addressed to Steven G. Leeds; steven.leeds@bswhealth.org

Academic Editor: Gabriel Sandblom

Laparoscopic sleeve gastrectomy (LSG) is the most common bariatric surgery performed for morbid obesity. Leaks of the vertical staple line can occur in up to 7% of cases and are difficult to manage. Endolumenal vacuum (EVAC) therapy and fistulojejunostomy (FJ) have separate documented uses to heal these complicated leaks. We aim to show the benefit of using EVAC with FJ in the treatment of LSG staple line leaks. The patient presented with an LSG chronic leak. EVAC therapy was initiated but failed to close the fistula after 101 days. EVAC therapy was abandoned, and FJ was performed to resolve the leak. Postoperatively, no leak was encountered requiring any additional procedures. Based on our findings, we conclude that EVAC therapy facilitates in resolving leaks that restore gastrointestinal continuity and maintain source control. It promotes healing and causes reperfusion of ischemic tissue and fistula cavity debridement.

1. Introduction

Laparoscopic sleeve gastrectomy (LSG) is used in the treatment of morbid obesity due to its perceived surgical simplicity and excellent outcomes [1]. A feared complication is a leak along the surgical staple line. These leaks have been reported in up to 7% of cases [2, 3]. Some current surgical interventions have been used to treat these leaks including Roux-en-Y fistulojejunostomy (FJ) [2, 3]. Our group has used endolumenal vacuum (EVAC) therapy to successfully heal leaks from sleeve gastrectomies [4]. We plan to discuss a case where FJ was used to treat a sleeve gastrectomy leak in conjunction with EVAC.

2. Case Presentation

We received Institutional Review Board approval for one patient that had a prolonged EVAC course for a chronic staple line fistula from SG, and EVAC was abandoned for surgical intervention with FJ. The EVAC therapy procedure used is described in depth in our previous publication [4]. In short, a nasogastric tube is used to deliver the negative pressure through the endosponge.

A 33-year-old female underwent an adjustable gastric band resulting in erosion, and three months later, she underwent SG. No endoscopic evaluation was done prior to proceeding with SG. She had a staple line leak (Figure 1(a)) on postoperative day 5 with associated septic shock. Laparotomy was performed for washout, omental patch, and a feeding jejunostomy tube. A stent was attempted, but migration resulted in stent removal, and EVAC therapy was initiated. The time from leak diagnosis to EVAC initiation was 84 days. Serial esophagogastroduodenoscopies with Endo-SPONGE removal failed to show resolution of the leak (Figure 1(b)). Laparoscopic FJ was performed 101 days following the initiation of EVAC (Figure 1(c)). She was discharged home 23 days after her surgery on a soft diet.

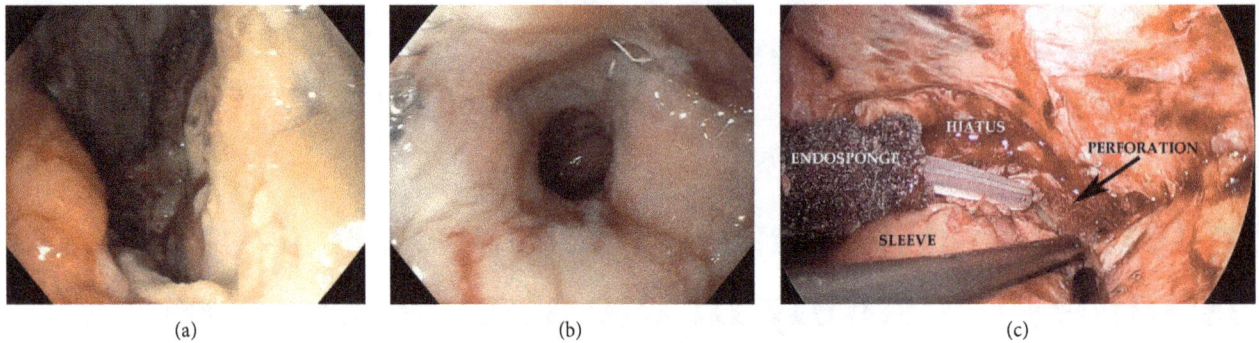

(a)   (b)   (c)

FIGURE 1: (a) View of the proximal sleeve perforation site prior to intervention. (b) View of the perforation after EVAC therapy. Cavity appears debrided, well perfused, and not infected. (c) Laparoscopic view of the hiatus at the time of FJ. Adhesions were taken down to see the proximal perforation site, and the Endo-SPONGE has been pulled through the perforation into the peritoneal cavity.

TABLE 1: Review of fistulojejunostomy in the literature.

	N	Time to FJ	Open versus Lap FJ	Resolution with FJ	Hospital LOS	Days to resolution after FJ	Fail endotherapy
Baltasar et al. [7]	1	7 weeks	Open	Yes	NR	NR	Yes
Zachariah et al. [6]	1	20 days	NR	NR	NR	NR	NR
Safadi et al. [5]	1	NR	NR	Yes	NR	NR	Yes
Vilallonga et al. [8]	18	NR	NR	Yes	18.4 days	13.5 days	Yes
Chouillard et al. [2]*	27	NR	27 Lap versus 3 open	Yes	NR	NR	Yes
Total	48						
P1	1	190 days	Lap	Yes	161 days	23 days	Yes
P2	1	509 days	Lap	No	34 days	74 days	Yes

*Interval report of midterm results for the cohort. Three patients lost to follow-up following their surgery; Lap FJ, laparoscopic fistulojejunostomy; LOS, length of stay; NR, not reported.

3. Discussion

The case presented here is an introduction to EVAC therapy and its effects on contaminated tissue during a gastrointestinal leak following bariatric surgery. The patient that underwent EVAC therapy for 101 days and was taken for FJ after being considered an EVAC failure revealed some interesting characteristics about EVAC therapy. Following that procedure, the patient had an upper gastrointestinal exam that demonstrated no leak and was started on a diet. We are proposing that the use of EVAC therapy can be used in conjunction with FJ creation and facilitate healing.

We are projecting that the chronic nature of the fistula [1] in this patient would have had a poorer outcome if EVAC was not used. We compare this to our experience using FJ without EVAC therapy. We have had similar patients that have undergone FJ without EVAC and had a postoperative leak requiring further intervention with a stent to resolve the leak.

A chronic leak of greater than 90 days will undoubtedly have a lining to the fistula tract and cavity, making it difficult to resolve with endoscopic stent placement alone and needing some surgical intervention. In a separate study, we have shown that EVAC therapy alone can heal fistulas in our own case series of nine patients [4], but with a prolonged hospital course of mean time of healing being 50 days. If EVAC and FJ are used together, as described here, we can likely avoid prolonged healing times and hospital stays. EVAC

therapy can debride the fistula cavity and tract and prepare the tissue for definitive surgical therapy with FJ, while maintaining source control. We are proposing that using these two techniques together in a chronic fistula, existing greater than 90 days, can assist in healing, disposition, and return to a diet faster than when EVAC is used alone.

There are five published reports describing FJ usage in 48 patients (Table 1) [2, 5–9]. The largest series by Chouillard et al. showed 27 patients with complete resolution of the chronic fistula; 3 patients were lost to follow-up. Vilallonga et al. showed 18 patients with chronic fistulas and a mean time of total hospital length of stay at 18.4 days [8]. The other three publications had one patient in each report, all demonstrating the feasibility and usage of FJ. Duration of healing of the fistula after FJ is reported only in the Vilallonga et al. series with a mean duration of healing after FJ at 13.5 days and a standard deviation of 10.3 days [8].

References

[1] R. J. Rosenthal, A. A. Diaz, D. Arvidsson, R. S. Baker, and N. Basso, "International Sleeve Gastrectomy Expert Panel Consensus Statement: best practice guidelines based on experience of >12,000 cases," *Surgery for Obesity and Related Diseases*, vol. 8, no. 1, pp. 8–19, 2012.

[2] E. Chouillard, E. Chahine, N. Schoucair et al., "Roux-En-Y fistulo-jejunostomy as a salvage procedure in patients with post-sleeve gastrectomy fistula," *Surgical Endoscopy*, vol. 28, no. 6, pp. 1954–1960, 2014.

[3] N. R. Smallwood, J. W. Fleshman, S. G. Leeds, and J. S. Burdick, "The use of endoluminal vacuum (E-Vac) therapy in the management of upper gastrointestinal leaks and perforations," *Surgical Endoscopy*, vol. 30, no. 6, pp. 2473–2480, 2016.

[4] S. G. Leeds and J. S. Burdick, "Management of gastric leaks after sleeve gastrectomy with endoluminal vacuum (E-Vac) therapy," *Surgery for Obesity and Related Disease*, vol. 12, no. 7, pp. 1278–1285, 2016.

[5] B. Y. Safadi, G. Shamseddine, E. Elias, and R. S. Alami, "Definitive surgical management of staple line leak after sleeve gastrectomy," *Surgery for Obesity and Related Diseases*, vol. 11, no. 5, pp. 1037–1043, 2015.

[6] P. J. Zachariah, W. J. Lee, K. H. Ser, J. C. Chen, and J. J. Tsou, "Laparo-endoscopic gastrostomy (LEG) decompression: a novel one-time method of management of gastric leaks following sleeve gastrectomy," *Obesity Surgery*, vol. 25, no. 11, pp. 2213–2218, 2015.

[7] A. Baltasar, R. Bou, M. Bengochea, C. Serra, and L. Cipagauta, "Use of a Roux limb to correct esophagogastric junction fistulas after sleeve gastrectomy," *Obesity Surgery*, vol. 17, no. 10, pp. 1408–1410, 2007.

[8] R. Vilallonga, J. Himpens, and S. van de Vrande, "Laparoscopic Roux limb placement for the management of chronic proximal fistulas after sleeve gastrectomy: technical aspects," *Surgical Endoscopy*, vol. 29, no. 2, pp. 414–416, 2015.

[9] C. Elie, Y. Antoine, A. Mubarak et al., "Roux-en-Y fistulo-jejunostomy as a salvage procedure in patients with post-sleeve gastrectomy fistula: mid-term results," *Surgical Endoscopy*, vol. 30, no. 10, pp. 4200–4204, 2016.

46

Laparoscopic Common Bile Duct Exploration for Retrieval of Impacted Dormia Basket following Endoscopic Retrograde Cholangiopancreatography with Mechanical Failure: Case Report with Literature Review

J. W. O'Brien,[1] R. Tyler,[1] S. Shaukat,[2] and A. M. Harris[1]

[1]*Department of Laparoscopic and Upper Gastro-Intestinal Surgery, Hinchingbrooke Healthcare NHS Trust, Hinchingbrooke Park, Huntingdon PE29 6NT, UK*
[2]*Department of Gastroenterology, Hinchingbrooke Healthcare NHS Trust, Hinchingbrooke Park, Huntingdon PE29 6NT, UK*

Correspondence should be addressed to J. W. O'Brien; james.obrien1@nhs.net

Academic Editor: Imran Hassan

Dormia baskets are commonly used during endoscopic retrograde cholangiopancreatography (ERCP). One complication is basket retention, through impaction with a gallstone or wire fracture. We describe a case where the external handle of the basket snapped causing retained basket plus large gallstone impacted in the common bile duct (CBD). Following laparoscopic cholecystectomy, laparoscopic CBD exploration allowed direct stone fragmentation under vision with the choledochoscope. Fragments were removed using a choledochoscopic basket and Fogarty catheter, and the basket was withdrawn. Literature search identified 114 cases of retained baskets with management including shockwave lithotripsy (27%), papillary balloon dilatation (22%), open CBD exploration (11%), and one laparoscopic case.

1. Introduction

ERCP is used for relieving biliary obstruction caused by choledocholithiasis [1, 2]. Stone removal can be performed with a Dormia basket or balloon catheter, an approach that extracts up to 90% of CBD stones successfully [3, 4]. Dormia baskets most commonly consist of four stainless steel wires arranged at 90 degrees radially that are opened onto a stone to allow capture. When a stone is too big to be removed via the papillary orifice, some models permit mechanical lithotripsy, and rescue mechanical lithotripters are available for impaction. This has a success rate of 79% to 92% [5–8]. Overall complications of mechanical lithotripsy are between 6% and 13%, with basket impaction or wire fracture contributing up to 4% [5, 6, 9]. Retention of a Dormia basket in the biliary tree is a recognised complication [2]. This may be due to capture of a stone that is too large to permit removal, with subsequent impaction of the basket and stone. Alternatively, retention through loss of

the ability to manipulate the basket can occur through fracture of the wires of the Dormia basket itself or fracture of a mechanical lithotripter, which can occur at an extra- or intracorporeal level. The impacted Dormia can cause cholangitis, pancreatitis, or migration, and no consensus exists on the optimal technique for removal [10]. We present laparoscopic management for a case of retained Dormia and review the available literature.

2. Case Report

A 67-year-old Caucasian female with a body mass index of 30 was referred to clinic with symptoms of biliary colic. Past medical history included type 2 diabetes mellitus, hypertension, asthma, and previous total abdominal hysterectomy. Regular medications included bendroflumethiazide, metformin, omeprazole, ramipril, salbutamol, and simvastatin. She was a nonsmoker with minimal alcohol intake. Abdominal examination was normal and there were no signs

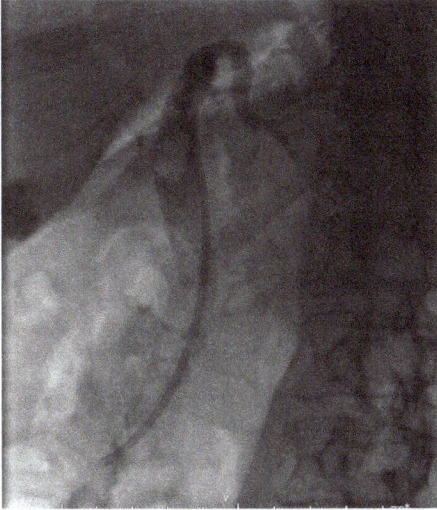

FIGURE 1: Gallstone seen near top of common bile duct.

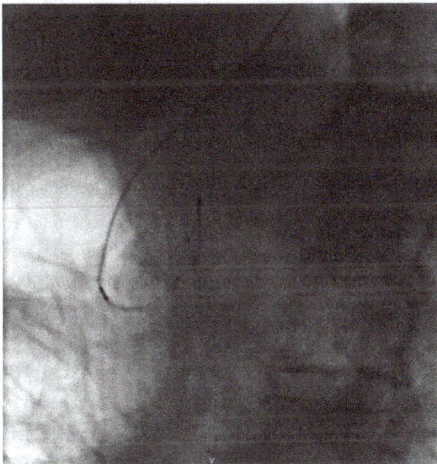

FIGURE 2: Dormia basket in CBD, after handle has broken (endoscope has been removed pending urgent surgery).

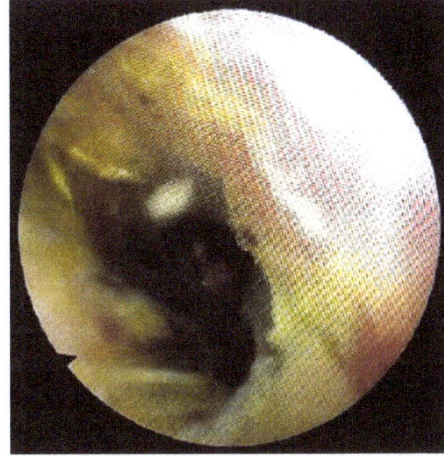

FIGURE 3: Choledochoscopic view of distal CBD. Large stone is seen within impacted ERCP Dormia basket.

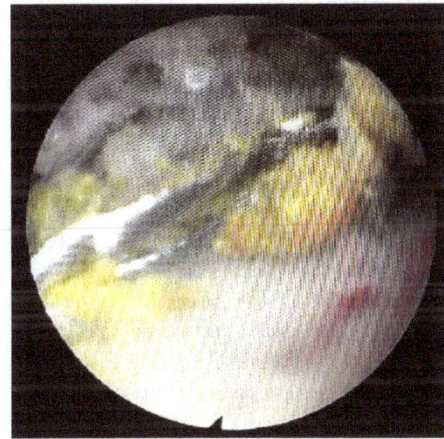

FIGURE 4: Debulked ERCP Dormia basket now collapsed and ready for removal, with few remaining stone fragments.

of jaundice or anaemia. Ultrasound imaging revealed a common bile duct diameter of 13 mm, containing a 12 mm stone. Liver function tests showed bilirubin 13 (<21 mg/dl), alanine transaminase 26 (≤34 IU/L), and alkaline phosphatase 46 (20–140 IU/L). She underwent an ERCP with sphincterotomy, placement of a straight stent, and removal of several stones. One large stone that could not be removed with the Dormia basket was left in situ. During repeat ERCP three weeks later the large CBD stone (Figure 1) was engaged in a Dormia basket for mechanical lithotripsy but on cranking the lithotripter handle the wires snapped externally at the mouth (Figure 2). The patient was referred to upper gastrointestinal surgery and was taken as an emergency to the operating theatre the same day. A two-stage approach was taken following laparoscopic cholecystectomy. A 5 mm choledochoscope was introduced via a longitudinal choledochotomy and confirmed the presence of an impacted basket plus large stone at the ampulla (Figure 3). The choledochoscope itself was

gently used to fragment the engaged stone into smaller pieces under direct vision. Next, a Fogarty balloon catheter and second Dormia basket *(Cook Medical, Ireland)* were used via the choledochoscope to remove most of the stone fragments laparoscopically. Having debulked the stone load (Figure 4), it was then possible to gently deliver the ERCP Dormia basket back into the duodenum without complication, which could then be removed orally. CBD clearance was confirmed and the choledochotomy closed with a 3-0 Vicryl continuous suture. After ERCP the patient was readmitted with acute pancreatitis and was hospitalised for 10 days, following which she made a full recovery.

3. Discussion

An extensive search of the English language literature in PubMed and MEDLINE® from 1950 onwards, including references, was carried out to obtain all published cases of retained biliary extraction baskets during ERCP for biliary or pancreatic stones. Search terms were "Dormia" or "basket" and "endoscopic retrograde cholangiopancreatography" or "ERCP". 46 publications were identified, which included a total of 114 cases. One large case series by Thomas et al. (31 patients) [9] was not included in the following calculation because management of additional non-Dormia related complications was not described separately, leaving 83 cases. There were 42 (51%) cases of retention due to basket impaction on an impacted stone, without any wire fracture. There were 41 (49%) cases of basket retention due to wire fracture. 14 (34%) of the wire fractures were described subsequent to basket impaction. The wire fractures occurred extracorporeally, at the handle of a mechanical lithotripter in 13 (32%) and intracorporeally, along the guide wire or basket wires in 28 (68%), 25 of which were mechanical lithotripter wires. When specified, the CBD was the site of retention in 83% of cases.

The retained baskets were retrieved by a variety of strategies: extracorporeal shockwave lithotripsy (22), balloon dilatation (18), open surgery (9), a second Dormia basket (10), rescue mechanical lithotripter (5), exchange of metal wires (5), conservative management (2), exchange of metal sheaths (2), extension of sphincterotomy (2), laparoscopic surgery (2), laser lithotripsy (2), rat tooth forceps (2), goose neck snare (1), and papillotome to the stone (1). Each patient underwent an average of 1.4 procedures (including the original ERCP). In 33 papers (42 patients) definitive management of the common bile duct was described. 28 (67%) of these patients needed at least one further procedure to manage their choledocholithiasis following the ERCP, and 6 (14%) needed more than one further procedure. The average total number of extra procedures required to definitively manage choledocholithiasis per patient following ERCP was 0.67.

Recent case series report impaction of a Dormia basket during ERCP in as few as 0.6% and 0.8% of cases. Previously, it was reported in as many as 5.9% of cases [11–15]. Certain techniques increase the risk of basket retention. In one multicentre study of 31 patients, overall complications were three times higher following mechanical lithotripsy for pancreatic stones (11.6%) compared to biliary stones (3.6%), with fracture of the basket the most common complication [9]. Stone impaction, stone size, and a stone to bile duct diameter ratio greater than one are predictors of failed mechanical lithotripsy [5, 13]. Stone size over 20 mm is suggested as a contraindication for ERCP by some authors [16], but others suggest the ratio, which is increased by previous cholecystitis and cholangitis, is as important [5]. In such cases, García-Gallont et al. recommend using alternative methods as soon as the Dormia basket begins to deform in the stiffened common bile duct [17]. Typically basket impaction is encountered at the ampulla but case of impaction at the distal pancreatic duct in chronic pancreatitis is described [18] and less commonly the hepatic ducts [19] and a single case within the gallbladder itself [20].

The most commonly described management of an impacted Dormia basket is extracorporeal shock wave lithotripsy, perhaps reflecting the high proportion of cases reported from European centres. This results in high clearance after one session (92%), but subsequent endoscopy may be necessary to remove stone fragments and achieve definitive duct clearance [9, 12]. In the event of failure of laser lithotripsy, repeat laser shock wave lithotripsy is required with surgical exploration recommended if further lithotripsy fails [21]. Although the basket is visible under fluoroscopy, if cannulation of the bile duct is necessary for visualisation, this can be difficult if an impacted Dormia with stone is obstructing the distal bile duct. Importantly, such techniques are only available in certain centres, which can result in delays whilst the patient is transferred. Any delay in management can increase the severity of any subsequent pancreatitis, cholangitis and sepsis.

Rescue papillary balloon dilatation is an option if it has not already been carried out prior to basket impaction. The overall rate of bleeding following ERCP is 1.3% [22] and meta-analyses describe a similar 1.2% rate following combined sphincterotomy and balloon dilatation [23]. In a small case series six impacted baskets were successfully managed with balloon dilatation [15]. All six were done by the same tertiary centre endoscopist. Given the risk of perforation previously reported following balloon dilatation [24], this highlights the importance of specialist ERCP referral in such cases. Extreme care needs to be taken when using monopolar devices to extend the sphincterotomy in order to deliver an impacted basket, due to the risk of thermal injury caused by heat conduction through exposed basket wires [25].

Rescue mechanical lithotripsy was utilised successfully in five cases of retained Dormia. One centre describes four cases of impacted stone and Dormia successfully managed with "through the endoscope" rescue lithotripsy [26]. However, mechanical lithotripsy itself is associated with basket retention and wire fracture. 89% of intracorporeal wire fractures occurred along mechanical lithotripsy wires, and, similar to the case we report, there were 12 cases reporting lithotripsy handle fracture. Equipment failures occurred during use of "through the endoscope" and external or rescue mechanical lithotripters. There are not enough equipment details supplied in the literature to attempt subanalysis.

In 1993 Ng et al. described laparoscopic retrieval (via cholecystotomy) of a basket inadvertently impacted within the gallbladder itself but suggested that retention in the biliary tree was not amenable to laparoscopic rescue [20]. Laparoscopic common bile duct exploration, conducted in experienced centres, established itself in the late 1990s, showing similar success rates and morbidity to ERCP [27, 28]. Laparoscopic retrieval was first described in 2000 by Ainslie et al. [29]. This is only the second case to describe successful laparoscopic rescue. There was no mortality reported following open surgical management of a retained basket, which was the third most common method of retrieval in the literature.

4. Conclusion

This review describes the established risk of basket retention in the bile duct when using mechanical lithotripsy during therapeutic ERCP and further highlights a range of scenarios which may present to the endoscopist, including basket retention due to wire fracture. In centres with appropriate equipment, extracorporeal shockwave lithotripsy and papillary balloon dilatation for retained baskets are described in the literature, with minimal further procedures required to ensure treatment of choledocholithiasis. We describe a single operative treatment whereby, following laparoscopic cholecystectomy, laparoscopic CBD exploration via choledochotomy allowed retrieval of the retained basket and confirmation of duct clearance with choledochoscopy. We have shown the approach to be both feasible and safe and, where surgical expertise permits, can reduce the risk of further treatment sessions to manage residual common bile duct stones or debris. When encountering difficult (large or impacted) common bile duct calculi the endoscopist should consider which options are available at their institution in the event that a basket complication is encountered.

References

[1] D. G. Adler, T. H. Baron, R. E. Davila et al., "ASGE guideline: the role of ERCP in diseases of the biliary tract and the pancreas," *Gastrointestinal Endoscopy*, vol. 62, no. 1, pp. 1–8, 2005.

[2] D. G. Adler, J. D. Conway, F. A. Farraye et al., "Biliary and pancreatic stone extraction devices," *Gastrointestinal Endoscopy*, vol. 70, no. 4, pp. 603–609, 2009.

[3] N. Fujita, H. Maguchi, Y. Komatsu et al., "Endoscopic sphincterotomy and endoscopic papillary balloon dilatation for bile duct stones: a prospective randomized controlled multicenter trial," *Gastrointestinal Endoscopy*, vol. 57, no. 2, pp. 151–155, 2003.

[4] D. L. Carr-Locke, "Therapeutic role of ERCP in the management of suspected common bile duct stones," *Gastrointestinal Endoscopy*, vol. 56, no. 6, pp. S170–S174, 2002.

[5] P. K. Garg, R. K. Tandon, V. Ahuja, G. K. Makharia, and Y. Batra, "Predictors of unsuccessful mechanical lithotripsy and endoscopic clearance of large bile duct stones," *Gastrointestinal Endoscopy*, vol. 59, no. 6, pp. 601–605, 2004.

[6] W.-H. Chang, C.-H. Chu, T.-E. Wang, M.-J. Chen, and C.-C. Lin, "Outcome of simple use of mechanical lithotripsy of difficult common bile duct stones," *World Journal of Gastroenterology*, vol. 11, no. 4, pp. 593–596, 2005.

[7] J. C. Vij, M. Jain, K. K. Rawal, R. A. Gulati, and A. Govil, "Endoscopic management of large bile duct stones by mechanical lithotripsy," *Indian J Gastroenterology*, vol. 14, no. 4, pp. 122-123, 1995.

[8] M. J. Shaw, R. D. Mackie, J. P. Moore et al., "Results of a multicenter trial using a mechanical lithotripter for the treatment of large bile duct stones," *Am J Gastroenterology*, vol. 88, no. 5, pp. 730–733, 1993.

[9] M. Thomas, D. A. Howell, D. Carr-Locke et al., "Mechanical lithotripsy of pancreatic and biliary stones: Complications and

available treatment options collected from expert centers," *American Journal of Gastroenterology*, vol. 102, no. 9, pp. 1896–1902, 2007.

[10] P. Ranjeev and K.-L. Goh, "Retrieval of an impacted Dormia basket and stone in situ using a novel method," *Gastrointestinal Endoscopy*, vol. 51, no. 4, part 1, pp. 504–506, 2000.

[11] M. U. Schneider, W. Matek, R. Bauer, and W. Domschke, "Mechanical lithotripsy of bile duct stones in 209 patients—effect of technical advances," *Endoscopy*, vol. 20, no. 5, pp. 248–253, 1988.

[12] G. Sauter, M. Sackmann, J. Holl, J. Pauletzki, T. Sauerbruch, and G. Paumgartner, "Dormia baskets impacted in the bile duct: Release by extracorporeal shock-wave lithotripsy," *Endoscopy*, vol. 27, no. 5, pp. 384–387, 1995.

[13] S. H. Lee, J. K. Park, W. J. Yoon et al., "How to predict the outcome of endoscopic mechanical lithotripsy in patients with difficult bile duct stones?" *Scandinavian Journal of Gastroenterology*, vol. 42, no. 8, pp. 1006–1010, 2009.

[14] W. H. Schreurs, J. R. Juttmann, W. N. H. M. Stuifbergen, H. J. M. Oostvogel, and T. J. M. V. Vroonhoven, "Management of common bile duct stones: short- and long-term results with selective endoscopic retrograde cholangiography and endoscopic sphincterotomy," *Surgical Endoscopy and Other Interventional Techniques*, vol. 16, no. 7, pp. 1068–1072, 2002.

[15] P. Katsinelos, K. Fasoulas, A. Beltsis et al., "Large-balloon dilation of the biliary orifice for the management of basket impaction: A case series of 6 patients," *Gastrointestinal Endoscopy*, vol. 73, no. 6, pp. 1298–1301, 2011.

[16] N. Fukino, T. Oida, A. Kawasaki et al., "Impaction of a lithotripsy basket during endoscopic lithotomy of a common bile duct stone," *World Journal of Gastroenterology*, vol. 16, no. 22, pp. 2832–2834, 2010.

[17] R. García-Gallont, J. S. Velasquez, and W. Duarte, "Surgical removal of a severed Dormia basket from the bile duct," *Endoscopy*, vol. 46, no. 1, pp. E20–E21, 2014.

[18] A. F. Cutler, W. Mark Hassig, and T. T. Schubert, "Basket impaction at the pancreatic head," *Gastrointestinal Endoscopy*, vol. 38, no. 4, pp. 520-521, 1992.

[19] J. Sheridan, T. M. Williams, E. Yeung, C. Ho, and W. Thurston, "Percutaneous transhepatic management of an impacted endoscopic basket," *Gastrointestinal Endoscopy*, vol. 39, no. 3, pp. 444–446, 1993.

[20] W. Ng, M. Yiu, and K. Lee, "Impaction of a stone basket in the gallbladder with laparoscopic rescue," *Gastrointestinal Endoscopy*, vol. 39, no. 2, pp. 217-218, 1993.

[21] T. Attila, G. R. May, and P. Kortan, "Nonsurgical management of an impacted mechanical lithotriptor with fractured traction wires: endoscopic intracorporeal electrohydraulic shock wave lithotripsy followed by extra-endoscopic mechanical lithotripsy," *Canadian Journal of Gastroenterology*, vol. 22, no. 8, pp. 699–702, 2008.

[22] A. Andriulli, S. Loperfido, G. Napolitano et al., "Incidence rates of post-ERCP complications: a systematic survey of prospective studies," *The American Journal of Gastroenterology*, vol. 102, no. 8, pp. 1781–1788, 2007.

[23] G. C. Meine and T. H. Baron, "Endoscopic papillary large-balloon dilation combined with endoscopic biliary sphincterotomy for the removal of bile duct stones (with video)," *Gastrointestinal Endoscopy*, vol. 74, no. 5, pp. 1119–1126, 2011.

[24] Y. S. Lee, J. H. Moon, B. M. Ko et al., "Endoscopic closure of a distal common bile duct perforation caused by papillary

dilation with a large-diameter balloon (with video)," *Gastrointestinal Endoscopy*, vol. 72, no. 3, pp. 616–618, 2010.

[25] F. Ekız, O. Yüksel, O. Üsküdar, İ. Yüksel, A. Altinbaş, and Ö. Başar, "Successful endoscopic removal of fractured basket traction wire during mechanical lithotripsy," *Turk J Gastroenterology*, vol. 22, no. 2, pp. 233-234, 2011.

[26] M. Matsushita, H. Takakuwa, Y. Matsubayashi et al., "Through-the-endoscope technique for retrieval of impacted biliary baskets with trapped stones," *American Journal of Gastroenterology*, vol. 99, no. 6, pp. 1198-1199, 2004.

[27] M. Rhodes, L. Sussman, L. Cohen, and M. P. Lewis, "Randomised trial of laparoscopic exploration of common bile duct versus postoperative endoscopic retrograde cholangiography for common bile duct stones," *The Lancet*, vol. 351, no. 9097, pp. 159–161, 1998.

[28] A. Cuschieri, E. Lezoche, M. Morino et al., "E.A.E.S. multicenter prospective randomized trial comparing two-stage vs single-stage management of patients with gallstone disease and ductal calculi," *Surgical Endoscopy*, vol. 13, no. 10, pp. 952–957, 1999.

[29] W. Ainslie, J. Reed, and M. Larvin et al., "Successful laparoscopic rescue of an impacted lithotriptor basket from the common bile duct," *Endoscopy*, vol. 32, 2000.

Thoracoscopic Surgery in a Patient with Multiple Esophageal Carcinomas after Surgery for Esophageal Achalasia

Yuki Yamasaki, Tomoya Tsukada, Tatsuya Aoki, Yusuke Haba, Katsuhisa Hirano, Toshifumi Watanabe, Masahide Kaji, and Koichi Shimizu

Department of Surgery, Toyama Prefectural Central Hospital, 2-2-78 Nishinagae, Toyama, Toyama 930-0975, Japan

Correspondence should be addressed to Yuki Yamasaki; yuki_in_lily@yahoo.co.jp

Academic Editor: Shin-ichi Kosugi

We present a case in which we used a thoracoscopic approach for resection of multiple esophageal carcinomas diagnosed 33 years after surgery for esophageal achalasia. A 68-year-old Japanese man had been diagnosed with esophageal achalasia and underwent surgical treatment 33 years earlier. He was examined at our hospital for annual routine checkup in which upper gastrointestinal endoscopy showed a "0-IIb+IIa" lesion in the middle esophagus. Iodine staining revealed multiple irregularly shaped iodine-unstained areas, the diagnosis of which was esophageal carcinoma. Thoracoscopic subtotal esophagectomy was performed. Esophageal carcinoma may occur many years after surgery for esophageal achalasia, even if the passage symptoms have improved. So, long-term periodic follow-up is necessary for detection of carcinoma at an earlier stage.

1. Introduction

Esophageal achalasia (EA) is an idiopathic primary esophageal motor disorder characterized by impaired relaxation of the lower esophageal sphincter (LES) and loss of esophageal peristalsis [1]. The classic symptom of EA is dysphagia associated with regurgitation of undigested food. Some patients also experience weight loss, coughing, and chest pain. Although there is no definitive cure, current treatments aim to reduce LES pressure in order to relieve symptoms, improve esophageal emptying, and prevent further esophageal dilation [2]. Treatments include balloon dilation and Heller myotomy with Dor fundoplication.

Patients with EA are at an increased risk for developing squamous cell carcinoma (SCC) of the esophagus, which is thought to be caused by continuous exposure to stagnant ingested food [3]. It has been reported that the frequency of esophageal carcinoma (EC) decreases after surgery for EA [4], but there are several reports of patients diagnosed with EC even after undergoing surgery for EA [5–7]. To the best of our knowledge, this is the first case report of EC treated with thoracoscopic surgery after Heller-Dor procedure.

2. Case Presentation

A 68-year-old Japanese man diagnosed with EA underwent surgical treatment 33 years ago. During an annual checkup, endoscopy revealed a "0-IIb+IIa" lesion in the middle esophagus (Figure 1(a)). The patient was referred to our hospital for further evaluation. Iodine staining revealed multiple irregularly shaped iodine-unstained areas spreading to the cervical esophagus (Figure 1(b)). These areas were biopsied and diagnosed as EC with invasion of the submucosal layer. Barium esophagram (Figure 2) showed esophageal dilation with a gradual tapering down to the gastroesophageal junction. Emptying of barium to the stomach was normal, owing to the previous surgery. There was a superficial protruding lesion in the midthoracic esophagus (arrowhead). A chest contrast-enhanced computerized tomography scan and positron emission tomography scan showed no lymph node or distant metastases. Early EC (clinical stage I; T1b(SM2)N0M0) was diagnosed based on the 11th edition of the Japanese Classification of Esophageal Carcinoma [6].

Thoracoscopic esophagectomy and open gastric pull-up reconstruction were planned. The thoracic procedure was

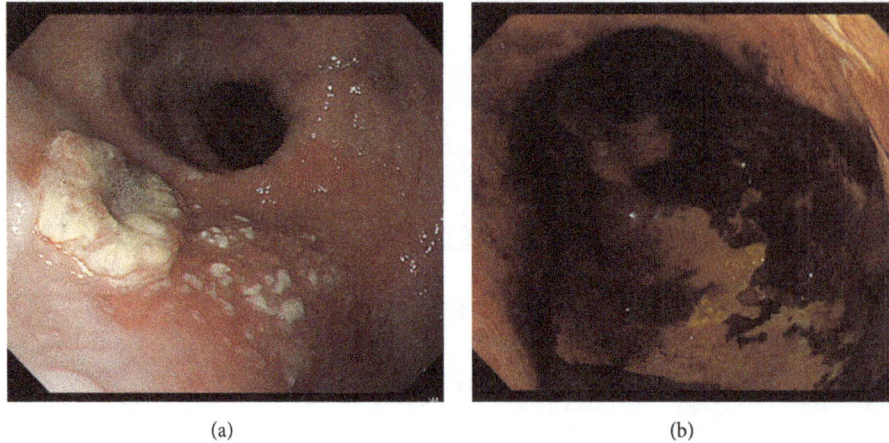

(a)
(b)

FIGURE 1: Upper gastrointestinal endoscopy showed a "0-IIb+IIa" lesion in the middle esophagus (a). Iodine staining revealed multiple irregularly shaped iodine-unstained areas (b).

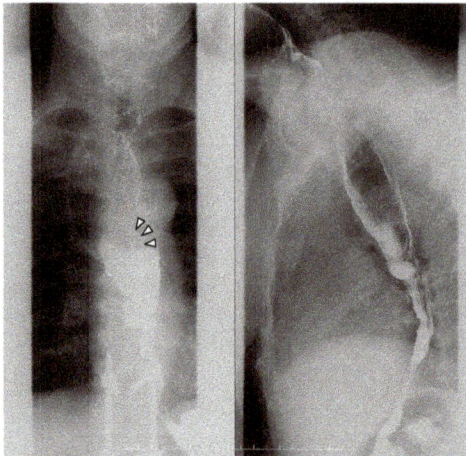

FIGURE 2: Barium esophagram showed esophageal dilation with a gradual tapering down to the gastroesophageal junction. There was a superficial protruding lesion in the midthoracic esophagus (arrowhead).

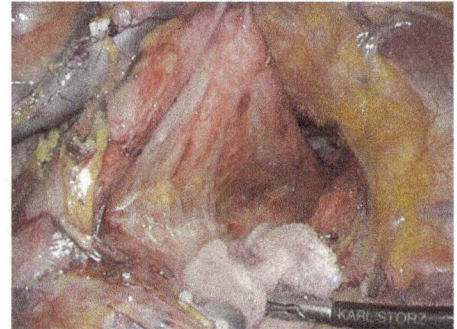

FIGURE 3: Intraoperative findings showed dilated esophagus. We secured the surgical field by elevating the esophagus dorsally and pushing down the trachea ventrally.

performed with the patient in the prone position. Mediastinal lymph node dissection was performed, and the esophagus was resected to a level lower than the lesion. Dilation of the esophagus resulted in difficulty with securing the surgical field, but we were able to manage by changing the grasping parts frequently (Figure 3). The patient was then placed in the supine position and laparotomy was performed. Adhesions were encountered between the lateral segment of the liver and the lesser curvature of the stomach, likely a consequence of the previous abdominal surgery. Through a cervical neck incision, the proximal gastric pull-up was retrieved in the posterior mediastinal pathway and a cervical esophagogastric anastomosis was performed. Additionally, an enteral feeding tube was placed. The total surgical time was 464 minutes and the total estimated blood loss was 100 ml.

Histopathology showed a moderately differentiated SCC invading the submucosal layer (Figures 4(a)① and 4(b)), as well as two SCC invading the mucosal layer (Figure 4(a)②, ③). There were no lymph node metastases. The final stage was T1b(SM2)N0M0, stage IA. Other histopathologic findings included marked dilation of the upper-middle esophagus and loss of ganglion cells in the myenteric plexus throughout the length of the resected esophagus (Figure 4(c)) (Grade III at both the dilated part and the nondilated part, according to descriptive rules for achalasia of the esophagus [1]).

The patient's postoperative course was uneventful with the exception of mild left recurrent laryngeal nerve paralysis (Clavien-Dindo Grade I). He was discharged on postoperative day 20. Ten months after the surgery, the patient was well without evidence of disease recurrence.

All diagnostic procedures and therapy concerning the patient were carried out after informed consent had been obtained.

3. Discussion

EA is a primary disorder of esophageal motility and is regarded as a risk factor for SCC [3]. In a prospective study, Leeuwenburgh et al. reported that carcinoma develops on

(a)

(b)

(c)

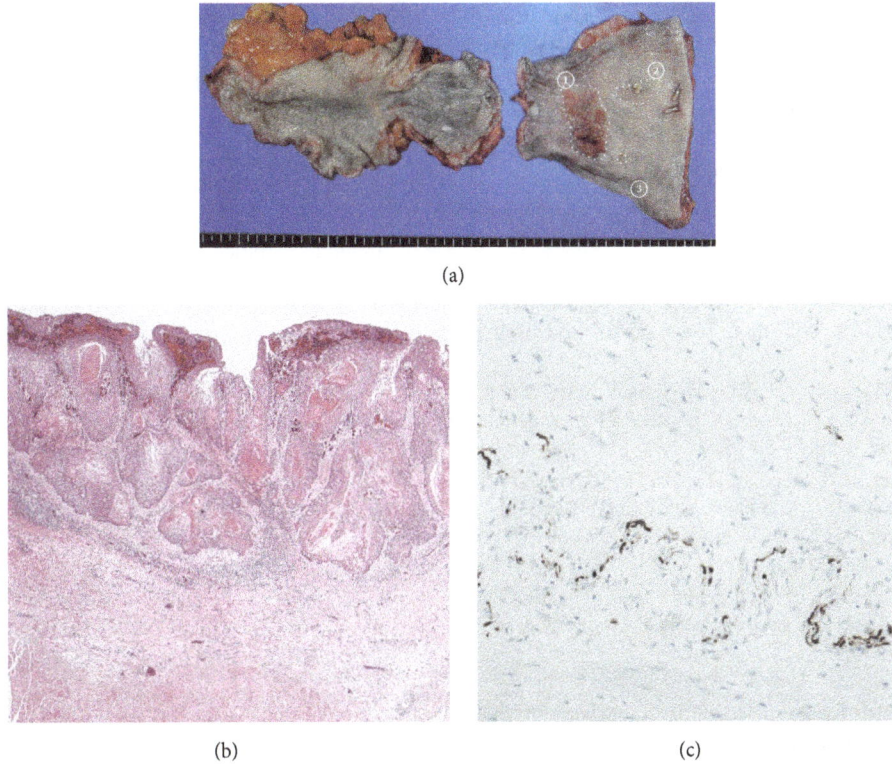

FIGURE 4: Resected specimen (a). There are three lesions (①–③) in the markedly dilated esophagus. Moderately differentiated SCC cells invaded the submucosal layer at elevated lesion (b). Loss of ganglion cells in the myenteric plexus throughout the length of the resected esophagus (c).

average 24 years (range: 10–43) after symptom onset [6]. However, there have been few reports on the results of follow-up after curative surgery for EA and it is unclear whether EC is frequent when EA has been treated successfully. Ellis Jr. et al. reported that the incidence of EC decreased to 0.3% in patients undergoing a second surgery for EA [4]. However, other reports have found that the incidence of carcinoma remained high despite surgery. For example, Arima et al. and Leeuwenburgh et al. reported that, respectively, 15.1 years and 11 years elapsed until the occurrence of EC after surgery for EA [7, 8]. Furthermore, Ota et al. reported the results of follow-up after curative surgery for EA. Thirty-two patients underwent long-term and periodic endoscopic follow-up. Esophageal SCC was detected in six patients (18%) and the average duration of follow-up until EC was seen after surgery for EA was 14.3 (5–40) years [5]. Carter and Brewer III reported that EC occurred early (15 months) after surgery for EA, but they considered that it was due to insufficient muscle layer incision [9]. These reports indicate that EC can occur many years after appropriate surgery for EA. In these patients including our case, the Heller-Dor operation was performed as surgical treatment for EA and no patient complained of passage symptoms. This suggests that the potential for malignant transformation persists even after surgery improves passage symptoms. Ribeiro Jr. et al. reported that the esophageal mucosa itself in EA appeared to be associated with malignant potential [10]. Also in our case, passage symptoms are improved after surgery for EA,

but barium esophagram showed that esophageal spasm was diffusely observed in the middle and lower esophagus and the dilation of the upper esophagus still remained. From these findings of the barium esophagram, this case is presumed to be Chicago classification type III EA. In addition, ganglion cells were not observed in the myenteric plexus throughout the length of the resected esophagus, which suggests that this case is type III achalasia. Pandolfine et al., who proposed the Chicago classification by high resolution manometry (HRM), reported that type III EA is the most resistant to treatment [11]. Considering these facts, we cannot deny the possibility that chronic inflammation caused by asymptomatic stagnation of food and saliva has remained. HRM was not conducted in our case, but even in EA after surgery, HRM may be useful for monitoring the effect of the surgical treatment and as a predictor of EC. From this point of view, the possibility that food and liquid, including saliva, were retained in the esophagus with no symptoms and that EC occurred on the background of chronic inflammation cannot be denied.

Even after surgery for EA, in many cases, we consider that superficial EC (especially T1a-epithelium or T1a-lamina propria mucosae) can be treated with endoscopic submucosal dissection (ESD). There are several reports on ESD for early EC after surgery for EA [7, 12]. Our case was not considered for ESD, because there were multiple lesions spread across a wide area, and part of the lesion invaded deeply. There had been no report on thoracoscopic esophagectomy for EC after surgery for EA, but we could perform it in the prone position and open gastric pull-up reconstruction safely in the present case.

It is important to discover malignancy at earlier stage due to recognition of the risk of developing EC in the patients after surgery for EA and long-term periodic follow-up.

References

[1] The Japan Esophageal Society, *Descriptive Rules for Achalasia of the Esophagus*, Kanehara Publication, Tokyo, Japan, 4th edition, 2012.

[2] J. T. Krill, R. D. Naik, and M. F. Vaezi, "Clinical management of achalasia: current state of the art," *Clinical and Experimental Gastroenterology*, vol. 9, pp. 71–82, 2016.

[3] B. L. D. M. Brücher, H. J. Stein, H. Bartels, H. Feussner, and J. R. Siewert, "Achalasia and esophageal cancer: incidence, prevalence, and prognosis," *World Journal of Surgery*, vol. 25, no. 6, pp. 745–749, 2001.

[4] F. H. Ellis Jr., R. E. Crozier, and S. P. Gibb, "Reoperative achalasia surgery," in *The Journal of Thoracic and Cardiovascular Surgery*, vol. 92, pp. 859–865, 1986.

[5] M. Arima, T. Kouzu, H. Arima et al., "Superficial esophageal cancer (m1) associated with postoperative achalasia of the esophagus, report of a case," *Stomach and Intestine*, vol. 30, pp. 1379–1385, 1995.

[6] I. Leeuwenburgh, P. Scholten, J. Alderliesten et al., "Long-term esophageal cancer risk in patients with primary achalasia: A prospective study," *American Journal of Gastroenterology*, vol. 105, no. 10, pp. 2144–2149, 2010.

[7] M. Ota, K. Narumiya, K. Kudo et al., "Incidence of esophageal carcinomas after surgery for achalasia: usefulness of long-term and periodic follow-up," *American Journal of Case Reports*, vol. 17, pp. 845–849, 2016.

[8] The Japan Esophageal Society, *Japanese Classification of Esophageal Cancer*, Kanehara Publication, Tokyo, Japan, 11st edition, 2015.

[9] R. Carter and L. A. Brewer III, "Achalasia and esophageal carcinoma. Studies in early diagnosis for improved surgical management," *The American Journal of Surgery*, vol. 130, no. 2, pp. 114–120, 1975.

[10] U. Ribeiro Jr., M. C. Posner, A. V. Safatle-Ribeiro, and J. C. Reynolds, "Risk factors for squamous cell carcinoma of the oesophagus," *British Journal of Surgery*, vol. 83, no. 9, pp. 1174–1185, 1996.

[11] J. E. Pandolfino, M. A. Kwiatek, T. Nealis, W. Bulsiewicz, J. Post, and P. J. Kahrilas, "Achalasia: a new clinically relevant classification by high-resolution manometry," *Gastroenterology*, vol. 135, no. 5, pp. 1526–1533, 2008.

[12] O. Chino, H. Shimada, Y. Kise et al., "Early carcinoma of the esophagus associated with achalasia treated by endoscopic mucosal resection," *The Tokai Journal of Experimental and Clinical Medicine*, vol. 33, pp. 13–16, 2008.

48

An Obstructing Small Bowel Phytobezoar in an Elderly Female Nigerian: A Case Report and Literature Review

O. S. Balogun, A. O. Osinowo, M. O. Afolayan, and A. A. Adesanya

General Surgery Unit, Department of Surgery, Faculty of Clinical Sciences, College of Medicine, University of Lagos, PMB 12003, Idi Araba, Lagos, Nigeria

Correspondence should be addressed to O. S. Balogun; drlanrebalogun@gmail.com

Academic Editor: Claudio Feo

Small bowel obstruction secondary to phytobezoars is an unusual presentation in surgery. We present a case of an elderly female patient with an insidious onset of abdominal pain, abdominal distension, and bilious vomiting diagnosed radiologically to be small bowel obstruction. Exploratory laparotomy revealed a trapped mass of vegetable matter in the distal ileum. She had enterotomy with primary closure for removal of obstructing ileal phytobezoars. Her postoperative recovery was uneventful.

1. Introduction

Bezoar is a general term that describes entrapment of a mass of materials of different sources within the lumen of the gastrointestinal tract. Phytobezoars comprise aggregates of indigestible plant materials and mucus which can be an unusual cause of intestinal obstruction. Small intestinal obstruction due to bands, adhesions, hernias, and tumours is more commonly encountered in surgical practice.

Phytobezoars may account for about 0.4–4% of cases of acute mechanical intestinal obstruction although there is no real consensus on its exact incidence [1, 2]. Predisposing factors for phytobezoars include previous surgery on the stomach, poor mastication and edentulous jaws, rapid swallowing of large amounts fruits and vegetables, intestinal stenosis, and systemic diseases impairing gastrointestinal motility.

We present a case report of an elderly female Nigerian with normal dentition who had surgery for an obstructing small bowel phytobezoar following ingestion of large amounts of vegetable matter. We also conduct a review of literature on the management of phytobezoars.

2. Case Presentation and Management

78-year-old known hypertensive woman was referred from a Private Hospital to the emergency room of Lagos University Teaching Hospital with an insidious onset of colicky right lower abdominal pain of 6-day duration and recurrent copious nonprojectile bilious vomiting of 5-day duration. She last opened bowel 5 days before presentation. She had developed abdominal distension and anorexia since the onset of her symptoms. She had no history of weight loss or jaundice. There was a history of high intake of vegetables based on advice from her friends.

Examination at presentation revealed an ill-looking elderly woman with a respiratory rate of 28 cycles per minute and pulse rate of 100 beats per minute. Her blood pressure was 157/100 mmHg. Her oxygen saturation (SPO2) was 98%. Her chest was clinically clear. However, her abdomen was distended. There was right lower quadrant tenderness but no guarding or rebound tenderness. Bowel sounds were hyperactive. Rectal examination was normal. A working clinical diagnosis of intestinal obstruction secondary to possible right sided colonic tumor was made.

Her full blood count and white cell count, differentials, and platelets counts were within normal range. Her renal function was normal except for the finding of hypokalemia of 3.0 mmol/l.

Computed tomography scan (Figures 1 and 2) revealed grossly dilated edematous small bowel loops and stomach with fluid distension. Chest X-ray showed evidence of left ventricular hypertrophy. Her electrocardiogram revealed features of sinus tachycardia, left axis deviation, and left ventricular hypertrophy.

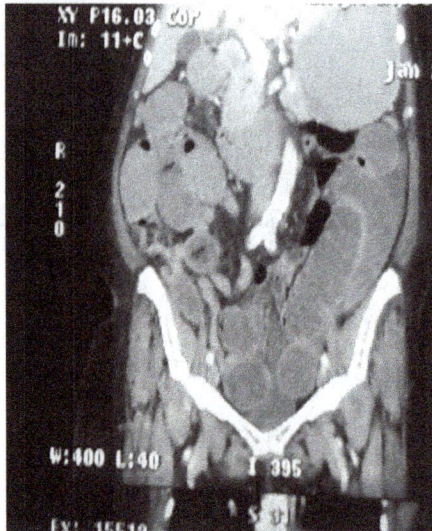

FIGURE 1: Coronal view of the computed tomography (CT) of the abdomen showing grossly dilated thickened small bowel loops up to the region of right iliac fossa.

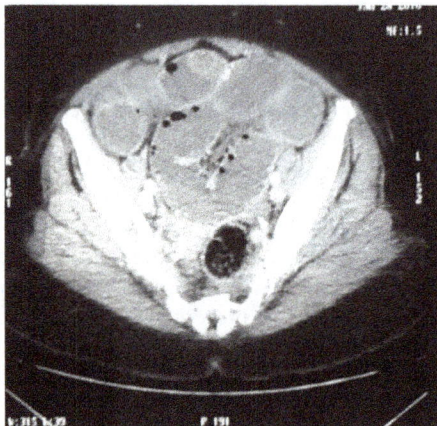

FIGURE 2: Axial view of computed tomography (CT) of the abdomen showing grossly dilated, thick-walled small bowel loops up to the region of the pelvis.

Patient was resuscitated and optimized for surgery. Exploratory laparotomy revealed dilated small bowel loop with a compressible obstructing mass (transition zone) at 50 cm from the ileocecal junction. The small bowel loop bowel distal to the transition zone was collapsed (Figure 3). Enterotomy of the transition zone revealed an 8 cm by 6 cm egg-shaped accretion of vegetable matter (Figure 3). Enterotomy was closed after removal of the phytobezoar. Postoperative period was uneventful. She was discharged home 5 days after surgery and was subsequently followed up at regular intervals as an outpatient.

3. Discussion

Mechanical intestinal obstruction in the elderly is a common presentation and indication for surgical intervention

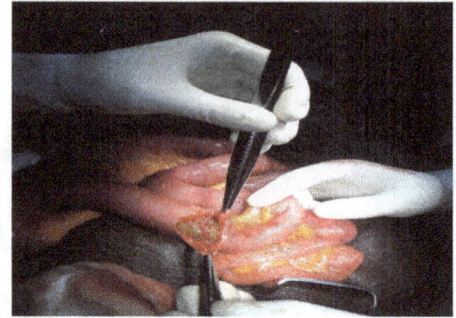

FIGURE 3: Obstructing distal ileal phytobezoar seen at laparotomy.

in surgery. Common intraluminal causes include tumours, gallstones, and foreign bodies. Bezoar-induced intestinal obstruction is rare. Bezoar is described according to its component and the location within the gastrointestinal tract. Four major types of bezoars include phytobezoar (derived from plant materials), trichobezoar (hair ball), lactobezoar (milk-curds), and pharmacobezoar (medications).

Gastric bezoars are found commonly in patients with poor mastication, poor gastric motility, and previous gastric surgery. Small and large bowel bezoars are uncommon. Phytobezoars are the most common bezoars encountered in surgical practice and are usually made up of concretions of plant cellulose, mucin, pectin, tannins, and mucins derived from ingested fruits and vegetables. Plant materials can aggregate to form an impacted bolus of material within the gastrointestinal tract resulting in acute intestinal obstruction. Persimmon fruit phytobezoar is the most common type reported in a series [3]. Our patient had a history of frequent ingestion of large amount of vegetable matter weeks prior to onset of her symptoms; otherwise, we found no other predisposing factors.

Clinical presentation in patients with phytobezoars depends on the type, location within the gastrointestinal tract, and presence of predisposing factors. Gastric bezoars can present with epigastric discomfort and nonspecific abdominal pains.

Small bowel phytobezoar usually presents with abdominal pain and distension, vomiting, and constipation. The principal symptoms of small bowel phytobezoars reported in a review are abdominal pain (49–100%), epigastric distress (80%), and vomiting and nausea (35–78%). Features of small bowel obstruction were found in 94.73% of cases. Less common symptoms include sensation of fullness or bloating, dysphagia, anorexia with weight loss, and even gastrointestinal hemorrhage [2, 4]. These findings support the notion that primary small bowel phytobezoar is usually obstructive in nature with average duration of 1–5 days between onset of abdominal symptoms and hospitalization [5, 6].

Diagnosing phytobezoar-induced small bowel obstruction can be challenging preoperatively. Plain abdominal X-ray showing evidence of mechanical small bowel obstruction can be seen in most patients but is not specific. Abdominal computed tomography (CT) scan is 90% sensitive and 57%

specific in excluding other differential diagnoses of bezoar-induced ileus [7]. According to Zissin et al. [7], faecal matter in the small bowel on abdominal CT may appear like a bezoar. Unlike bezoar, impacted faeces tend to appear in a longer transition zone of dilated segment of small bowel proximal to the site of obstruction.

Treatment options for phytobezoar can be conservative, medical, or surgical. Conservative approach may be reasonable if the presenting symptoms resolve while the patient is being resuscitated or prepared for a more definitive treatment. Endoscopic fragmentation and extraction as well as chemical dissolution and lavage have been used in the treatment of gastric bezoars. However, surgical intervention is often required in the management of small bowel phytobezoars. Both open and laparoscopic approaches are described in the literature. Samdani et al. [8] reported a case of small bowel obstruction due to impacted apricot fruit which was successfully treated by laparoscopy. Compared to open approach, laparoscopy has benefits of less postoperative complications and shorter hospital stay. However, laparoscopy is less suitable when bowel loops are grossly dilated due to risk of enteric injury.

Definitive diagnosis of phytobezoars is often made at laparotomy. The most common site of impaction is the distal ileum at 50–70 cm proximal to ileocaecal valve [9]. This is because of relatively small diameter and reduced peristalsis of bowel content in this segment and increased water absorption [9, 10]. In our patient, obstructing phytobezoar was found at 50 cm from the ileocaecal valve.

Distal ileal phytobezoars may be fragmented manually at laparotomy and milked into the caecum [10]; more often an enterotomy with primary closure is required for definitive diagnosis and treatment [2]. Rarely, bowel resection and anastomosis are indicated for impacted bezoar with bowel ischaemia [8]. In most cases, surgical treatment of small bowel obstruction can be accomplished successfully. General preventive measures include avoidance of high fiber diet, more water consumption, proper mastication, and treatment of underlying gastrointestinal motility disorders.

4. Conclusion

Small bowel phytobezoar is an uncommon cause of acute intestinal obstruction in the elderly with a virgin abdomen. Preoperative aetiologic diagnosis based on history and physical examination may be difficult. Plain abdominal X-ray and ultrasound findings are that of nonspecific small bowel obstruction. Abdominal CT scan is invaluable in excluding other differential diagnoses. Surgery is often required in resolving the diagnostic puzzle and for definitive treatment. Recurrence following treatment is common and can be prevented by appropriate dietary habits and control of underlying factors.

References

[1] B. M. Hall, M. J. Shapiro, J. A. Vosswinkel, S. Meisel, and N. Curci, "Phytobezoar as a Cause of Intestinal Obstruction," *Journal of Gastrointestinal Surgery*, vol. 15, no. 12, pp. 2293–2295, 2011.

[2] K. Erzurumlu, Z. Malazgirt, and A. Bektas, "Gastrointestinal bezoars: a retrospective analysis of 34 cases," *World Journal of Gastroenterology*, vol. 11, no. 12, pp. 1813–1817, 2005.

[3] M. M. Krausz, E. Z. Moriel, A. Ayalon, D. Pode, and A. L. Durst, "Surgical aspects of gastrointestinal persimmon phytobezoar treatment," *The American Journal of Surgery*, vol. 152, no. 5, pp. 526–530, 1986.

[4] A. G. Verstandig, B. Klin, R. A. Bloom, I. Hadas, and E. Libson, "Small bowel phytobezoars: detection with radiography," *Radiology*, vol. 172, no. 3, pp. 705–707, 1989.

[5] S. Yakan, A. Şirinocak, K. E. Telciler, M. T. Tekeli, and A. G. Deneçli, "A rare cause of acute abdomen: Small bowel obstruction due to phytobezoar," *Ulusal Travma ve Acil Cerrahi Dergisi*, vol. 16, no. 5, pp. 459–463, 2010.

[6] H. Bedioui, A. Daghfous, M. Ayadi et al., "A report of 15 cases of small-bowel obstruction secondary to phytobezoars: Predisposing factors and diagnostic difficulties," *Gastroenterologie Clinique et Biologique*, vol. 32, no. 6-7, pp. 596–600, 2008.

[7] R. Zissin, A. Osadchy, V. Gutman, V. Rathaus, M. Shapiro-Feinberg, and G. Gayer, "CT findings in patients with small bowel obstruction due to phytobezoar," *Emergency Radiology*, vol. 10, no. 4, pp. 197–200, 2004.

[8] T. Samdani, T. Singhal, S. Balakrishnan, A. Hussain, S. Grandy-Smith, and S. El-Hasani, "An apricot story: view through a keyhole," *World Journal of Emergency Surgery*, vol. 2, no. 1, article 20, 2007.

[9] K. G. Spyridon, N. Zikos, C. Charalampous, K. Christodoulou, L. Sakkas, and N. Katsamakis, "Management of gastrointestinal bezoars: an analysis of 23 cases," *International Surgery*, vol. 93, no. 2, pp. 95–98, 2008.

[10] S. S. Das, M. Husain, A. Bhat, and F. F. Hajini, "Phytobezoar causing terminal ileal obstruction can enterotomy be avoided?" *JSM Clinical Case Reports*, vol. 2, no. 2, p. 1024, 2014.

49

Concurrent Occurrence of Tumor in Colon and Small Bowel following Intestinal Obstruction: A Case Report and Review of the Literature

Seyed Mohammad Reza Nejatollahi[1] and Omid Etemad[2]

[1]The Division of Hepatobiliary & Organ Transplantation, Taleghani Hospital, Shahid Beheshti University of Medical Sciences, Tehran, Iran
[2]Shahid Beheshti University of Medical Sciences, Tehran, Iran

Correspondence should be addressed to Omid Etemad; rasaeti@yahoo.com

Academic Editor: Alexander R. Novotny

An intestinal obstruction occurs when either the small or large intestine is partly or completely blocked so it prevents passing the food or fluid through the small/large bowel. This blockage is due to the existence of a mechanical obstruction such as foreign material, mass, hernia, or volvulus. Common symptoms include cramping pain, nausea and vomiting, changes in bowel habits, inability to pass stool, and lack of gas. We present a case of an 83-year-old man who had been referred to Taleghani Hospital with symptoms of bowel obstruction. He underwent the surgery. The findings of exploration of the entire abdomen showed two types of mass separately in two different organs. In postoperative workup, pathology reported two types of tumors (adenocarcinoma and neuroendocrine tumors).

1. Introduction

An Intestinal obstruction occurs when either the small or large intestine is partly or completely blocked so it prevents passing the food or fluid through the small/large bowel. This condition would cause inability to pass food, fluid, and gas in the digestive tract. The obstacle could be a foreign material or the result of volvulus, hernia, or tumor growth [1].

Bowel obstruction could also be a result of abdominal infection or inflammation caused by conditions such as diverticulitis. In patients with Crohn's disease or peritoneal carcinomatosis, the risk of bowel obstruction may arise [2].

Some symptoms of this disease include abdominal cramping, abdominal distension, diarrhea, or inability to have bowel habits [3]. Cancer is suspected in patients older than 60 years who have experienced changes in their bowel habits for more than six weeks [4], with nausea, vomiting, and inability to pass gas or stool [5]. In such cases, first the mechanical factors and then nonmechanical factors must be examined. For this aim, physical examinations, X-ray, CT scan, and lab test are used.

Intravenous hydration and correcting electrolyte levels are the first treatment for such patients and then, according to the nature of bowel obstruction, the curative treatment will be begun [1].

2. Case Report

This is reportage of an 83-year-old man who had experienced changes in bowel habits with feeling of diffuse abdominal pain aggravated by eating and relieved by passing stool from 5 months before. Due to these symptoms, colonoscopy was planned for him, but because of the lack of consent, CT scan of the abdomen/pelvis was performed. As you can see in Figure 1, the CT scan reported significant thickening in the sigmoid colon.

Due to increasing abdominal pain, nausea, vomiting, and inability to pass gas and stool for six days, the patient was referred to Taleghani Hospital of Tehran. In Figure 2, the abdominal X-ray showed multiple air-fluid levels. After precise examination and diagnosis of bowel obstruction, the patient underwent surgery.

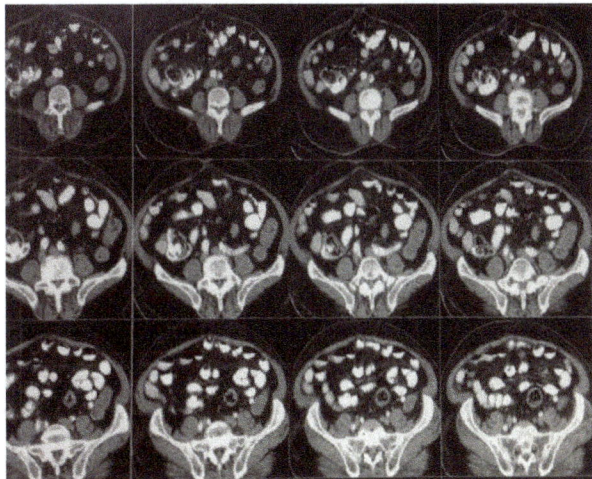

FIGURE 1: CT scan 5 months before surgery.

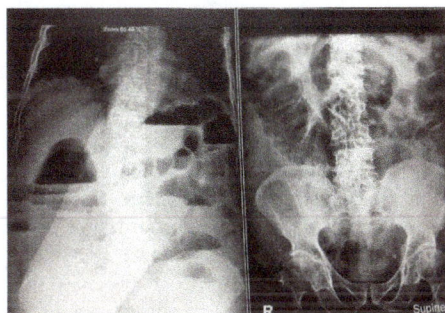

FIGURE 2: Abdominal X-ray (supine and upright) just before surgery.

Intraoperative findings indicated bowel obstruction due to a mass that was located at a distance of 20 cm from the rectosigmoid junction in the sigmoid region, dilation of the colon and small intestine, and another mass with dimensions of 2 × 2 cm that was located at a distance of 80 cm from the ileocecal valve in the ileum region.

The patient underwent the small bowel segmental resection and primary anastomosis and total abdominal colectomy because of the severe dilatation of the proximal part of the colon and ischemic changes of the cecum with ileorectal anastomosis (end-to-end) was done for him. In postoperative workup, there was no sign of metastasis and he was discharged from the hospital after six days with good general conditions. Figure 3 shows the resected colon after total colectomy.

3. Pathologic Findings

The pathologic findings showed existence of two tumors as the following.

(1) The small bowel wall was infiltrated by a neoplasm composed of monotonous small round cells with small nucleoli, salt and pepper chromatin, and moderated finely granular cytoplasm arranged in nesting and trabecular structure.

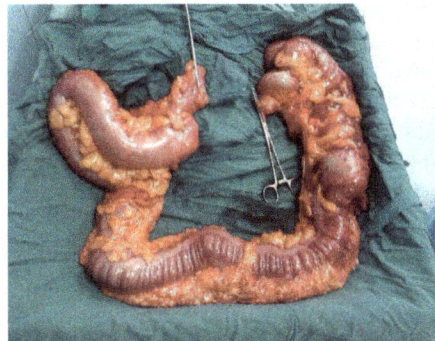

FIGURE 3: Total colectomy.

Well-differentiated neuroendocrine tumor with lymphovascular invasion and size of 2 cm with greatest dimension and mitotic rate of less than 1/10 hpf was seen in the ileum site. Tumor invades the subserosa tissue without involvement of the visceral peritoneum (pT3).

(2) There was a well-differentiated adenocarcinoma with lymphovascular invasion and size of 5.5 cm in the greatest dimension in the sigmoid-colon region with microsatellite instability and mucinous production (20% of tumor). Tumor invades the subserosal tissue and 21 lymph nodes were removed (T3 N0).

Due to the existence of an obstructive tumor and lymphovascular invasion, the patient was a candidate for chemotherapy. But because of some factors such as age and his disability to tolerate the conditions of chemotherapy, chemotherapy was not done for him.

4. Discussion

More than 575.000 people die of cancer and more than 1.5 million people are diagnosed with cancer every year in the USA. According to the World Health Organization (WHO), the numbers of new cancer cases are expected to be raised by about 70% over the next 20 years [6]. Surgery is a preferred treatment for many types of cancer.

According to studies in the USA, each year an estimated 8.000 people in the USA are diagnosed with a neuroendocrine tumor that starts in the gastrointestinal tract which includes the stomach, intestine, appendix, colon, or rectum [7].

Well-differentiated neuroendocrine tumors have cells that do not look very abnormal and are not multiplying rapidly and sometimes the only way to know that a mass is a neuroendocrine cancer is when it spreads to the other organs or tissues [8].

In some cases, there is a possibility of existence of some other benign tumor in the other organs. Accordingly the surgeon must check the possibility of other masses in the abdomen [9]. Studies show neuroendocrine tumors in the rectum and colon are rare [10]. Studies have estimated the annual incidence of clinically significant neuroendocrine tumors is approximately 2.5–5 per 100,000 [11]. More prevalence of neuroendocrine tumors is in the small bowel and often in the ileum (about 70%) [12].

The synchronous occurrence of two differentiated tumors in a single patient is rare. So far, there are several reported cases that had two differentiated tumors in two or several other organs simultaneously [8, 13–15].

Ferrando Marco and his colleagues reported the case of a 64-year-old man with periampullary collision tumor, in which a duodenal-wall carcinoid and an adenocarcinoma of the head of the pancreas coexisted [9].

Akiba and his colleagues reported a case of a 64-year-old man who was found to have EEBV-associated gastric carcinoma with primary gastric extranodal marginal zone lymphoma of mucosa-associated lymphoid tissue [16].

Kleist and his colleagues reported two collision tumors containing a gastrointestinal stromal tumor with intermingling elements of gastric adenocarcinoma [17].

Jang and his colleagues reported a case of a 70-year-old man found to have two separated masses which were observed in the proximal ascending colon containing two separated well-differentiated neuroendocrine tumors with necrosis and increased mitosis [18].

Singh and his colleagues reported a case of a 52-year-old found to have a mass at the base of the appendix. On microscopic examination of the tumor, mixed adenocarcinoma and carcinoid were identified [19].

Van Kerkhóve and his colleagues reported a case of a 72-year-old female found to have a rare ileal collision tumor consisting of an adenocarcinoma and a small cell neuroendocrine tumor with peritoneal metastasis of neuroendocrine origin and coincidental benign lesions on both ovaries [20].

According to the studies, 15–35% of patients with neuroendocrine cancer in the ileum had more than one tumor and 50–60% of them survived about 5 years after surgery (85% if the tumor was confined to the bowel wall and 5% in case of serosal invasion) [21].

In 15–30% of cases with ileum neuroendocrine tumor, there is more than one tumor, and 15–29% of tumors are associated with other noncarcinoid malignancies [22].

5. Conclusion

Neuroendocrine tumors are neoplasms that are raised from cells of endocrine and nervous system. They could be malignant or benign and most commonly occur in the intestine and will spread to other organs. Ileal neuroendocrine tumors often grow in the distal part of the ileum. In 15–30% of cases, there is more than one tumor, and 15–29% of tumors are associated with the other noncarcinoid malignancies.

Diagnosis must be done by using laboratory tests, X-ray, CT scan, and endoscopy. Surgery is a definitive treatment in the early stages. Patient's age, the exact location, dimension and differentiation of tumor, and lymphovascular invasion are parameters which affect the progression of the disease.

In this case report, the patient with diagnosis of the bowel obstruction underwent surgery and we found a mass in the sigmoid region with pathologic diagnosis of adenocarcinoma and another mass in the ileum region with pathologic diagnosis of a neuroendocrine tumor.

Due to the increased prevalence of malignant tumors, checking the entire of the digestive system according to existing protocols in similar cases and not forgetting to consider the possibility of coexisting malignant tumors to find and treat them at an early stage are recommended.

Competing Interests

The authors declare that they have no competing interests.

References

[1] Amber Erickson Gabbey, Ileus, Medically Reviewedby George Krucik, MD, MBA, June 18, 2013.

[2] J. T. Dunn, J. M. Halls, and T. V. Berne, "Roentgenographic contrast studies in acute small-bowel obstruction," *Archives of Surgery*, vol. 119, no. 11, pp. 1305–1308, 1984.

[3] B. Culhane, "Constipation," in *Guidelines for Cancer Care: Symptom Management*, J. Yasko, Ed., pp. 184–187, Reston Publishing Company, Reston, Va, USA, 1983.

[4] B. G. Hampton and R. A. Bryant, Eds., *Ostomies and Continent Diversions: Nursing Management*, Mosby, St. Louis, Mo, USA, 1992.

[5] *Referral for Suspected Cancer*, NICE Clinical Guideline, National Institute for Health and Care Excellence, 2005.

[6] P. Crosta, "Medical News Today," September 2008.

[7] American Society of Cancer.

[8] http://www.cancer.org .

[9] J. Ferrando Marco, A. Pallas Regueira, D. Moro Valdezate, and C. Fernández Martínez, "Collision tumor of the ampulla of Vater: carcinoid and adenocarcinoma," *Revista Espanola de Enfermedades Digestivas*, vol. 99, no. 4, pp. 235–238, 2007.

[10] L. Peng and R. E. Schwarz, "Collision tumor in form of primary adenocarcinoma and neuroendocrine carcinoma of the duodenum," *Rare Tumors*, vol. 4, no. 2, article e20, 2012.

[11] K. Öberg and D. Castellano, "Current knowledge on diagnosis and staging of neuroendocrine tumors," *Cancer and Metastasis Reviews*, vol. 30, supplement 1, pp. 3–7, 2011.

[12] K. Y. Bilimoria, D. J. Bentrem, J. D. Wayne, C. Y. Ko, C. L. Bennett, and M. S. Talamonti, "Small bowel cancer in the United States: changes in epidemiology, treatment, and survival over the last 20 years," *Annals of Surgery*, vol. 249, no. 1, pp. 63–71, 2009.

[13] S.-J. Ni, W.-Q. Sheng, and X. Du, "Pathologic research update of colorectal neuroendocrine tumors," *World Journal of Gastroenterology*, vol. 16, no. 14, pp. 1713–1719, 2010.

[14] I. M. Modlin, K. D. Lye, and M. Kidd, "A 5-decade analysis of 13,715 carcinoid tumors," *Cancer*, vol. 97, no. 4, pp. 934–959, 2003.

[15] I. M. Modlin and A. Sandor, "An analysis of 8305 cases of carcinoid tumors," *Cancer*, vol. 79, no. 4, pp. 813–829, 1997.

[16] J. Akiba, T. Nakane, F. Arakawa, K. Ohshima, and H. Yano, "Collision of EBV-associated gastric carcinoma and primary gastric extranodal marginal zone lymphoma of mucosa-associated lymphoid tissue in the remnant stomach," *Pathology International*, vol. 60, no. 2, pp. 102–106, 2010.

[17] B. Kleist, J. Lasota, and M. Miettinen, "Gastrointestinal stromal tumor and gastric adenocarcinoma collision tumors," *Human Pathology*, vol. 41, no. 7, pp. 1034–1039, 2010.

[18] K. Y. Jang, W. S. Moon, H. Lee, C. Y. Kim, and H. S. Park, "Gastric collision tumor of large cell neuroendocrine carcinoma and adenocarcinoma-a case report," *Pathology Research and Practice*, vol. 206, no. 6, pp. 387–390, 2010.

[19] N. G. Singh, A. A. S. R. Mannan, M. Kahvic, and A. M. Nur, "Mixed adenocarcinoma-carcinoid (collision tumor) of the appendix," *Medical Principles and Practice*, vol. 20, no. 4, pp. 384–386, 2011.

[20] F. Van Kerkhóve, K. Coenegrachts, L. Steyaert, I. Van Den Berghe, and J. W. Casselman, "Collision tumor in the ileum: a rare combination of an adenocarcinoma and small cell neuroendocrine tumor," *JBR-BTR*, vol. 89, no. 5, pp. 258–260, 2006.

[21] M. D. Hanni Gulwani, "Small bowel (small intestine) other malignancies carcinoid tumor," PathologyOutlines.com, August 2012.

[22] B. Eriksson, G. Klöppel, E. Krenning et al., "Consensus guidelines for the management of patients with digestive neuroendocrine tumors—well-differentiated jejunal-ileal tumor/carcinoma," *Neuroendocrinology*, vol. 87, no. 1, pp. 8–19, 2008.

A Case of Laparoscopic Resection for Carcinoma of the Gastric Remnant following Proximal Gastrectomy Reconstructed with Jejunal Interposition

Kazuhito Yajima, Yoshiaki Iwasaki, Ken Yuu, Ryouki Oohinata, Misato Amaki, Yoshinori Kohira, Souichiro Natsume, Satoshi Ishiyama, and Keiichi Takahashi

Department of Surgery, Tokyo Metropolitan Cancer and Infectious Diseases Center, Komagome Hospital, 3-18-22 Honkomagome, Bunkyo-ku, Tokyo 113-8677, Japan

Correspondence should be addressed to Kazuhito Yajima; yajikazu@nifty.com

Academic Editor: Boris Kirshtein

A 72-year-old Japanese man had a history of proximal gastrectomy for early gastric cancer located in the upper third of the stomach in 2007. Our usual treatment strategy for early gastric cancer in the upper third of the stomach in 2007 was open proximal gastrectomy reconstructing by jejunal interposition with a 10 cm single loop. Upper gastrointestinal fiberscopy for annual follow-up revealed a type 0-IIc-shaped tumor with ulcer scar, 4.0 cm in size, located in the gastric remnant near the jejunogastrostomy. A clinical diagnosis of cancer of the gastric remnant, clinical T1b(SM)N0M0, Stage IA, following the proximal gastrectomy was made and a laparoscopic approach was selected because of the cancer's early stage. Remnant total gastrectomy with D1 plus lymphadenectomy was carried out with five ports by a pneumoperitoneal method. Complete resection of the reconstructed jejunum was undergone along with the jejunal mesentery. Reconstruction by the Roux-en-Y method via the antecolic route was selected. Total operative time was 395 min and blood loss was 40 mL. Our patient was the first successful case of resection for carcinoma of the gastric remnant following proximal gastrectomy reconstructed with jejunal interposition in a laparoscopic approach.

1. Introduction

Laparoscopic gastrectomy has become widely used for the treatment of early gastric cancer in Japan; the feasibility of laparoscopic distal gastrectomy in particular has been assessed in several studies [1–3]. However, laparoscopic procedures are more challenging in patients with previous abdominal surgery because of a higher risk of enteric injury, technical difficulties associated with adhesions, and longer operative times. In terms of the recent advantages of the laparoscopic technique, several reports have presented the usefulness of the laparoscopic approach for patients with remnant gastric cancer following radical distal gastrectomy [4–12]. We here present a case of laparoscopic resection for carcinoma of the gastric remnant following proximal gastrectomy reconstructed with jejunal interposition.

2. Case Presentation

A 72-year-old Japanese man had a history of proximal gastrectomy for early gastric cancer located in the upper third of the stomach in 2007. Our usual treatment strategy for early gastric cancer in the upper third of the stomach at this time was open proximal gastrectomy reconstructing by jejunal interposition with a 10 cm single loop. In this patient, interposed jejunum was approached via the retrocolic route. Lymphadenectomy was D1 (station numbers 1, 2, 3a, 4sa, 4sb, and 7) according to the Japanese Gastric Cancer Association (JGCA) guidelines for initial proximal gastrectomy [13]. Upon physical examination, he was found to be 165 cm in height and weighed 55 kg. There was an upper middle operative scar, 17 cm in length, in his abdomen. All of the laboratory data were within the normal range and the tumor markers

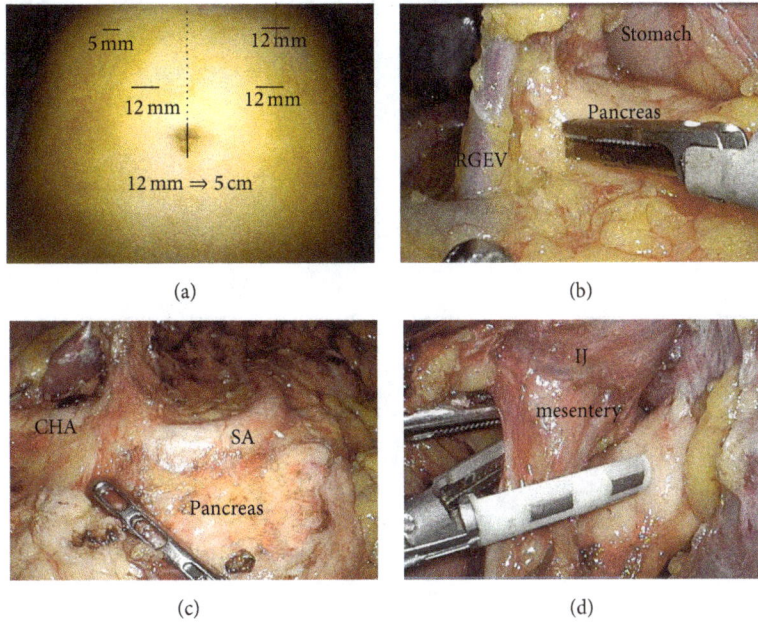

FIGURE 1: Port sites and lymphadenectomy at laparoscopic remnant total gastrectomy. (a) The port sites and scar of initial gastrectomy (dotes line). (b) Station number 6 lymph nodes were completely removed (RGEV; right gastroepiploic vein). (c) The suprapancreatic lymph nodes (station numbers 8a, 9, and 11p) were dissected en bloc (CHA; common hepatic artery, SA; splenic artery). (d) The mesentery of the interposed jejunum (IJ) was transected using a vessel sealing system (LigaSure™ Blunt Tip 5 mm–37 mm, Covidien, Tokyo, Japan).

CEA and CA 19-9 were 7.4 ng/mL and 9.7 U/mL, respectively. Upper gastrointestinal fiberscopy for annual follow-up revealed a type 0-IIc-shaped tumor with ulcer scar, 4.0 cm in size, located in the gastric remnant near the jejunogastrostomy (Figure 1). Biopsy specimen showed well-differentiated adenocarcinoma. A clinical diagnosis of early gastric cancer according to the Japanese Classification of Gastric Carcinoma [14], T1b(SM)N0M0, Stage IA, following the proximal gastrectomy was made. A laparoscopic approach was selected for remnant gastrectomy because of the cancer's early stage.

Surgery was carried out with five ports by the pneumoperitoneal method using our usual laparoscopic technique (Figure 1(a)). The lateral segment of the liver was retracted using a Nathanson Liver Retractor (Cook Surgical, Bloomington, Indianapolis, USA). At initial laparoscopy, there was a little adhesion in the median abdominal incision. At first, adhesion was removed as much as possible and omentum was dissected to open the bursa. The tightest adhesion in this operation was that between the lateral segment of the liver and the dissected lesser curvature of the remnant stomach. The right gastroepiploic artery and vein were clipped and divided, and station number 6 lymph nodes were completely removed (Figure 1(b)). After dividing the right gastric artery (station number 5), the duodenum was transected using a linear stapler (GIA™ Tri-Staple™ 60 mm, purple 60 mm, Covidien, Tokyo, Japan). The suprapancreatic lymph nodes (station numbers 8a, 9, and 11p) could be easily dissected en bloc because these regions were not dissected at initial proximal gastrectomy (Figure 1(c)). After gastrectomy, the reconstructed jejunum was resected. The mesentery of the interposed jejunum was transected using a vessel sealing system (LigaSure™ Blunt Tip 5 mm–37 mm, Covidien)

(Figure 1(d)). After the abdominal esophagus had been scarified circumferentially, the esophagus was transected using a linear stapler on the proximal side of the anastomosis of the esophagojejunostomy at initial proximal gastrectomy (Figure 2(a)). The remnant stomach and interposed jejunum were successfully reduced back into the peritoneal cavity through the umbilical port-side. A minilaparotomy incision of about 5 cm was made in the umbilical port site, for an Alexis® Wound Retractor S (Applied Medical Resources Co., Tokyo, Japan). Reconstruction using the Roux-en-Y method via the antecolic route was performed. At first, jejunojejunostomy was carried out by side-to-side anastomosis using a linear stapler extracorporeally (Figure 2(b)). Next, esophagojejunostomy was performed by an end-to-side anastomosis using a circular stapler (DST Series™ EEA™ Staplers, 25 mm, Covidien) (Figures 2(c) and 2(d)). Total operative time was 395 min and blood loss was 40 mL.

The postoperative course was uneventful and the patient was discharged on the 10th postoperative day. The resected stomach contained a superficial depressed-type tumor, 37 × 17 mm in size (Figure 3, black arrowhead). Histological examination revealed well-differentiated adenocarcinoma to the depth of the mucosa, with no lymph node metastasis, which was pathologically classified as Stage IA.

3. Discussion

We have described a 72-year-old Japanese man who underwent a laparoscopic approach for carcinoma of the gastric remnant following proximal gastrectomy reconstructed with jejunal interposition. To the best of our knowledge, this is

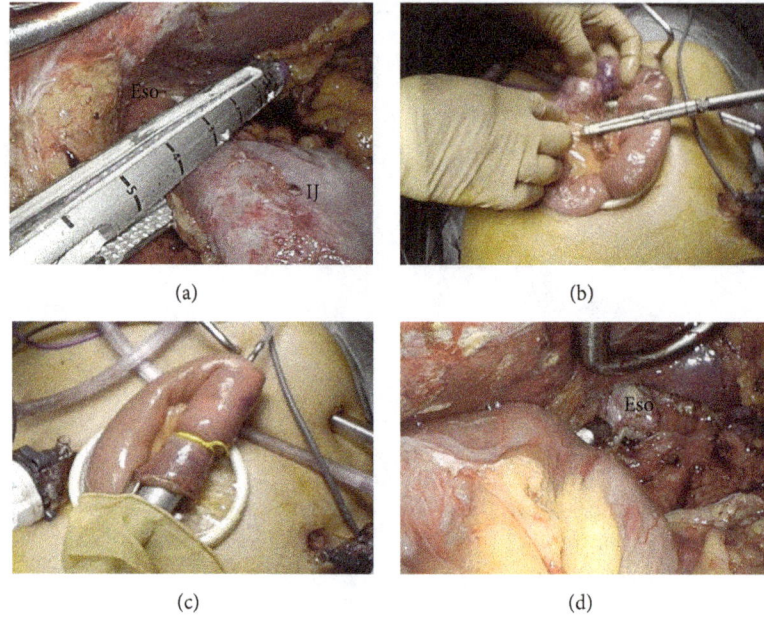

FIGURE 2: Reconstruction at laparoscopic remnant total gastrectomy. (a) The esophagus was transected using a linear stapler (GIA Tri-Staple 60 mm, purple 60 mm, Covidien) on the proximal side of the anastomosis of the esophagojejunostomy at initial proximal gastrectomy. (b) Jejunojejunostomy was carried out by side-to-side anastomosis using a linear stapler extracorporeally. (c, d) Esophagojejunostomy was performed by an end-to-side anastomosis using a circular stapler (DST Series EEA Staplers, 25 mm, Covidien) intracorporeally (IJ; interposes jejunum, Eso; esophagus).

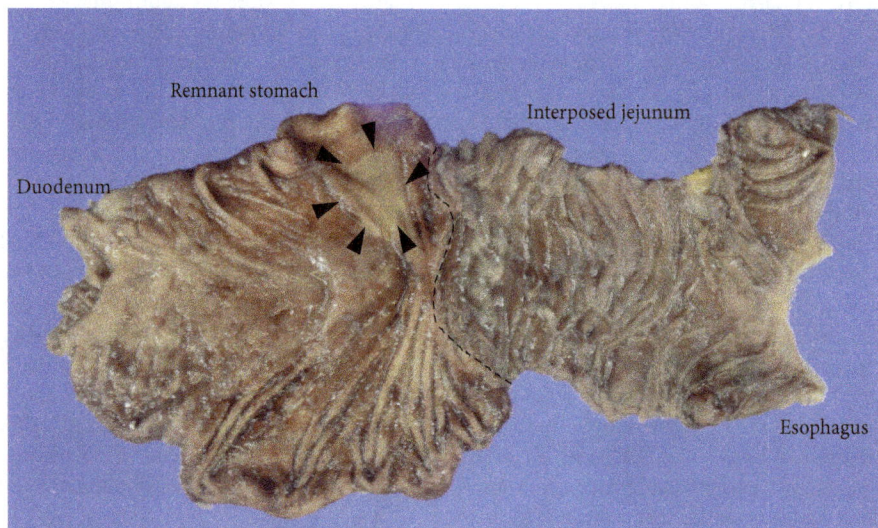

FIGURE 3: Resected specimen. The resected stomach contained a superficial depressed-type tumor, 37 × 17 mm in size (black arrowhead). The black dote line showed the jejunogastrostomy at initial gastrectomy.

the first reported case of laparoscopic resection for remnant stomach reconstructed by jejunal interposition in the English language literature. In our case, the remnant total gastrectomy with *en bloc* lymphadenectomy could be completed easily and safely using a laparoscopic approach.

Remnant gastric cancer was originally defined as gastric cancer arising after distal gastrectomy for benign disease. More recently, remnant gastric cancer has been used to refer to all cancers arising in the remnant stomach, regardless of

initial disease or operation. According to previous reports, with proximal gastrectomy becoming a conventional type of gastrectomy, the incidence of remnant cancer following proximal gastrectomy is increasing [15]. Ohyama et al. reported that gastric stump carcinoma following proximal gastrectomy occurred at a high frequency of 5.4% of initial resections and the time interval between the initial gastrectomy and the treatment of gastric stump cancer was within 5 years in 3 patients, within 5–10 years in 8, and after 10 years in 6. In our case, the occurrence of gastric remnant cancer was 7 years after the initial surgery.

Yamada et al. [4] first reported a laparoscopy-assisted complete gastrectomy for patients with early gastric remnant cancer in 2005. Since then, there have been increasing reports of successful laparoscopy-assisted gastrectomy for gastric remnant cancer. To date, just a hundred patients have undergone it by a laparoscopic approach for remnant gastric cancer [12]. Among these, laparoscopic total gastrectomy following proximal gastrectomy was reported in only three cases [8, 9, 12]. Proximal gastrectomy is performed widely as a function-preserving operation for early gastric cancer located in the upper third of the stomach. In terms of reconstruction after proximal gastrectomy, three reconstruction methods are mainly used: esophagogastrostomy [16, 17], jejunal interposition [18–20], and double-tract method [21]. To avoid reflux esophagitis after proximal gastrectomy, jejunal interposition has been selected for the reconstruction method in our department since 1973 and, to date, more than 200 cases have undergone this surgical procedure [22]. All of the three reported cases [8, 9, 12] were initial reconstruction of esophagogastrostomy; this is the first reported case of laparoscopic resection for remnant stomach reconstructed by jejunal interposition in the English language literature.

Cases of resection for remnant stomach reconstructed by jejunal interposition have been rarely reported, even in open surgery. Nozaki et al. reported five cases with removal of remnant gastric cancer following proximal gastrectomy with jejunal interposition [23]. The unique technique of Nozaki et al. was preserving the interposed jejunum for re-reconstruction by Roux-en-Y anastomosis. In our case, removal of the total gastric remnant with radical lymphadenectomy was the same as that of Nozaki et al. On the other hand, the interposed jejunum was totally removed at the same time. In our case, the first reason for the total removal of interposed jejunum was the difficulty of safely preserving the vessels feeding the interposed jejunum owing to severe adhesions. The second reason for the total removal of interposed jejunum was that esophagojejunostomy was a usual and safe anastomotic technique after laparoscopy-assisted total gastrectomy or proximal gastrectomy. Accordingly, we selected total removal of the gastric remnant with interposed jejunum and re-reconstruction by the Roux-en-Y method.

The selected surgical approach after major surgery for intra-abdominal malignancies has usually been the conventional open method. Kwon et al. [10] and Son et al. [9] reported a comparison of the surgical outcomes between an open approach group and a minimally invasive approach group for patients with remnant gastric cancer. In their report, compared with the open approach group, the minimally invasive approach group for remnant gastric cancer demonstrated better short-term outcome and comparable oncologic results. On the other hand, eight of 17 patients (47.1%) required conversion to open surgery because of the presence of severe intra-abdominal adhesions [9]. Adhesion formation is one of the major concerns in patients who undergo major abdominal surgery. In laparoscopic surgery after major abdominal surgery, the first key to a safe procedure is the insertion of the first trocar in an area free from

adhesion. In our case, the first trocar was inserted from the left lower oblique to an open method. The second key was careful lysis of adhesion from the abdominal wall. If all trocars are inserted at the same site of laparoscopic gastrectomy, removal of remnant stomach, and lymphadenectomy, reconstruction might be performed by the usual method easily.

4. Conclusion

We have described a good result of a laparoscopic approach for early gastric remnant cancer following radical proximal gastrectomy. A review of the literature supports a minimally invasive approach for this procedure, showing that it is safe, effective, and technically feasible.

References

[1] I. Uyama, A. Sugioka, J. Fujita et al., "Completely laparoscopic extraperigastric lymph node dissection for gastric malignancies located in the middle or lower third of the stomach," *Gastric Cancer*, vol. 2, pp. 186–190, 1999.

[2] S. Kitano, N. Shiraishi, I. Uyama, K. Sugihara, and N. Tanigawa, "A multicenter study on oncologic outcome of laparoscopic gastrectomy for early cancer in Japan," *Annals of Surgery*, vol. 245, no. 1, pp. 68–72, 2007.

[3] H. Katai, M. Sasako, H. Fukuda et al., "Safety and feasibility of laparoscopy-assisted distal gastrectomy with suprapancreatic nodal dissection for clinical stage I gastric cancer: a multicenter phase II trial (JCOG 0703)," *Gastric Cancer*, vol. 13, no. 4, pp. 238–244, 2010.

[4] H. Yamada, K. Kojima, T. Yamashita, T. Kawano, K. Sugihara, and Z. Nihei, "Laparoscopy-assisted resection of gastric remnant cancer," *Surgical Laparoscopy, Endoscopy and Percutaneous Techniques*, vol. 15, no. 4, pp. 226–229, 2005.

[5] F. Corcione, F. Pirozzi, E. Marzano, D. Cuccurullo, A. Settembre, and L. Miranda, "Laparoscopic approach to gastric remnant-stump: our initial successful experience on 3 cases," *Surgical Laparoscopy, Endoscopy and Percutaneous Techniques*, vol. 18, no. 5, pp. 502–505, 2008.

[6] H. J. Cho, W. Kim, H. Hur, and H. M. Jeon, "Laparoscopy-assisted completion total gastrectomy for gastric cancer in remnant stomach: report of 2 cases," *Surgical Laparoscopy, Endoscopy and Percutaneous Techniques*, vol. 19, no. 2, pp. e57–e60, 2009.

[7] T. Shinohara, N. Hanyu, Y. Tanaka, K. Murakami, A. Watanabe, and K. Yanaga, "Totally laparoscopic complete resection of the remnant stomach for gastric cancer," *Langenbeck's Archives of Surgery*, vol. 398, no. 2, pp. 341–345, 2013.

[8] E. Nagai, K. Nakata, K. Ohuchida, Y. Miyasaka, S. Shimizu, and M. Tanaka, "Laparoscopic total gastrectomy for remnant gastric cancer: feasibility study," *Surgical Endoscopy and Other Interventional Techniques*, vol. 28, no. 1, pp. 289–296, 2014.

[9] S.-Y. Son, C. M. Lee, D.-H. Jung et al., "Laparoscopic completion total gastrectomy for remnant gastric cancer: a single-institution experience," *Gastric Cancer*, vol. 18, no. 1, pp. 177–182, 2015.

[10] I. G. Kwon, I. Cho, A. Guner et al., "Minimally invasive surgery for remnant gastric cancer: a comparison with open surgery," *Surgical Endoscopy and Other Interventional Techniques*, vol. 28, no. 8, pp. 2452–2458, 2014.

[11] H. S. Kim, B. S. Kim, I. S. Lee, S. Lee, and J. H. Yook, "Laparo-scopic gastrectomy in patients with previous gastrectomy for gastric cancer: a report of 17 cases," *Surgical Laparoscopy, Endoscopy, and Percutaneous Techniques*, vol. 24, no. 2, pp. 177–182, 2014.

[12] S. Tsunoda, H. Okabe, E. Tanaka et al., "Laparoscopic gastrec-tomy for remnant gastric cancer: a comprehensive review and case series," *Gastric Cancer*, vol. 19, no. 1, pp. 287–292, 2016.

[13] Japanese Gastric Cancer Association, "Japanese gastric cancer treatment guidelines 2010, ver. 3," *Gastric Cancer*, vol. 14, pp. 113–123, 2011.

[14] Japanese Gastric Cancer Association, "Japanese classification of gastric carcinoma. 3rd English edition," *Gastric Cancer*, vol. 14, no. 2, pp. 101–112, 2011.

[15] S. Ohyama, M. Tokunaga, N. Hiki et al., "A clinicopathological study of gastric stump carcinoma following proximal gastrec-tomy," *Gastric Cancer*, vol. 12, no. 2, pp. 88–94, 2009.

[16] S. Sakuramoto, K. Yamashita, S. Kikuchi et al., "Clinical experience of laparoscopy-assisted proximal gastrectomy with Toupet-like partial fundoplication in early gastric cancer for preventing reflux esophagitis," *Journal of the American College of Surgeons*, vol. 209, no. 3, pp. 344–351, 2009.

[17] Y. Adachi, T. Katsuta, M. Aramaki, A. Morimoto, N. Shi-raishi, and S. Kitano, "Proximal gastrectomy and gastric tube reconstruction for early cancer of the gastric cardia," *Digestive Surgery*, vol. 16, no. 6, pp. 468–470, 1999.

[18] I. Uyama, A. Sugioka, J. Fujita, Y. Komori, H. Matsui, and A. Hasumi, "Completely laparoscopic proximal gastrectomy with jejunal interposition and lymphadenectomy," *Journal of the American College of Surgeons*, vol. 191, no. 1, pp. 114–119, 2000.

[19] H. Katai, T. Sano, T. Fukagawa, H. Shinohara, and M. Sasako, "Prospective study of proximal gastrectomy for early gastric cancer in the upper third of the stomach," *British Journal of Surgery*, vol. 90, no. 7, pp. 850–853, 2003.

[20] T. Kinoshita, N. Gotohda, Y. Kato, S. Takahashi, M. Konishi, and T. Kinoshita, "Laparoscopic proximal gastrectomy with jejunal interposition for gastric cancer in the proximal third of the stomach: a retrospective comparison with open surgery," *Surgical Endoscopy and Other Interventional Techniques*, vol. 27, no. 1, pp. 146–153, 2013.

[21] S.-H. Ahn, D. H. Jung, S.-Y. Son, C.-M. Lee, D. J. Park, and H.-H. Kim, "Laparoscopic double-tract proximal gastrectomy for proximal early gastric cancer," *Gastric Cancer*, vol. 17, no. 3, pp. 562–570, 2014.

[22] T. Suzuki, Y. Awane, M. Kitamura, T. Konishi, K. Arai, and G. Kosaki, "Indication of proximal gastrectomy for gastric cancer," *Japanese Society of Gastroenterological Surgery*, vol. 19, no. 1, pp. 1–11, 1986 (Japanese).

[23] I. Nozaki, S. Hato, and A. Kurita, "A new technique for resecting gastric remnant cancer after proximal gastrectomy with jejunal interposition," *Surgery Today*, vol. 42, no. 11, pp. 1135–1138, 2012.

51

Transanal Drainage of Coloanal Anastomotic Leaks

Bradley Sherman,[1] Mark Arnold,[2] and Syed Husain ⓘ[2]

[1]Department of Surgery, OhioHealth Doctors Hospital, 5100 West Broad Street, Columbus, OH 43228, USA
[2]Division of Colon and Rectal Surgery, Wexner Medical Center, The Ohio State University, N737 Doan Hall, 410 West 10th Avenue, Columbus, OH 43210, USA

Correspondence should be addressed to Syed Husain; syed.husain@osumc.edu

Academic Editor: Nisar A. Chowdri

The conventional operative intervention for leaks following coloanal anastomoses has been proximal fecal diversion with or without take-down of anastomosis. A few of these cases are also amenable to percutaneous drainage. Ostomies created in this situation are often permanent, specifically in cases where coloanal anastomoses are taken down at the time of reoperation. We present two patients who developed perianastomotic pelvic abscesses that were treated with transanal large bore catheter drainage resulting in successful salvage of coloanal anastomoses without the need for a laparotomy or ostomy creation. We propose this to be an effective therapeutic approach to leaks involving low coloanal anastomoses in the absence of generalized peritonitis.

1. Introduction

Anastomotic leaks carry a reported mortality of 6 to 39% [1]. Majority of these patients require a reoperation with complete take-down of anastomosis and fecal diversion. Take-down of coloanal anastomosis presents a unique challenge as pelvic scarring, and absence of distal bowel segment precludes restoration of bowel continuity at a later day.

We present two patients managed with a transanal drainage following coloanal anastomotic dehiscence.

2. Case 1

An 86-year-old female underwent uncomplicated Altemeier procedure for rectal prolapse and was discharged on postoperative day (POD) 5. She presented to the emergency department two days after her discharge with fevers up to 102.6°F, pelvic pain, fatigue, and anorexia.

On exam, she was febrile to 101.6°F, pulse was 79, and blood pressure was 117/58. Her abdominal exam did not reveal any evidence of generalized peritonitis, and lower abdominal tenderness was present. Her WBC count was 13.1. Imaging demonstrated a large fluid collection and gas within the pelvis that tracked cephalad in the retroperitoneum.

She was admitted, made NPO, and started on antibiotics. Interventional radiology deemed the abscess not amenable to percutaneous drainage. Thus, we proceeded with an anorectal examination under anesthesia for surgical drainage of the area and stoma creation, if needed. She was noted to have a grossly intact anastomosis. A vaginal exam demonstrated fluctuant swelling in the posterior vaginal vault, and a 18-gauge needle was used to aspirate 30 mL of clear straw-colored fluid and air. A diagnostic laparoscopy was then performed demonstrating normal-appearing bowel and pelvis without evidence of fecal matter. We felt that the collection represented a post-op seroma, and operation was concluded at this time.

The patient was maintained on empiric IV antibiotics, and her diet was resumed. She remained hemodynamically stable however continued to experience ongoing fevers. A CT scan was repeated on hospital day 6 (Figure 1), demonstrating an enlarging fluid collection containing enteric contrast measuring 5.8 × 7.5 cm, previously 5.4 × 6.4 cm.

Once again, interventional radiology determined that the collection was not suitable for percutaneous approach, and she was taken back to the operating room. We were unsuccessful in accessing the abscess cavity via a skin incision on the right lateral aspect of coccyx. An anorectal exam

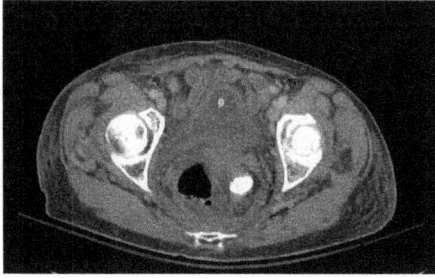

FIGURE 1: Perirectal fluid collection with contrast in the rectal lumen.

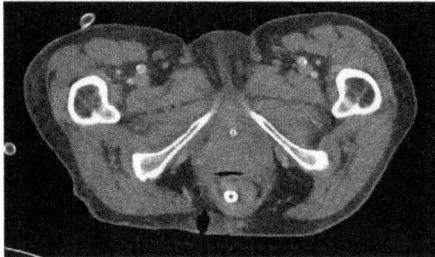

FIGURE 3: CT on day 15 after drainage demonstrating resolution of abscess with transanal drain in place.

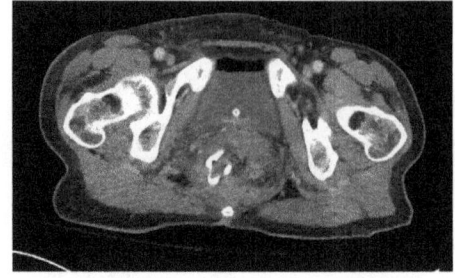

FIGURE 2: CT on day 7 after drainage demonstrating resolution of abscess with transanal drain in place.

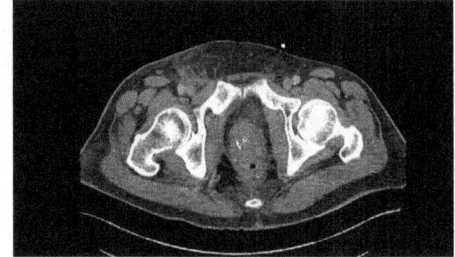

FIGURE 4: Postdrainage resolution of perirectal collection.

under anesthesia revealed anastomotic defect extending about 1.5 proximally. The abscess cavity was suctioned out via this defect, and a 26-French Malecot drain was placed in the cavity transanally. The drain was then secured to perianal skin via two nylon sutures.

Repeat CT scans done on 7 and 15 days after the drainage demonstrated resolving fluid collections (Figures 2 and 3). The patient did well and was discharged on hospital day 19 with a plan to maintain the drain for 4–6 weeks to allow complete collapse of abscess cavity.

The patient presented again two weeks later after spontaneous removal of Malecot drain. An exam under anesthesia was performed revealing involution of abscess cavity into fibrotic sinus tract. This tract was incorporated into the bowel lumen by dividing the septum with LigaSure device precluding the possibility of recurrent abscess caused by the presence of a narrow sinus tract.

The patient was seen in follow-up in the office two months after her last procedure. She reported minimal residual rectal discomfort, was continent without recurrent prolapse, and endorsed normal bowel function.

3. Case 2

A 61-year-old male underwent low anterior resection for rectal cancer. He was discharged on postoperative day 11 after recovering from post-op ileus. Six days later, he presented to the emergency department with acute onset of abdominal pain. He was afebrile, had normal heart rate, and was mildly hypertensive on presentation. Although diffuse abdominal tenderness was present, there were no signs of peritonitis on exam. WBC count was 11.8K. CT scan demonstrated possible dehiscence at the anastomotic site

and presence of enteric contrast in a pelvic collection measuring 4×5.1 cm without gross contamination of peritoneal cavity.

He was taken to the operating room as the abscess was determined inaccessible via percutaneous route. The exam revealed a small posterior disruption of coloanal anastomosis. The cavity was suctioned out, and a transanal 26-French Malecot drain was placed.

Diet was resumed a week after drainage, and drain was removed prior to his discharge on day 10. Follow-up CT scan demonstrated near resolution of the previously visualized fluid collection and a smaller cavity that communicated with the rectum (Figure 4). The patient was seen in follow-up about four months after his last surgery and reported a complete recovery.

4. Discussion

Abdominal wash out with stoma creation is the treatment of choice for an anastomotic dehiscence in presence of peritonitis. Many of these patients also require a complete takedown of anastomosis [2]. The reported healing rates after diversion are widely variable, and this approach obviously subjects the patient to another abdominal surgery [3]. Contrary to leaks presenting with peritonitis, anastomotic dehiscence leading to localized peritoneal contamination and walled off abscess can often be treated with intravenous antibiotics with or without placement of interventional radiology-guided percutaneous drains.

Restoration of bowel continuity may not be possible after take-down of coloanal anastomosis; however, these leaks carry the benefit of accessibility via transanal route, which in select cases may allow for preservation of the anastomosis.

It is imperative to note that both of our cases were hemodynamically stable and did not exhibit any signs of generalized peritonitis. Furthermore, anastomotic failures encompassed a small portion of anastomotic circumference. We strongly caution against employment of this technique in patients with frank peritonitis, hemodynamic instability, or major anastomotic disruption which, in our opinion, are best managed with fecal diversion and anastomotic take-down.

Several previous publications have addressed the issue of anastomotic preservation with or without proximal diversion. Out of the techniques described, perhaps the most similar to our proposed method is the vacuum-assisted closure anastomotic leaks. Weidenhagen et al. [4] reported a success rate of 28 out of 29 patients treated with endoscopic suction-assisted drainage of anastomotic leaks after low anterior resections. Contrary to our patients, overwhelming majority of patients in this cohort had proximal fecal diversion, and only four patients were managed without a stoma. Other authors have described similar success rates with this technique; however, common to these reports is the need for frequent, multiple procedures due to the need for repeated debridements and sponge replacements [5, 6]. Verlaan et al. [7] reported successful management of five out of six colorectal anastomotic leaks using a modification of this technique combining endosponge placement with closure of anastomotic defect using sutures or an endoscopic clip. Finally, Gardenbroek et al. [8] compared endoscopic vacuum closure to conventional treatment for management of ileoanal pouch leaks. The authors reported similar results and concluded that vacuum-assisted closure of anastomotic leaks was a highly effective method of managing ileoanal pouch anastomotic leaks. While the above-described reports testify the effectiveness of suction-assisted closure of low anastomotic leaks, we feel that our proposed method offers a simple, low-cost alternative.

Possible complications of proposed approach include anal pain, poor bowel function, and compromised fecal continence. Many patients go on to develop a chronic sinus that could lead to fistula formation [9] as witnessed in one of our patients.

Our case report demonstrates that transanal drainage is a viable option that allows anastomotic preservation while avoiding fecal diversion in selected patients with low anastomotic leaks.

References

[1] Z. A. Murrell and M. J. Stamos, "Reoperation for anastomic failure," *Clinics in Colon and Rectal Surgery*, vol. 19, no. 4, pp. 213–216, 2006.

[2] P. B. Soeters, J. P. de Zoete, C. H. Dejong, N. S. Williams, and C. G. Baeten, "Colorectal surgey and anastomotic leakage," *Digestive Surgery*, vol. 19, no. 2, pp. 150–155, 2002.

[3] Y. Parc, P. Frileux, G. Schmitt, N. Dehni, J. M. Ollivier, and R. Parc, "Management of postoperative peritonitis after anterior resection: experience from a referral intensive care unit," *Diseases of the Colon & Rectum*, vol. 43, no. 5, pp. 579–587, 2000.

[4] R. Weidenhagen, K. U. Gruetzner, T. Wiecken, F. Spelsberg, and K. W. Jauch, "Endoscopic vacuum-assisted closure of anastomotic leakage following anterior resection of the rectum: a new method," *Surgical Endoscopy*, vol. 22, no. 8, pp. 1818–1825, 2008.

[5] A. Glitsch, W. von Bernstorff, U. Seltrecht, I. Partecke, H. Paul, and C. D. Heidecke, "Endoscopic transanal vacuum-assisted rectal drainage (ETVARD): an optimized therapy for major leaks from extraperitoneal rectal anastomoses," *Endoscopy*, vol. 40, no. 3, pp. 192–199, 2008.

[6] A. Arezzo, A. Miegge, A. Garbarini, and M. Morino, "Endoluminal vacuum therapy for anastomotic leaks after rectal surgery," *Techniques in Coloproctology*, vol. 14, no. 3, pp. 279–281, 2010.

[7] T. Verlaan, S. A. Bartels, M. I. van Berge Henegouwen, P. J. Tanis, P. Fockens, and W. A. Bemelman, "Early, minimally invasive closure of anastomotic leaks: a new concept," *Colorectal Disease*, vol. 13, no. 7, pp. 18–22, 2011.

[8] T. J. Gardenbroek, G. D. Musters, C. J. Buskens et al., "Early reconstruction of the leaking ileal pouch-anal anastomosis: a novel solution to an old problem," *Colorectal Disease*, vol. 17, no. 5, pp. 426–432, 2015.

[9] J. Blumetti and H. Abcarian, "Management of low colorectal anastomic leak: preserving the anastomosis," *World Journal of Gastrointestinal Surgery*, vol. 7, no. 12, pp. 378–383, 2015.

52

First Video Case Report of Chronic Retrograde Jejunojejunal Intussusception after Subtotal Gastrectomy with Braun's Anastomosis

Savaş Bayrak,[1] **Hasan Bektaş,**[1] **Necdet Derici,**[2] **Ekrem Çakar,**[1] **and Şükrü Çolak**[1]

[1]*Department of General Surgery, Istanbul Training and Research Hospital, Istanbul, Turkey*
[2]*Private Ataköy Hospital, Istanbul, Turkey*

Correspondence should be addressed to Savaş Bayrak; savasbayrak74@gmail.com

Academic Editor: Giovanni Mariscalco

Intussusception, which is seen rarely in adults, is defined as the pulling or invagination of a part of the intestine into another segment of the intestine. In this case report we present chronic retrograde jejunojejunal intussusception following gastric surgery with Braun's anastomosis in adult with video presentation. A 66-year-old woman, who had undergone gastric surgery 39 years ago and cholecystectomy 20 years ago, was admitted to our clinic with the complaints about weight loss, abdominal pain, nausea, and vomiting. Upper gastrointestinal endoscopy (UGISE) was applied, and patient was treated with surgery. This case report indicates that intussusception should be considered in the presence of clinical complaints following gastric surgery, as well as importance of endoscopy in diagnosis.

1. Introduction

Intussusception is defined as the pulling or invagination of a part of the intestine into another segment of the intestine. Childhood cases are often idiopathic whereas intussusception seen in adults usually has different causes including benign and malign conditions such as lipoma, submucosal fibroids, gastrointestinal stromal tumors, and adenocarcinoma. Patients can also develop intussusception in the postoperative period. In adults, the complaints related to intussusception can be acute or chronic with nonspecific findings being predominant in the latter, which is one of the major factors that delay diagnosis [1, 2].

To the best of our knowledge, this is the first video case report in the literature presenting a case of chronic retrograde jejunojejunal intussusception following gastric surgery with Braun's anastomosis.

2. Case Report

A 66-year-old woman was admitted to our clinic with the complaints of weight loss, abdominal pain, nausea, and vomiting. She reported that she had undergone gastric surgery 39 years earlier and cholecystectomy 20 years before. She also stated that she had consulted several physicians about this problem; however, the prescribed medication did not relieve her symptoms.

For diagnostic purposes, abdominal computed tomography (CT) and upper gastrointestinal endoscopy (UGISE) were planned. The results of UGISE revealed a large amount of bilious gastric content as well as intestinal lumen with a mass at the previous Braun's anastomotic site. As the UGISE procedure progressed, the lesion was identified as an approximately 10–15 cm jejunal segment that developed due to retrograde jejunojejunal intussusception of the efferent loop at the Braun anastomotic site. This part of the intestine was observed to have spontaneously reduced. The whole procedure was video-recorded (Video 1; see Supplementary Material available online at: https://doi.org/10.1155/2017/6945017).

Following informed consent given by the patient, the surgery was performed. Since the patient history included subtotal gastrectomy, antecolic gastrojejunostomy, and Braun's anastomosis, first, the previous anastomosis was removed and the passage was unobstructed using Roux-en-Y gastrojejunostomy (Video 2). The patient did not develop any early postoperative complications and was thus discharged on the sixth day after surgery. No problem was observed over the 5-year routine follow-up by the hospital.

3. Discussion

The term intussusception was first defined by John Hunter in 1789 as one part of the intestine folding into another part of the intestine. Although the first case of intussusception following gastric surgery was reported by Bozzi as early as 1914, the mechanism of this condition has not yet been clarified. However, it is believed that the process starts when a lesion in the intestinal wall or an irritant in the lumen changes the intestinal peristalsis [3–5].

Intussusception is classified as "antegrade" if it is directed towards the physiological peristalsis and "retrograde" if the movement is in the opposite direction [6]. It is mostly seen in newborns and children with only 5% of all cases belonging to adults. In adult intussusception cases, 70–90% have organic causes, of which more than half are malignant [7, 8]. Intussusception is rare in the postoperative period with an incidence of less than 0.1% [2].

In the literature, five forms of intussusception are described: Type 1 is the antegrade intussusception of the afferent loop and is commonly seen with an incidence of 5.5%. Type 2, the most frequent form (75.5%), is further divided into two as follows: Type 2a, which are the retrograde intussusceptions of the efferent loop, and Type 2b efferent-efferent intussusceptions. Type 3 is the combination of the first two types and is seen in 6.5% of patients. The last form, Type 4, is the intussusception at the site of Braun's anastomosis and has an 8% incidence [9]. As can be seen in Video 2, the case presented here was identified as Type 4 characterized by chronic retrograde jejunojejunal intussusception at the anastomotic site. We think that the reader is better able to understand the subject with visual materials. This makes the article different from other similar manuscripts.

In the literature, several factors have been reported to contribute to the development of intussusception, including adhesions in the suture line, making long intestinal loops during surgery, increased intra-abdominal pressure, reverse peristalsis, and short jejunal mesentery [3]. In the present case, no mechanical or functional cause was identified. The acute form presents with symptoms associated with a high level of intestinal obstruction including severe epigastric pain, sensitivity, nausea, vomiting, hematemesis, and palpable masses. These complaints may lead to serious complications such as strangulation and incarceration. In the presence of these symptoms particularly in those patients with a history of gastric surgery, an intussusception diagnosis should be considered. The treatment for intussusception is emergency surgery. Although the chronic form of the condition has similar symptoms in essence, it has certain differences in terms of the symptoms being recurrent, long-term, and spontaneous with less clamorous manifestations [5]. In the present case, gastric complaints began following gastric surgery and increased significantly within the previous 3-4 years.

Since intussusception is rarely seen in adults, it is difficult to diagnose. Therefore, given the presence of clinical suspicion, further examination is necessary with UGISE, ultrasonography (US), barium swallow tests, and abdominal CT being conventionally used in the diagnosis of intussusception [10]. In the present study, the diagnosis was made following endoscopy. Since there is no single treatment option that can be used for all patients, the chosen method should be specific to the individual. In the literature, a frequently recommended method is the reduction or resection of the affected part of the intestine to unblock it, closing previous anastomoses and performing reanastomosis. However, Ozdogan et al. suggested that, in cases presenting with normal intestinal viability, manual reduction is sufficient [11].

To date, several methods have been proposed to prevent the recurrence of intussusception following treatment, including but not limited to suturing the jejunum or mesentery to the neighboring tissue, fixing the afferent loop mesentery to the efferent loop and converting Billroth II to Billroth I [12]. The complaints of the present case had persisted for a long time; therefore, resection Roux-en-Y gastrojejunostomy was performed on the patient. Since no complication was observed in the early postoperative period, the patient was discharged on the sixth day after surgery.

4. Conclusion

Intussusception should be considered in the presence of clinical complaints following gastric surgery and diagnosed using appropriate diagnostic tools to reduce the morbidity and mortality associated with this condition.

Competing Interests

The authors declare that there is no conflict of interests regarding the publication of this paper.

References

[1] S. I. Kang, J. Kang, M. J. Kim et al., "Laparoscopic-assisted resection of jejunojejunal intussusception caused by a juvenile polyp in an adult," *Case Reports in Surgery*, vol. 2014, 4 pages, 2014.

[2] S. Yakan, C. Caliskan, O. Makay, A. G. Denecli, and M. A. Korkut, "Intussusception in adults: clinical characteristics, diagnosis and operative strategies," *World Journal of Gastroenterology*, vol. 15, no. 16, pp. 1985–1989, 2009.

[3] J. M. Kwak, J. Kim, and S. O. Suh, "Anterograde jejunojejunal intussusception resulted in acute efferent loop syndrome after subtotal gastrectomy," *World Journal of Gastroenterology*, vol. 16, no. 27, pp. 3472–3474, 2010.

[4] E. Bozzi, "Annotation," *Bulletin of the Academy of Medicine*, vol. 122, pp. 3–4, 1914.

[5] A. J. Archimandritis, N. Hatzopoulos, P. Hatzinikolaou et al., "Jejunogastric intussusception presented with hematemesis: a case presentation and review of the literature," *BMC Gastroenterology*, vol. 1, article 1, 2001.

[6] D. B. O'Connor, R. Ryan, D. O'Malley, and E. MacDermott, "Retrograde intussusception 5 years after Roux-en-Y gastric

bypass for morbid obesity," *Irish Journal of Medical Science*, vol. 181, no. 3, pp. 419–421, 2012.

[7] T. Azar and D. L. Berger, "Adult intussusception," *Annals of Surgery*, vol. 226, no. 2, pp. 134–138, 1997.

[8] B. Y. Huang and D. M. Warshauer, "Adult intussusception: diagnosis and clinical relevance," *Radiologic Clinics of North America*, vol. 41, no. 6, pp. 1137–1151, 2003.

[9] S. Brynitz and E. Rubinstein, "Hematemesis caused by jejuno-gastric intussusception," *Endoscopy*, vol. 18, no. 4, pp. 162–164, 1986.

[10] S. H. Lee, I. G. Kwon, S. W. Ryu, and S. S. Sohn, "Jejunogastric intussusception: a rare complication of gastric cancer surgery," *International Journal of Clinical and Experimental Medicine*, vol. 7, no. 11, pp. 4498–4502, 2014.

[11] M. Ozdogan, E. Hamaloglu, A. Ozdemir, and A. Ozenc, "Ante-grade jejunojejunal intussusception after roux-en-Y esophago-jejunostomy as an unusual cause of postoperative intestinal obstruction: report of a case," *Surgery Today*, vol. 31, no. 4, pp. 355–357, 2001.

[12] K. H. Kim, M. K. Jang, H. S. Kim et al., "Intussusception after gastric surgery," *Endoscopy*, vol. 37, no. 12, pp. 1237–1243, 2005.

53

Primary Hepatic Lymphoma Mimicking a Hepatocellular Carcinoma in a Cirrhotic Patient: Case Report and Systematic Review of the Literature

Ali Bohlok ⓘ,[1] Thierry De Grez,[2] Fikri Bouazza,[1] Roland De Wind,[3] Melody El-Khoury,[1] Deborah Repullo,[1] and Vincent Donckier[1]

[1]Service de Chirurgie, Institut Jules Bordet, Université Libre de Bruxelles (ULB), Bruxelles, Belgium
[2]Service de Gastroentérologie, CHR Sambre et Meuse, Namur, Belgium
[3]Service d'Anatomie Pathologique, Institut Jules Bordet, Université Libre de Bruxelles (ULB), Bruxelles, Belgium

Correspondence should be addressed to Ali Bohlok; ali.bohlok@bordet.be

Academic Editor: Paola De Nardi

Introduction. Primary hepatic lymphomas (PHLs) are rare liver tumors, frequently misdiagnosed preoperatively. As these tumors could be successfully treated with chemotherapy, their early recognition is essential, potentially, to avoid useless surgery. We report on the case of a cirrhotic patient with hemochromatosis who presented a PHL, initially diagnosed as a hepatocellular carcinoma (HCC), and we analyze recent data from the literature on this subject. *Case Presentation and Review of the Literature.* A 45 mm liver tumor was found is a 68-year-old man with alcohol cirrhosis and hemochromatosis. At imaging, the diagnosis of HCC was suspected according to vascular characteristics and the presence of cirrhosis. FDG PET scan showed a solitary hypermetabolic liver tumor. Tumor markers were negative. Surgery consisted in left lateral hepatectomy. At pathology, the diagnosis of the primary hepatic marginal zone B cell lymphoma of mucosa-associated lymphoid tissue (MALT) type was demonstrated. Twenty-two articles reporting 33 cases of true PHL of MALT type were found. Presentation lacked specific symptoms (70% asymptomatic). Half of patients were suspected to have other etiologies of liver mass (HCC, intrahepatic cholangiocarcinoma), and thus diagnosis was established postoperatively. In the patient, diagnosis was made by preoperative biopsy, and chemotherapy was first-line treatment. *Discussion.* Preoperative diagnosis of PHL, and particularly of primary hepatic MALT lymphoma, is challenging. This case illustrates that PHL remains to be considered among the differential diagnosis of isolated solid liver tumors. Further, it indicates that biopsy could be still indicated in case of suspected HCC in cirrhotic patients, particularly in the presence of unusual findings such as the combination of a FDG PET scan positive tumor in the absence of elevated alpha-fetoprotein.

1. Introduction

Primary hepatic lymphoma (PHL) represents less than 10% of space occupying focal hepatic lesion [1]. Among lymphoma, PHLs represent 0.4% of all extranodal lymphomas and 0.016% of all non-Hodgkin lymphomas [2]. Primary hepatic marginal zone B cell lymphoma of mucosa-associated lymphoid tissue (MALT) is extremely rare, representing 3% of PHL [3]. Because of this rarity and in the absence of specific symptoms and imaging characteristics, the early recognition of PHL is a challenge and most of the diagnoses are established on operative specimen [4]. Multiple treatment modalities depending on the timing of

diagnosis of PHL include chemotherapy and surgery associated or not with chemotherapy [5]. Therefore, preoperative recognition of PHL could be critical, as it may avoid unnecessary liver resection or reduce the extent of liver resection in case of response to preoperative chemotherapy [6, 7]. Herein, we present a case of surgically resected primary hepatic MALT lymphoma mimicking HCC on preoperative imaging, a review of literature of primary hepatic MALT lymphoma, and further discuss on the need for additional tools to establish such diagnosis preoperatively. In addition, we review recent data from the literature in order to identify potential recommendations for the diagnosis and the treatment in these cases.

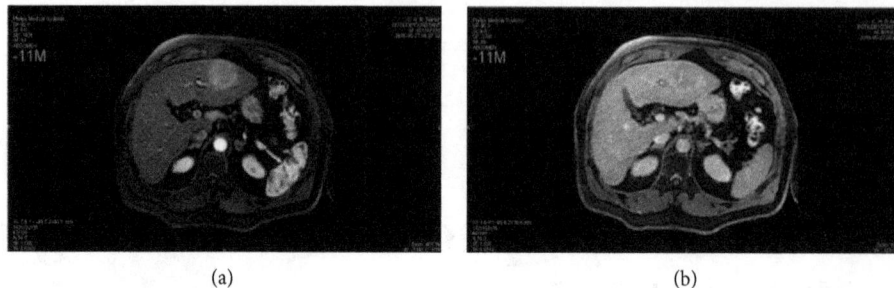

(a)   (b)

FIGURE 1: Liver MRI showing the segment III lesion, enhancing at the arterial phase (a) with rapid washout on the portal phase (b).

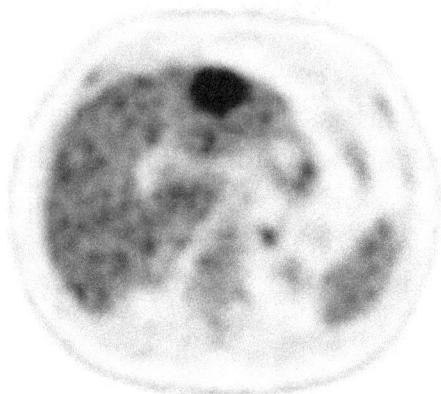

FIGURE 2: FDG PET-CT showing the hypermetabolic segment III liver lesion (SUV max: 7.3).

2. Materials and Methods

We performed a systematic review of the literature using two databases (PubMed and Scopus). In the PubMed search, we used the following search terms ("Liver Neoplasms" [Mesh]) AND "Lymphoma, B-Cell, Marginal Zone" [Mesh]. Free terms included ("Liver OR hepatic" AND "Lymphoma, B-Cell, Marginal Zone"). In the Scopus database search, we used the terms TITLE-ABS-KEY ("Lymphoma, B-Cell, Marginal Zone" AND " liver" OR" hepatic").

The search strategy had no publication date or publication type restriction. In addition, the reference lists of relevant reviews or included articles were also searched to find other eligible studies. We included only studies published in English.

Study characteristics such as patient age, sex, and presenting symptoms, associated liver disease and lesions, the presence of cirrhosis, associated liver lesions, timing of diagnosis (preoperative biopsy or postoperatively), type of treatment, and outcome were evaluated.

3. Case Presentation

A 68-year-old male patient with hemochromatosis and Child A cirrhosis due to alcohol consumption was referred to our department for a liver tumor. The patient is known to have a Child A cirrhosis without any previous episode of liver decompensation. Physical examination was normal, and laboratory tests showed a minimal elevation of transaminases levels. Serologies for hepatitis B and C and tumor

markers, including alpha-fetoprotein (AFP) and CA19.9, were negative. Contrast-enhanced liver MRI showed a 46 mm tumor in segment III with arterial wash in and portal phase washout (Figures 1(a) and 1(b)). Liver morphology, and particularly irregular hepatic surface, confirmed the presence of cirrhosis. On this basis, the diagnosis of hepatocellular carcinoma (HCC) on cirrhotic liver was proposed. A FDG PET scan showed a hypermetabolic liver tumor in segment III, without extrahepatic lesion (Figure 2). Bone scintigraphy and chest CT scan showed no distant metastases, and gastroscopy showed no esophageal varices. Accordingly, a left lateral liver R0 resection was performed. Postoperative course was uneventful, and the patient was discharged at day 4 after surgery. Pathological examination demonstrated the diagnosis of MALT lymphoma (Figures 3(a) and 3(b)). Small-to-middle-sized lymphocytes formed lymphoepithelial lesions on some bile capillaries (Figure 4(a)). Immunohistochemical stains were positive for CD20 (++) (Figure 4(b)), CD3 (+), CD5 (+), CD43 (+), CD10 (+), Ki67 (10%) anti BCL-6 (+), MUM-1 (+), and CD138 (+), whereas they were negative for CD1. PCR amplification showed monoclonal Ig λ and IG κ (kappa). The pathology of the nontumor liver confirmed the presence of cirrhosis.

The patient's disease was classified as Ann Arbor stage IE (stage I extranodal), and no adjuvant therapy was proposed.

4. Systematic Literature Review

4.1. Study Selection. A total of 158 articles were identified from the PubMed and Scopus. After removing duplicated articles, 124 articles were assessed further assessment. A total of 92 articles were excluded on the basis of the titles and the abstracts. Only true cases of primary hepatic MALT were included (Ann Arbor stage IE). All cases of extrahepatic biliary tract MALT were excluded. Of the remaining 32 articles, only 22 articles had full text published in English. After full-text review of these remaining articles, they were all eligible and included in the systematic review (Figure 5).

4.2. Patient and Tumor Characteristics. A total of 22 articles (Table 1) reporting 33 cases of primary hepatic MALT were found [8–29]. The statistical analysis of all patient characteristics is summarized in Table 1.

There were 17 male (51.5%) and 16 female (48.5%) patients with a mean age of 61.7 years (range 36 to 85 years). Twenty-one patients (63.6%) were asymptomatic at presentation, 3 had

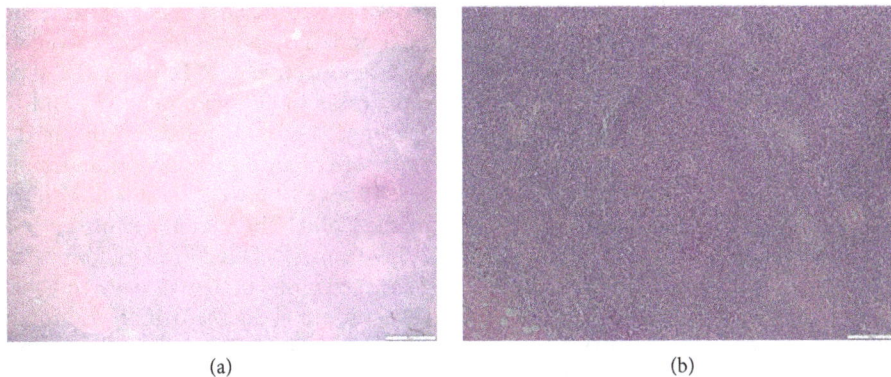

FIGURE 3: (a) Lymphoid infiltration (bluish discoloration) in hepatocellular parenchyma and (b) germinal center (×100).

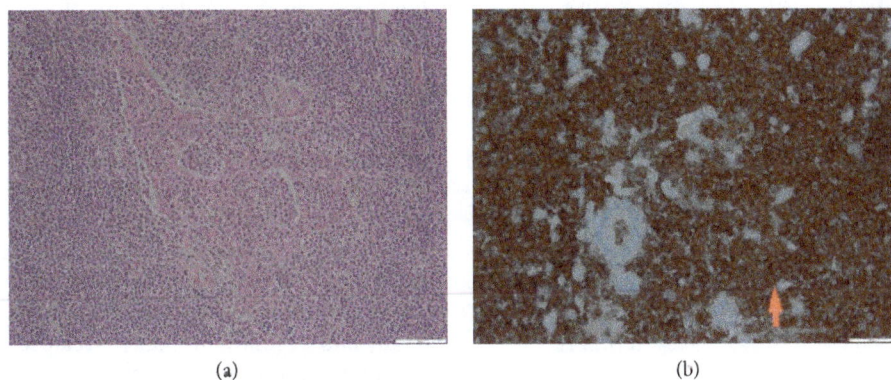

FIGURE 4: Lymphoepithelial complex in hematoxylin eosin stain (×200) (a) and CD20 staining (×400) (b).

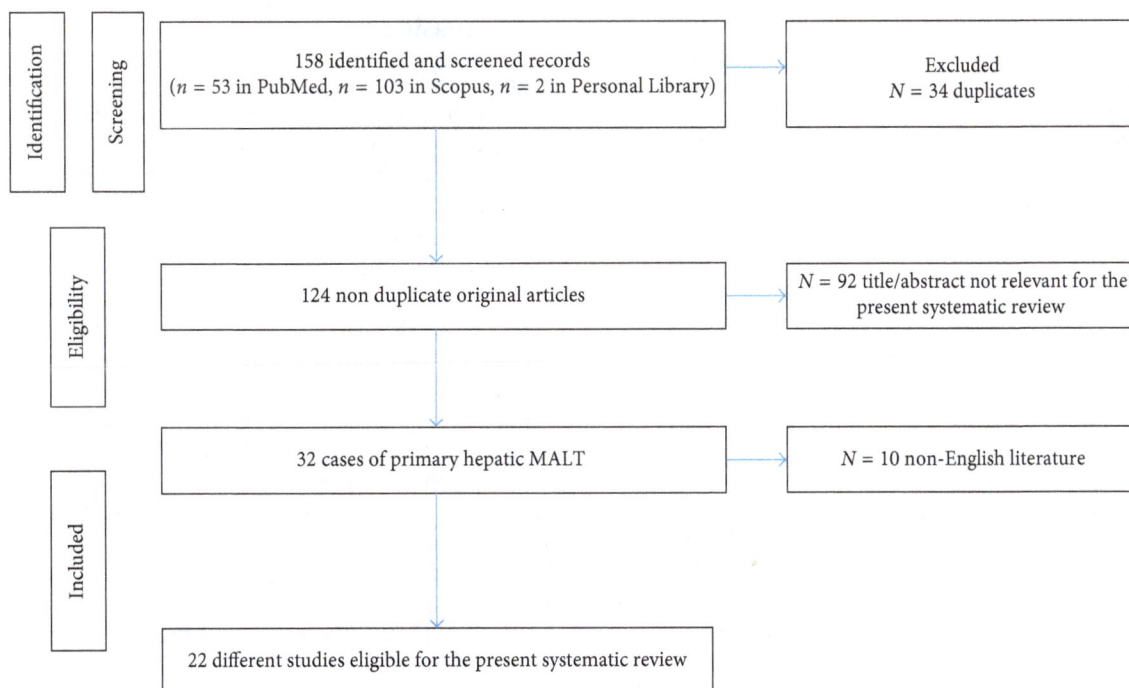

FIGURE 5: Prisma guidelines for the selection of eligible articles of primary hepatic MALT lymphoma.

TABLE 1: Patient characteristics.

Characteristics	
Number	
Age	61.67 range (36–85) median: 61 y
Sex	
Male	17 (51.5%)
Female	16 (48.5%)
Presenting symptom	
Asymptomatic	21 (63.6%)
Abdominal pain	3 (9.1%)
Elevated liver enzymes	2 (6.1%)
Generalized weakness	1 (3%)
Cough	1 (3%)
NA	5 (15.2%)
Preexisting liver disease	
HCV	7 (21.2%)
HBV	6 (18.2%)
Primary biliary cirrhosis	1 (3%)
Old HAV	1 (3%)
None	16 (48.5%)
NA	2 (7.1%)
Cirrhosis	
Yes	7 (21.2%)
No	26 (78.8%)
Associated HCC	2 (6.1%)
Number	1.34 range (1–6) median 1
Size (cm)	35.61 mm range (15–90) median: 30 mm
Available MRI description	6 (18.2%)
Available CT scan description	7 (21.2%)
Available FDG PET	5 (15.2%)
Mean SUV max	5.5 (3.5–8.2)
Diagnosis	
Preoperative biopsy	15 (45.5%)
After surgery	16 (48.5%)
NA	2 (6.1%)
Type of treatment	
Resection	12 (36.4%)
Transplantation	4 (12.1%)
Chemotherapy	6 (18.2%)
Radiotherapy	2 (6.1%)
Surgery + chemotherapy	5 (15.2%)
Surgery + antiviral treatment	1 (3%)
Surgery + radiotherapy	1 (3%)
No treatment	2 (6.1%)
Outcome	
Disease free survival at the last follow-up (9 months–5 years)	21 (63.6%)
Relapse at 30–51 months	3 (9.1%)
Death	2 (6.1%)
Lost to follow-up	2 (6.1%)
NA	5 (15.2%)

NA: non available; HCV: hepatitis C virus; HBV: hepatitis B virus; HAV: hepatitis A virus; HCC: hepatocellular carcinoma; MRI: magnetic resonance imaging; CT: computed tomography; FDG PET: 2-deoxy-2[F-18]fluoro-D-glucose positron emission tomography; SUV: standardized uptake value.

abdominal pain (9.1%), and 2 had elevated liver enzymes (6.1%). Fifteen patients had associated liver disease. Cirrhosis was documented in 7 cases (21.2%) including hepatitis C and B and primary biliary origins. Two patients

(6.1%) had associated HCC lesion at the time of diagnosis. MRI and CT scan reports were available in only 6 and 7 cases, respectively. PHL of MALT type was described in most cases to be hypointense T1 and iso- or hyperintense T2 on MRI and hypodense with variable enhancement on contrast-enhanced CT. The number of hepatic MALT lesions ranged between 1 and 6 with a mean of 1.34 and median of 1. The mean size of the lesions was 35.61 mm (15–90 mm). Detailed FDG PET report was available in only 1 case series of 5 patients, suggesting that these tumors only show minimal increase in FDG uptake, as indicated by mean SUV of 5.5 (3.5–8.2) [28]. In another case, the tumor was reported as hypermetabolic but no SUV max result was described [26].

Primary hepatic MALT was diagnosed based on biopsy in 15 cases (45.5%) and postoperatively in 16 (48.5%) cases. Treatment options varied depending on the timing of diagnosis. Exclusive chemotherapy (most had R-CHOP), and exclusive radiotherapy were administered in 6 patients (18.2%) and 2 patients (6.1%), respectively. Tumors were resected in 23 patients (70%); of these, 4 were diagnosed posthepatic transplantation (12.1%), and the remaining had surgical resection of the tumor.

Adjuvant therapy was administered in 8 patients and consisted of chemotherapy, antiviral treatment, *Helicobacter pylori* eradication treatment, radiotherapy in 5 (15.2%), 1 (3%), 1 (3%), and 1 (3%), respectively. The follow-up period ranged between 9 months and 5 years with a median of 24 months. At the end of follow-up, only 3 relapses (9.1%) were noted and they were treated by chemotherapy (R-CHOP) in 2 patients [24] and radiotherapy in 1 patient [28]. In operated patients, no correlation could be established between the risk of recurrence and the use of adjuvant chemotherapy or radiotherapy.

5. Discussion

In this case, the initial presentation was highly suggestive for the diagnosis of HCC, according to vascular imaging features, the presence of cirrhosis, and for the diagnosis of hemochromatosis. On this basis, in the presence of Child A cirrhosis without significant portal hypertension, surgical resection was decided, without preoperative biopsy [30, 31]. On pathological specimen, the unexpected diagnosis of PHL of MALT subtype was found. In fact, such diagnosis could have change dramatically the treatment plan if it has been obtained preoperatively. Indeed, these tumors are chemosensitive and recent studies reported major response rates using rituximab with cyclophosphamide, doxorubicin, vincristine, and prednisone (R-CHOP), leading to complete remission in more than 80% of the cases [5–7]. The clinical presentation of PHL is variable from incidental discovery in asymptomatic patient, to nonspecific symptoms such as fatigue, night sweats, weight loss, night fever or jaundice, abdominal pain, and hepatomegaly in case of massive liver involvement [32]. The laboratory tests are poorly contributive, and tumor markers, including CEA, AFP, and CA19.9, are usually negative [33]. Among PHL, hepatic MALT lymphoma may arise as solitary or multiple lesions, with variable imaging characteristics, including enhancement on the arterial phase and late washout, as in HCC [34] The definitive diagnosis of MALT is based on pathology, showing CD20 positivity on immunohistochemistry and the presence of the lymphoepithelial complexes [35]. As a consequence, PHLs are rarely diagnosed preoperatively and most frequently confounded with other malignant lesions [7]. In the present case, however, the absence of elevated AFP together with a positive FDG PET scan might have served as an alert, to consider alternative diagnosis to HCC. Separately, neither normal AFP level nor hypermetabolic tumor on FDG PET scan may exclude the diagnosis of HCC. However, while the overall sensitivity of FDG PET scan for the diagnosis of HCC is approximately of 50% [36], it has been shown that HCC could be FDG positive mostly in case of large tumor, superior to 50 mm, corresponding to moderately or poorly differentiated tumor and associated with high AFP levels [37]. Accordingly, in the present case, even if not recommended in current algorithms for tumor superior to 20 mm with characteristic vascular imaging behavior on cirrhotic liver [30, 31] a liver biopsy could have been indicated, leading eventually to avoid first-line liver resection.

In conclusion, primary hepatic MALT lymphoma is an extremely rare tumor with poorly contributive clinical, laboratory, and imaging findings. Early recognition is infrequent, and the definite diagnosis is mostly based on histopathologic examination of operative specimen. The present case illustrates that this diagnosis should be kept in mind and that preoperative biopsy could be still indicated, particularly when the diagnosis of HCC is suspected but in presence of unusual findings such as the combination of positive FDG PET scan with normal AFP level.

According to literature review, the preoperative diagnosis of this tumor remains a challenge, due to the scarcity of specific clinical and imaging signs [8, 11, 14, 24]. In the cases where diagnosis could be established preoperatively, patients should be orientated first to chemotherapy (CHOP) as this treatment could be curative [13, 24, 25]. In the frequent cases where the diagnosis is established postoperatively and when surgical resection has been radical, the role for adjuvant chemotherapy remains unclear [8, 12, 14, 15, 17].

References

[1] M. Sans, V. Andreu, J. M. Bordas et al., "Usefulness of laparoscopy with liver biopsy in the assessment of liver involvement at diagnosis of Hodgkin's and non-Hodgkin's lymphomas," *Gastrointestinal Endoscopy*

[2] C. Loddenkemper and T. Longerich, "Lymphoma of the liver," in *Extranodal Lymphomas, Pathology and Management* H. Stein, and E. Zucca, Eds., pp. 277–288, CRC Press, Abingdon, UK, 2008.

[3] E. S. Jaffe, "Malignant lymphomas: pathology of hepatic involvement," *Seminars in Liver Disease*, vol. 7, no. 3, pp. 257–268, 1987.

[4] I. Serrano-Navarro, J. F. Rodríguez-López, and R. Navas-Espejo, "Primary hepatic lymphoma-favorable outcome with

chemotherapy plus rituximab," *Revista Española de Enfermedades Digestivas*, vol. 100, no. 11, pp. 724–728, 2008.

[5] A. W. Avolio, S. Agnes, R. Barbarino et al., "Post-transplant lymphoproliferative disorders after liver transplantation: analysis of early and end late cases in a 255 patient series," *Transplantation Proceedings*, vol. 39, no. 6, pp. 1956–1960, 2007.

[6] A. Masood, S. Kairouz, K. H. Hudhud, A. Z. Hegazi, A. Banu, and N. C. Gupta, "Primary non-Hodgkin lymphoma of liver," *Current Oncology*, vol. 16, no. 4, pp. 74–77, 2009.

[7] V. Noronha, N. Shafi, J. A. Obando, and S. Kummar, "Primary non-Hodgkin's lymphoma of the liver," *Critical Reviews in Oncology/Hematology*, vol. 53, no. 3, pp. 199–207, 2009.

[8] D. Nart, Y. Ertan, F. Yilmaz, G. Yüce, M. Zeytunlu, and M. Kilic, "Primary hepatic marginal zone B-cell lymphoma of mucosa-associated lymphoid tissue type in a liver transplant patient with hepatitis B cirrhosis," *Transplantation Proceedings*, vol. 37, no. 10, pp. 4408–4412, 2005.

[9] S. Y. Shin, J. S. Kim, J. K. Lim, J. S. Hahn, W. I. Yang, and C. O. Suh, "Longlasting remission of primary hepatic mucosa-associated lymphoid tissue (MALT) lymphoma achieved by radiotherapy alone," *Korean Journal of Internal Medicine*, vol. 21, no. 2, pp. 127–131, 2006.

[10] M. Q. Ye, A. Suriawinata, C. Black, A. D. Min, J. Strauchen, and S. N. Thung, "Primary hepatic marginal zone B-cell lymphoma of mucosa-associated lymphoid tissue type in a patient with primary biliary cirrhosis," *Archives of Pathology and Laboratory Medicine*, vol. 124, no. 4, pp. 604–608, 2000.

[11] M. Orrego, L. Guo, C. Reeder et al., "Hepatic B-cell non-Hodgkin's lymphoma of MALT type in the liver explant of a patient with chronic hepatitis C infection," *Liver Transplantation*, vol. 11, no. 7, pp. 796–799, 2005.

[12] F. Takeshima, M. Kunisaki, T. Aritomi et al., "Hepatic mucosa-associated lymphoid tissue lymphoma and hepatocellular carcinoma in a patient with hepatitis B virus infection," *Journal of Clinical Gastroenterology*, vol. 38, no. 9, pp. 823–826, 2004.

[13] S. Mehrain, W. Schima, A. Ba-Ssalamah, A. Kurtaran, and M. Raderer, "Primary MALT-lymphoma of the liver: multimodality imaging," *Critical Reviews in Computed Tomography*, vol. 44, no. 6, pp. 347–355, 2003.

[14] S. Mizuno, S. Isaji, M. Tabata, S. Uemoto, H. Imai, and K. Shiraki, "Hepatic mucosa-associated lymphoid tissue (MALT) lymphoma associated with hepatitis C," *Journal of Hepatology*, vol. 37, no. 6, pp. 872-873, 2002.

[15] K. Yago, H. Shimada, M. Itoh et al., "Primary low-grade B-cell lymphoma of mucosa-associated lymphoid tissue (MALT)-type of the liver in a patient with hepatitis C virus infection," *Leukemia & Lymphoma*, vol. 43, no. 7, pp. 1497–1500, 2002.

[16] J. Murakami, N. Fukushima, H. Ueno et al., "Primary hepatic low-grade B-cell lymphoma of the mucosa-associated lymphoid tissue type: a case report and review of the literature," *International Journal of Hematology*, vol. 75, no. 1, pp. 85–90, 2002.

[17] C. M. Kirk, D. Lewin, and J. Lazarchick, "Primary hepatic B-cell lymphoma of mucosa-associated lymphoid tissue," *Archives of Pathology and Laboratory Medicine*, vol. 123, no. 8, pp. 716–719, 1999.

[18] M. Maes, C. Depardieu, J. L. Dargent et al., "Primary low-grade B-cell lymphoma of MALT-type occurring in the liver: a study of two cases," *Journal of Hepatology*, vol. 27, no. 5, pp. 922–927, 1997.

[19] P. G. Isaacson, P. M. Banks, P. V. Best, S. P. McLure, H. K. Muller-Hermelink, and J. I. Wyatt, "Primary low-grade hepatic B-cell lymphoma of mucosa-associated lymphoid

tissue (MALT)-type," *American Journal of Surgical Pathology*, vol. 19, no. 5, pp. 571–575, 1995.

[20] S. Dong, L. Chen, Y. Chen, and X. Chen, "Primary hepatic extranodal marginal zone B-cell lymphoma of mucosa-associated lymphoid tissue type: a case report and literature review," *Medicine*, vol. 96, no. 13, p. e6305, 2017.

[21] L. X. Li, S. T. Zhou, X. Ji et al., "Misdiagnosis of primary hepatic marginal zone B cell lymphoma of mucosa associated lymphoid tissue type, a case report," *World Journal of Surgical Oncology*, vol. 14, no. 1, p. 69, 2016.

[22] R. CK. Chan, C. M. Chu, C. Chow, S. L. Chan, and A. WH. Chan, "A concurrent primary hepatic MALT lymphoma and hepatocellular carcinoma," *Pathology*, vol. 47, no. 2, pp. 178–181, 2015.

[23] Y. Zhong, X. Wang, M. Deng, H. Fang, and R. Xu, "Primary hepatic mucosa-associated lymphoid tissue lymphoma and hemangioma with chronic hepatitis B virus infection as an underlying condition," *BioScience Trends*, vol. 8, no. 3, pp. 185–188, 2014.

[24] B. Kiesewetter, L. Müllauer, B. Streubel et al., "Primary mucosa-associated lymphoid tissue (MALT) lymphoma of the liver: clinical, molecular, and microbiological aspects," *Annals of Hematology*, vol. 91, no. 11, pp. 1817-1818, 2012.

[25] P. Cabassa, M. Morone, and L. Matricardi, "An unusual liver mass," *Gastroenterology*, vol. 138, no. 2, pp. e7–e9, 2010.

[26] H. Doi, N. Horiike, A. Hiraoka et al., "Primary hepatic marginal zone B cell lymphoma of mucosa-associated lymphoid tissue type: case report and review of the literature," *International Journal of Hematology*, vol. 88, no. 4, pp. 418–423, 2008.

[27] K. Willenbrock, S. Kriener, S. Oeschger, and M. L. Hansmann, "Nodular lymphoid lesion of the liver with simultaneous focal nodular hyperplasia and hemangioma: discrimination from primary hepatic MALT-type non-Hodgkin's lymphoma," *Virchows Archiv*, vol. 448, no. 2, pp. 223–227, 2006.

[28] D. Albano, R. Giubbini, and F. Bertagna, "18F-FDG PET/CT and primary hepatic MALT: a case series," *Abdominal Radiology*, vol. 41, no. 10, pp. 1956-1959, 2016.

[29] S. Nagata, N. Harimoto, and K. Kajiyama, "Primary hepatic mucosa-associated lymphoid tissue lymphoma: a case report and literature review," *Surgical Case Reports*, vol. 1, no. 1, p. 87, 2015.

[30] A. Forner, M. Gilabert, J. Bruix, and J. L. Raoul, "Treatment of intermediate-stage hepatocellular carcinoma," *Nature Reviews Clinical Oncology*, vol. 11, no. 9, pp. 525–535, 2014.

[31] European Association for the Study of the Liver; European Organisation for Research and Treatment of Cancer, "EASL-EORTC clinical practice guidelines: management of hepatocellular carcinoma," *Journal of Hepatology*, vol. 56, no. 4, pp. 908–943, 2012.

[32] Y. K. Park, J. E. Choi, W. Y. Jung, S. K. Song, J. I. Lee, and C. W. Chung, "Mucosa-associated lymphoid tissue (MALT) lymphoma as an unusual cause of malignant hilar biliary stricture: a case report with literature review," *World Journal of Surgical Oncology*, vol. 14, no. 1, p. 167, 2016.

[33] G. Ugurluer, R. C. Miller, Y. Li et al., "Primary hepatic lymphoma: a retrospective, multicenter rare cancer network study," *Rare Tumors*, vol. 8, no. 3, pp. 118–123, 2016.

[34] J. Lee, K. S. Park, M. H. Kang et al., "Primary hepatic peripheral T-cell lymphoma mimicking hepatocellular carcinoma: a case report," *Annals of Surgical Treatment and Research*, vol. 93, no. 2, pp. 110–114, 2017.

[35] J. Jaso, L. Chen, S. Li et al., "CD5-positive mucosa-associated lymphoid tissue (MALT) lymphoma: a clinicopathologic study of 14 cases," *Human Pathology*, vol. 43, no. 9, pp. 1436–1443, 2012.

[36] M. A. Khan, C. S. Combs, E. M. Brunt et al., "Positron emission tomography scanning in the evaluation of hepatocellular carcinoma," *Journal of Hepatology*, vol. 32, no. 5, pp. 792–797, 2000.

[37] J. Trojan, O. Schroeder, J. Raedle et al., "Fluorine-18 FDG positron emission tomography for imaging of hepatocellular carcinoma," *American Journal of Gastroenterology*, vol. 94, no. 11, pp. 3314–3319, 1999.

54

Hem-o-lok Clips Migration: An Easily Neglected Complication after Laparoscopic Biliary Surgery

Jun-wen Qu, Gui-yang Wang, Zhi-qing Yuan, and Ke-wei Li

Department of Biliary-Pancreatic Surgery, Renji Hospital, School of Medicine, Shanghai Jiao Tong University, No. 160, Pujian Road, Pudong New Area, Shanghai 200127, China

Correspondence should be addressed to Ke-wei Li; keweipig@126.com

Academic Editor: Mehrdad Nikfarjam

Clip migration into the common bile duct (CBD) is a rare but well-established phenomenon of laparoscopic biliary surgery. The mechanism and exact incidence of clip migration are both poorly understood. Clip migration into the common bile duct can cause recurrent cholangitis and serve as a nidus for stone formation. We present a case, a 54-year-old woman, of clip-induced cholangitis resulting from surgical clip migration 12 months after laparoscopic cholecystectomy and laparoscopic common bile duct exploration (LC+LCBDE) with primary closure.

1. Introduction

Laparoscopic cholecystectomy and laparoscopic common bile duct exploration (LC+LCBDE) is currently a widely use technology for patients with gallstone and choledocholithiasis. Clip migration into the common bile duct (CBD) is a rare complication of laparoscopic biliary surgery. Surgical clip migration into the common bile duct can cause recurrent cholangitis and serve as a nidus for stone formation. Up to date, few cases of surgical clip migration have been reported in the literature. The etiology and exact incidence of clip migration are both unclear. We report a case of Hem-o-lok clips migration 1 year after laparoscopic cholecystectomy and laparoscopic common bile duct exploration (LC+LCBDE) with primary closure. The patient was successfully treated with endoscopic sphincterotomy plus balloon dilation (ESBD) and Hem-o-lok clips extraction. The patient improved uneventfully following the procedure. We hope that this case draws laparoscopic surgeon's attention to this rare phenomenon.

2. Case Presentation

A 54-year-old woman had undergone a successful LC+LCBDE in our hospital on December, 2015. The operation had been performed without difficulty and we had used 2 Hem-o-lok for the duct/artery. Subsequently, primary closure of the incision of CBD was performed with an interrupted 5-0 absorbable suture. A bile leakage was detected on postoperative day 2 and spontaneously resolved after 18 days of conservative treatment. The patient was discharged uneventfully on postoperative day 20.

On January, 2017, this patient was readmitted for intermittent upper abdominal pain for a month without fever and jaundice. Physical examination revealed tenderness in the right upper quadrant of her abdomen. Laboratory examination showed no abnormal parameters. Abdominal US revealed a mildly dilated biliary tree with no visualized CBD stone. Magnetic resonance cholangiopancreatography (MRCP) showed a slightly dilated common bile duct with a low signal filling-defect in the distal common bile duct, considering CBD stone (Figure 1). During ERCP, only a single filling-defect was seen in the common bile duct (Figure 2). An endoscopic sphincterotomy with balloon dilation was carried out and two Hem-o-lok clips were successfully removed from the bile duct with an extraction balloon (Figure 3). An endoscopic nasobiliary drainage (ENBD) tube was inserted after extraction. At one-month follow-up the patient was symptom-free.

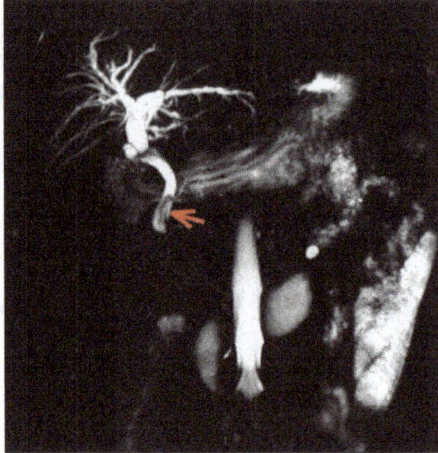

FIGURE 1: Magnetic resonance cholangiopancreatography (MRCP) showed a slightly dilated common bile duct with a low signal filling-defect in the distal common bile duct, considering CBD stone, with the filling-defect being represented by a red arrow.

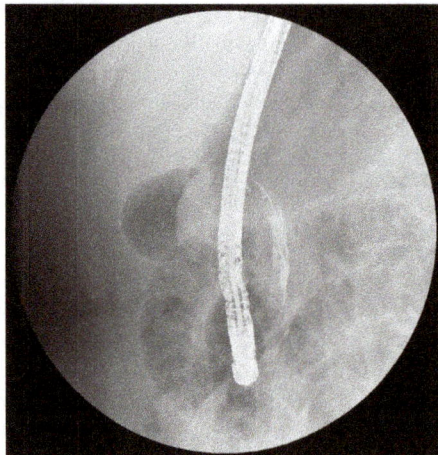

FIGURE 2: Endoscopic retrograde cholangiopancreatography demonstrates the filling-defect in the common bile duct.

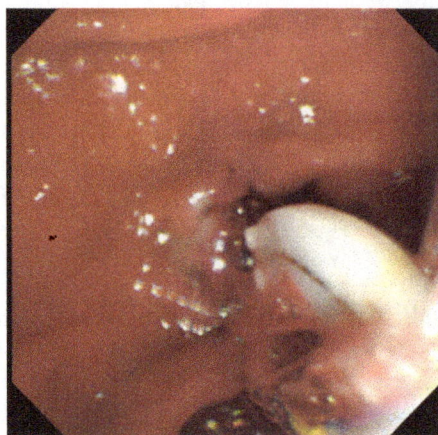

FIGURE 3: The extracted Hem-o-lok clip within the duodenal lumen.

3. Discussion

Advances in laparoscopy have made LC+LCBDE a widely accepted strategy for patients with gallstones and choledocholithiasis. The single-stage surgical strategy has been shown to be safe, effective, and cost-effective with shorter hospital stays [1]. Exposure of Calot's triangle and securing the gallbladder vessels and cystic duct are the key steps of the LC. Currently, Hem-o-lok clip is widely applied in the controlling of the cystic duct and artery.

Postoperative clip migration is a rare but well-established complication. Migration into the common bile duct after laparoscopic cholecystectomy was first reported in 1992 [2]. Although a huge number of LC have been performed worldwide up to 2016, less than 100 cases of clip migration after LC have been reported in the literature. Most of the cases are metal clips migration. Clip migration tends to develop from 11 days to 20 years; the median time was 26 months [3]. Apart from choledocholithiasis, clip migration may also lead to acute pancreatitis [4], duodenal ulcer [5], biliary-colonic fistula [6], subdiaphragmatic abscess [7], and so forth. To our knowledge, Hem-o-lok clips migration into CBD after LC+LCBDE with primary closure has not been previously reported.

However, the exact mechanism of this condition remains controversial. Multifactor may contribute to the process: the first possible pathogenesis is inappropriate application of clips including incomplete closure of cyst duct and incorrect placement of clips that result in biloma. The number of endoclips used during the initial operation is also an important factor [3, 8]. The second possible pathogenesis is bile leakage caused by intraoperative bile tract injury. In the present case, a primary closure of CBD was performed after LC+LCBDE. Bile leakage was detected after the surgery, and the subhepatic suction drained biliary fluid until it stopped spontaneously on postoperative day 18. We postulate that the subsequent adhesion and inflammation caused by bile leakage make surrounding tissues brittle and induced Hem-o-lok clips detachment and migration from the cystic duct/artery stump into the biliary tract through the incision of CBD mechanically. According to Rawal, the pressure exerted from intra-abdominal organ movements accelerates the process of clip migration [9]. Rejection response of human body to surgical clips may also contribute to the process.

To prevent the incidence of clip migration, all the technical factors in the surgery should be considered: confirming the relationship of Calot's triangle during dissection, minimizing the number of clips, and avoiding unnecessary surgical procedures [10]. The placement of clips should not be too close to the common bile duct. Absorbable clips seem to be a safe and effective method in providing hemostasis in the cystic artery and during ligation of the cystic duct [11]. In three studies, application of absorbable clips brings fewer complications compared to nonabsorbable clips [12–14]. Absorbable clips can burden a higher weight and intraluminal pressure. Furthermore, the biocompatible and nonallergic materials of absorbable clips seldom cause rejection response [11]. Absorbable sutures are also used to seal the cystic artery and duct in some studies [15, 16]. However, the knot is made totally intracorporeally that should be done by an experience surgeon. In spite of many advantages, Francesco Cetta indicated that absorbable clips and sutures are still a nidus for subsequent stones formation [10]. Besides, clipless cholecystectomy using ultrasound dissection technology is an alternative to standard clip of cystic duct and artery. Kandil and Kavlakoglu reported that harmonic scalpel has been proved to be as effective and safe as surgical clips in the ligation of the cystic duct after a period of training [17, 18]. Nonetheless, harmonic scalpel is an expensive device. From the health economics, the clinical application of harmonic scalpel cannot be routinely carried out currently. Primary closure of the CBD has been demonstrated to be a safe and feasible method with a similar rate of bile leaks and recurrent stones compared with that of the T-tube insertion [19]. Advanced laparoscopic skills and experience and appropriate patient selection are the main limitations of LCBDE with primary suture. In our view, further studies are needed to establish more effective and safe methods to prevent complications after LC and LCBDE.

Clinical manifestations of clip migration-induced cholangitis are similar to those of noniatrogenic ones, usually present with abdominal pain, fever, and obstructive jaundice. In our case, pure abdominal pain made us consider the postcholecystectomy syndrome at first. Thus, it emphasizes the importance of early recognition of this complication when patients present with upper abdominal pain or symptoms of biliary obstruction after LC. The diagnosis is suspected on the basis of noninvasive imaging. Ultrasonography is cheap, widely available, and safe and is recommended for patients with suspected foreign body. CT scan is widely used to investigate patients with pain or other abdominal symptoms. MRCP provides clear anatomy of biliary tree with a high sensitivity and specificity.

ERCP is a superior approach to manage the complication with a high success rate of about 85% [3]. In our case, limited endoscopic sphincterotomy with balloon dilation (ESBD) was performed to extract the Hem-o-lok clips. ESBD is a promising technique in treating common bile duct stones with a high success rate of stone extraction and a low risk of complications. Surgical procedures or percutaneous transhepatic cholangiography should be reserved as rescue procedures when ERCP fails [20]. In addition, spontaneous passage of clips through sphincter of Oddi after a failed ERCP extraction or LC had been also reported in some literatures [21, 22].

In conclusion, postoperative clip migration has been a well-recognized phenomenon ever since their first use in surgery, albeit rare. Patients who had LC and LCBDE should have a careful surveillance and strict follow-up to ensure the safety. The first investigation might be MRCP and then ERCP for subsequent management.

Acknowledgments

This paper is supported by Incubating Program for Clinical Research and Innovation of Ren Ji Hospital, School of Medicine, Shanghai Jiao Tong University (Grant no. PYZY16-011).

References

[1] H.-Y. Zhu, M. Xu, H.-J. Shen et al., "A meta-analysis of single-stage versus two-stage management for concomitant gallstones and common bile duct stones," *Clinics and Research in Hepatology and Gastroenterology*, vol. 39, no. 5, pp. 584–593, 2015.

[2] J. L. Raoul, J. F. Bretagne, L. Siproudhis, D. Heresbach, J. P. Campion, and M. Gosselin, "Cystic duct clip migration into the common bile duct: a complication of laparoscopic cholecystectomy treated by endoscopic biliary sphincterotomy," *Gastrointestinal Endoscopy*, vol. 38, no. 5, pp. 608–611, 1992.

[3] V. H. Chong and C. F. Chong, "Biliary complications secondary to post-cholecystectomy clip migration: a review of 69 cases," *Journal of Gastrointestinal Surgery*, vol. 14, no. 4, pp. 688–696, 2010.

[4] A. G. Antunes, B. Peixe, and H. Guerreiro, "Pancreatitis and cholangitis following intraductal migration of a metal clip 5 years after laparoscopic cholecystectomy," *Gastroenterologia y Hepatologia*, 2016.

[5] K. Soga, K. Kassai, and K. Itani, "Duodenal ulcer induced by Hem-o-Lok clip after reduced port laparoscopic cholecystectomy," *Journal of Gastrointestinal and Liver Diseases*, vol. 25, no. 1, article no. 14, pp. 95–98, 2016.

[6] T. Hong, X.-Q. Xu, X.-D. He, Q. Qu, B.-L. Li, and C.-J. Zheng, "Choledochoduodenal fistula caused by migration of endoclip after laparoscopic cholecystectomy," *World Journal of Gastroenterology*, vol. 20, no. 16, pp. 4827–4829, 2014.

[7] M. Little, P. C. Munipalle, and O. Nugud, "A rare late complication of laparoscopic cholecystectomy," *BMJ Case Reports*, 2013.

[8] C.-H. Tsai, M.-C. Tsai, and C.-C. Lin, "Unusual cause of abdominal pain after laparoscopic cholecystectomy," *Gastroenterology*, vol. 144, no. 7, pp. e8–e9, 2013.

[9] K. K. Rawal, "Migration of surgical clips into the common bile duct after laparoscopic cholecystectomy," *Case Reports in Gastroenterology*, vol. 10, no. 3, pp. 787–792, 2016.

[10] F. Cetta, C. Baldi, F. Lombardo, L. Monti, P. Stefani, and G. Nuzzo, "Migration of metallic clips used during laparoscopic cholecystectomy and formation of gallstones around them: surgical implications from a prospective study," *Journal of Laparoendoscopic & Advanced Surgical Techniques*, vol. 7, no. 1, pp. 37–46, 1997.

[11] F. Feroci, E. Lenzi, K. C. Kröning, and M. Scatizzi, "A single-institution review of the absorbable clips used in laparoscopic colorectal and gallbladder surgery: Feasibility, safety, and effectiveness," *Updates in Surgery*, vol. 63, no. 2, pp. 103–107, 2011.

[12] H. Yano, K. Okada, M. Kinuta et al., "Efficacy of absorbable clips compared with metal clips for cystic duct ligation in laparoscopic cholecystectomy," *Surgery Today*, vol. 33, no. 1, pp. 18–23, 2003.

[13] L. Bencini, B. Boffi, M. Farsi, L. J. Sanchez, M. Scatizzi, and R. Moretti, "Laparoscopic cholecystectomy: retrospective comparative evaluation of titanium versus absorbable clips," *Journal of Laparoendoscopic & Advanced Surgical Techniques*, vol. 13, no. 2, pp. 93–98, 2003.

[14] A. Rohatgi and A. L. Widdison, "An audit of cystic duct closure in laparoscopic cholecystectomies," *Surgical Endoscopy and Other Interventional Techniques*, vol. 20, no. 6, pp. 875–877, 2006.

[15] V. Golash, "An experience with 1000 consecutive cystic duct ligation in laparoscopic cholecystectomy," *Surgical Laparoscopy,*

Endoscopy and Percutaneous Techniques, vol. 18, no. 2, pp. 155-156, 2008.

[16] G. Suo and A. Xu, "Clipless minilaparoscopic cholecystectomy: a study of 1096 cases," *Journal of Laparoendoscopic and Advanced Surgical Techniques*, vol. 23, no. 10, pp. 849–854, 2013.

[17] T. Kandil, A. E. Nakeeb, and E. E. Hefnawy, "Comparative study between clipless laparoscopic cholecystectomy by harmonic scalpel versus conventional method: a prospective randomized study," *Journal of Gastrointestinal Surgery*, vol. 14, no. 2, pp. 323–328, 2010.

[18] B. Kavlakoglu, R. Pekcici, and S. Oral, "Clipless cholecystectomy: which sealer should be used?" *World Journal of Surgery*, vol. 35, no. 4, pp. 817–823, 2011.

[19] H.-W. Zhang, Y.-J. Chen, C.-H. Wu, and W.-D. Li, "Laparoscopic common bile duct exploration with primary closure for management of choledocholithiasis: a retrospective analysis and comparison with conventional T-tube Drainage," *American Surgeon*, vol. 80, no. 2, pp. 178–181, 2014.

[20] S. Ray and S. P. Bhattacharya, "Endoclip migration into the common bile duct with stone formation: a rare complication after laparoscopic cholecystectomy," *Journal of the Society of Laparoendoscopic Surgeons*, vol. 17, no. 2, pp. 330–332, 2013.

[21] P. Kissmeyer-Nielsen and J. Kiil, "Endoclip on the cystic duct after laparoscopic cholecystectomy," *Ugeskrift for Laeger*, vol. 167, no. 24, pp. 2657-2658, 2005.

[22] A. B. Lentsch, "Activation and function of hepatocyte NF-κB in postischemic liver injury," *Hepatology*, vol. 42, no. 1, pp. 216–218, 2005.

55

A Case Study of Severe Esophageal Dysmotility following Laparoscopic Sleeve Gastrectomy

Caroline E. Sheppard,[1] **Daniel C. Sadowski,**[2] **Richdeep Gill,**[3] **and Daniel W. Birch**[1]

[1]*Centre for the Advancement of Minimally Invasive Surgery, Royal Alexandra Hospital, University of Alberta, Rm 511 CSC, 10240 Kingsway Avenue, Edmonton, AB, Canada T6X 1R8*

[2]*Department of Medicine, Division of Gastroenterology, Zeidler Ledcor Centre, University of Alberta, Edmonton, AB, Canada T6G 2X8*

[3]*Rm 3656 West Wing, Peter Lougheed Hospital, 3500 26th Avenue NE, Calgary, AB, Canada T1Y 6J4*

Correspondence should be addressed to Caroline E. Sheppard; csheppar@ualberta.ca

Academic Editor: Boris Kirshtein

Following bariatric surgery, a proportion of patients have been observed to experience reflux, dysphagia, and/or odynophagia. The etiology of this constellation of symptoms has not been systematically studied to date. This case describes a 36-year-old female with severe esophageal dysmotility following LSG. Many treatments had been used over a course of 3 years, and while calcium channel blockers reversed the esophageal dysmotility seen on manometry, significant symptoms of dysphagia persisted. Subsequently, the patient underwent a gastric bypass, which seemed to partially relieve her symptoms. Her dysphagia was no longer considered to be associated with a structural cause but attributed to a "sleeve dysmotility syndrome." Considering the difficulties with managing sleeve dysmotility syndrome, it is reasonable to consider the need for preoperative testing. The question is whether motility studies should be required for all patients planning to undergo a LSG to rule out preexisting esophageal dysmotility and whether conversion to gastric bypass is the preferred method for managing esophageal dysmotility after LSG.

1. Introduction

Laparoscopic sleeve gastrectomy (LSG) is a commonly performed bariatric surgical procedure. LSG involves removal of approximately 75% of the stomach, leaving a narrow tubular stomach, similar in diameter to the esophagus. Following bariatric surgery, a proportion of patients have been observed to experience reflux, dysphagia, and/or odynophagia. The etiology of this constellation of symptoms has not been systematically studied to date. Often these symptoms are treated empirically with proton-pump inhibitors or dilation of strictures despite the lack of evidence for acid-peptic pathology or mechanical obstruction [1]. We present a case of severe esophageal dysmotility following LSG.

2. Case

A 36-year-old female with a BMI of 39.7 kg/m^2 underwent an uncomplicated laparoscopic sleeve gastrectomy using a 50 F bougie with dissection 6 cm proximal to the pylorus. Her prior medical history consisted of pulmonary embolism (PE), neurocardiogenic syncope, and back pain. She denied any symptoms of dysphagia or gastroesophageal reflux preoperatively. Three months after LSG, she developed recurrent mild retrosternal pain. Her imaging was negative for a PE, and she was treated with proton-pump inhibitors for presumed gastroesophageal reflux. She underwent gastroscopy, CT, and full cardiac work-up, which were unremarkable. No hiatal hernia, stricture, ulcer, leak, partial dilation of the sleeve, retained fundus, or abnormality in the gastroesophageal junction was observed. However, over the next 6 months the symptoms worsened, and she presented to hospital 8 times requiring admission for assessment of severe high epigastric pain.

One year after LSG, esophageal manometry and 24 h pH studies were performed to investigate a possible esophageal etiology of her pain. The manometry study demonstrated

TABLE 1: Changes in esophageal motility after 30 mg diltiazem QD therapy.

Esophageal manometry measurement	Before diltiazem	After diltiazem	Normal value
Completed peristalsis (%)	100	100	≥80%
LES pressure (mmHg)	40.5	10.8	13.0–43.0
LES residual pressure (mmHg)	13.4	4.0	<15.0
Contraction amplitude (mmHg)	210.4	76.6	30.0–180.0
High amplitude contraction (%)	100.0	0.0	—
Distal contractile integral (mmHg/s/cm)	5216.4	1481.7	500.0–5000.0

a pattern consistent with hypertensive peristalsis with an average distal contractile interval (DCI) of 5216 mmHg/sec/cm (normal DCI = 500–5000) with solicited swallows. The 24 h esophageal pH study was normal (DeMeester score of 15.0) with a negative Symptom Index score (0.0%) between acid reflux episodes and chest pain symptoms. Her symptoms of dysphagia continued, and she steadily declined in weight to a BMI of 27.8. To treat the hypertensive peristalsis, the patient was begun on therapy with diltiazem 30 mg QD.

Because of continuing symptoms while on diltiazem, further investigations were carried out one year later. A second manometry demonstrated weak lower esophageal sphincter pressure, with normalization of manometry parameters while on diltiazem (Table 1). An esophageal 24 h impedance study was normal (DeMeester score of 3.2). During the study a high number of nonacid reflux episodes occurred ($n = 71$), but this was not significantly linked to Symptom Association Probability (74%). She continued to have severe retrosternal chest pain and episodes of dysphagia with solids, despite evidence that the hypertensive peristalsis appeared to have improved with therapy. Botox injection of 100 units at the gastroesophageal junction was performed in order to attempt relieving the esophageal spasms. These appeared to have little effect on the patient's symptoms.

Dysphagia symptoms began to worsen to both liquids and solids, and multiple emergency room visits were again observed. More than 3 years after LSG, various treatments had been used to treat her esophageal spasms, including calcium channel blockers (diltiazem), LABA-2 (Symbicort), vasodilators (Nitrate), antispasmodic medication (Lyrica, Gabapentin, and Botox), analgesics (Tylenol 4, Tramadol, Butrans, oxyNEO, viscous lidocaine, Hydromorph contin, Fentanyl, Methadone, Dilaudid, Morphine, and Clonidine), muscle relaxants (Baclofen, Tizanidine, Zanaflex, and Cyclobenzaprine), antimigraine (Zomig), promotility (Domperidone), antiemetic medication (Zofran), antireflux medication (Nexium, Omeprazole, and Pantoloc), benzodiazepine (Ativan), nonbenzodiazepine hypnotics (Zopiclone), cannabinoid (Cesamet), tricyclic antidepressant (Nortriptyline, Elavil), serotonin norepinephrine reuptake inhibitor (Cymbalta), and selective serotonin reuptake inhibitors (Prozac). Proposed treatment options for this escalating esophageal pain included Botox injection to the pylorus, pyloromyotomy, partial esophageal myotomy, or a gastric bypass to try and reduce the hypothesized high-pressure

sleeve. As a last resort, some surgeons may also consider a total gastrectomy. After discussion with the patient, a laparoscopic Roux-en-Y gastric bypass was performed, which seemed to relieve the dysphagia and retrosternal pain.

After the gastric bypass, ER and outpatient visits both decreased twofold (0.5 versus 0.2 ER visits/month and 0.6 versus 0.3 outpatient visits/month) attributed to pain relief. Presently 5 years following LSG, pain symptoms are being managed with analgesics and neuropathic treatment is being considered. This complicated patient has had over 100 visits with specialists over the past 6 years to manage her obesity and chronic dysphagia. Her dysphagia is no longer considered to be associated with a structural cause but is now attributed to a "sleeve dysmotility syndrome."

3. Discussion

Esophageal dysmotility occurs when the muscles and sphincters of the esophagus have impaired coordination, altered contraction strength, and/or contractile duration causing impaired esophageal transit. The combination of these abnormalities after LSG has not yet been described.

Symptoms of foregut dysmotility are disconcerting when they arise following LSG. These symptoms are varied and include dysphagia, odynophagia, nausea, vomiting, heartburn, and pain.

Carabotti et al. found that dysphagia developed in 19.7% of patients after LSG, which manifested in retrosternal or throat discomfort when consuming solids or liquids [2]. A significant increase in dyspepsia (59.4%) was also attributed to increased pressure in the sleeve [2]. Kleidi et al. found a combination of reflux and dysphagia significantly increased after LSG [3]. Additional reports describe dysmotility after the laparoscopic adjustable gastric band as causing symptoms of dysphasia and reflux [4]. These symptoms normally resolve after adjustment or removal of the band. In contrast, dysmotility following LSG may be irreversible.

Our case demonstrated manometric evidence for hypertensive peristalsis. It is unclear if this disorder was present before LSG surgery, whether this was a preexisting condition that was exacerbated by the LSG, or whether the syndrome was created by the LSG. However, treatment with calcium channel blockers reversed the manometric abnormalities but failed to resolve symptoms. Sleeve dysmotility syndrome causes persistent dysphagia and reflux-like symptoms and may respond partially to gastric bypass.

It is difficult to determine whether technique contributes to this sleeve dysmotility syndrome, as many of these esophageal syndromes are idiopathic. Bougie size for LSG and its impact on leak rate and gastroesophageal reflux have been greatly discussed in the literature. Parikh et al. described in their meta-analysis using data from nearly 10,000 patients that a bougie size equal or greater to 40 F decreased the odds of developing a postoperative leak [5]. The literature on technique contributing to gastroesophageal reflux symptoms has many theories (i.e., retained fundus, blunted angle of His, bougie size, resection of antrum, high-pressure system, etc.). This patient was negative for both leak and acid reflux, which made it challenging to assess whether technique contributed to the patient's symptoms based on current literature. The patient had manometric abnormalities, and the causal relationship of LSG technique and esophageal dysmotility has yet to be defined.

The LSG has been described as creating a high-pressure system in the sleeve from simultaneous gastric and pyloric contractions [6]. When filled with saline, the intragastric pressure is increased after LSG (43 mmHg) compared to normal gastric anatomy (34 mmHg) [7]. By reducing the "high-pressure" system to a "low-pressure" system, that is, by gastric bypass, our hope was that this would alleviate the hypertensive esophagus and esophageal spasms. The gastric bypass has been successful for improving or resolving other gastroesophageal issues after the LSG, such as uncontrollable gastroesophageal reflux [8], and may be the preferential choice for managing dysmotility.

Preoperative manometry is used to avoid major postoperative issues of dysphagia before antireflux surgery. Concurrent 24 h pH testing is also used to confirm the presence of reflux. These results can detect an upper range of 1 of 14 patients being inappropriate for surgical intervention [9]. Consequently, preoperative manometry may be a method to screen patients with dysmotility in order to select an appropriate bariatric procedure. This would avoid significant postoperative complications and the ultimate need for reoperation.

This is a complicated question that has significant impact on the investigation burden placed on the patient. Considering the difficulties with managing sleeve dysmotility syndrome, it is reasonable to consider the need for preoperative testing. The question is whether motility studies should be required for all patients planning to undergo a LSG. Manometry results would identify patients that may not be able to tolerate a high-pressure sleeve from either esophageal spasms, hypertensive esophagus, achalasia, or scleroderma. Consequently, they may be better candidates for a gastric bypass.

Competing Interests

The authors declare that they have no competing interests.

References

[1] A. Keidar, L. Appelbaum, C. Schweiger, R. Elazary, and A. Baltasar, "Dilated upper sleeve can be associated with severe postoperative gastroesophageal dysmotility and reflux," *Obesity Surgery*, vol. 20, no. 2, pp. 140–147, 2010.

[2] M. Carabotti, G. Silecchia, F. Greco et al., "Impact of laparoscopic sleeve gastrectomy on upper gastrointestinal symptoms," *Obesity Surgery*, vol. 23, no. 10, pp. 1551–1557, 2013.

[3] E. Kleidi, D. Theodorou, K. Albanopoulos et al., "The effect of laparoscopic sleeve gastrectomy on the antireflux mechanism: can it be minimized?" *Surgical Endoscopy*, vol. 27, no. 12, pp. 4625–4630, 2013.

[4] M. Naef, W. G. Mouton, U. Naef, B. Van Der Weg, G. J. Maddern, and H. E. Wagner, "Esophageal dysmotility disorders after laparoscopic gastric banding-an underestimated complication," *Annals of Surgery*, vol. 253, no. 2, pp. 285–290, 2011.

[5] M. Parikh, R. Issa, A. McCrillis, J. K. Saunders, A. Ude-Welcome, and M. Gagner, "Surgical strategies that may decrease leak after laparoscopic sleeve gastrectomy: a systematic review and meta-analysis of 9991 cases," *Annals of Surgery*, vol. 257, no. 2, pp. 231–237, 2013.

[6] R. Weiner, I. El-Sayes, and S. Weiner, "LSG: complications—diagnosis and management," in *Obesity, Bariatric and Metabolic Surgery—A Practical Guide*, S. Agrawal, Ed., pp. 259–272, Springer, Basel, Switzerland, 1st edition, 2015.

[7] R. T. Yehoshua, L. A. Eidelman, M. Stein et al., "Laparoscopic Sleeve gastrectomy-volume and pressure assessment," *Obesity Surgery*, vol. 18, no. 9, pp. 1083–1088, 2008.

[8] F. B. Langer, A. Bohdjalian, S. Shakeri-Leidenmühler, S. F. Schoppmann, J. Zacherl, and G. Prager, "Conversion from sleeve gastrectomy to roux-en-Y gastric bypass—indications and outcome," *Obesity Surgery*, vol. 20, no. 7, pp. 835–840, 2010.

[9] W. W. Chan, L. R. Haroian, and C. P. Gyawali, "Value of preoperative esophageal function studies before laparoscopic antireflux surgery," *Surgical Endoscopy and Other Interventional Techniques*, vol. 25, no. 9, pp. 2943–2949, 2011.

Permissions

List of Contributors

Peter Waweru
Department of Surgery, St. Mary's Mission Hospital, Nairobi 00506, Kenya

David Mwaniki
Department of Surgery, The Karen Hospital, Nairobi 00200, Kenya

Konstantinos Blouhos, Konstantinos A. Boulas, Anna Konstantinidou, Ilias I. Salpigktidis, Stavroula P. Katsaouni, Konstantinos Ioannidis and Anestis Hatzigeorgiadis
Department of General Surgery, General Hospital of Drama, End of Hippokratous Street, 66100 Drama, Greece

Scott Samona and Richard Berri
General Surgery Department, St. John Hospital and Medical Center, Detroit, MI 48236, USA

Robert H. Krieger and Katherine M. Wojcicki
1Kansas City University of Medicine and Biosciences (KCU), 1750 E. Independence Avenue, Kansas City, MO 64106, USA

Andrew C. Berry
2Department of Internal Medicine, University of South Alabama, Mobile, AL 36608, USA

Warren L. Reuther III
3Department of Radiology, West Palm Hospital, West Palm Beach, FL 33407, USA

Kendrick D. McArthur
4Department of Surgery, West Palm Hospital, West Palm Beach, FL 33407, USA

MA Modi, SS Deolekar and AK Gvalani
Department of General Surgery, King Edward Memorial Hospital and Seth Gordhandas Sunderdas Medical College, Parel, Mumbai 400012, India

Dimitrios K. Manatakis, Ioannis Terzis, Ioannis D. Kyriazanos, Ioannis D. Dontas, Christos N. Stoidis, Nikolaos Stamos and Demetrios Davides
1st Surgical Department, Athens Naval and Veterans Hospital, 70 Deinokratous Street, 11521 Athens, Greece

OrhanHayri Elbir, Kerem Karaman, Ali Surmelioglu, Erdal Birol Bostanci and Musa Akoglu
Department of Gastroenterological Surgery, Turkiye Yuksek Ihtisas Teaching and Research Hospital, 06410 Sihhiye, Ankara, Turkey

K. Naidoo, S. Mewa Kinoo and B. Singh
Department of Surgery, Nelson R Mandela School of Medicine, University of KwaZulu-Natal, 719 Umbilo Road, Congella 4013, South Africa

Takeshi Matsutani, Tsutomu Nomura, Nobutoshi Hagiwara, Akihisa Matsuda and Eiji Uchida
Department of Gastrointestinal and Hepato-Biliary-Pancreatic Surgery, Nippon Medical School, 1-1-5 Sendagi, Bunkyo-ku, Tokyo 113-8603, Japan

Atsushi Hirakata and Hiroshi Yoshida
Department of Surgery, Nippon Medical School Tama-Nagayama Hospital, 1-7-1 Nagayama, Tama, Tokyo 206-8512, Japan

Mazen E. Iskandar, Fiona M. Chory, Elliot R. Goodman and Burton G. Surick
Department of Surgery, Mount Sinai Beth Israel Medical Center, New York, NY 10003, USA

Christian Grønhøj Larsen and Birgitte Charabi
Department of Otorhinolaryngology, Head and Neck Surgery and Audiology, Copenhagen University Hospital (Rigshospitalet), 2100 Copenhagen, Denmark

Sanoop Koshy Zachariah
Department of General, Laparoscopic and Gastrointestinal Surgery, MOSC Medical College Kolenchery, Cochin 682311, India

Rocio Santos-Rancaño and Esteban Martín Antona
Division of Hepatobiliopancreatic Surgery, Department of General Surgery, San Carlos Clinic Hospital of Madrid, Madrid, Spain

José Vicente Méndez Montero
Unit of Abdomen Imaging Diagnosis and Interventional Radiology, Department of Radiology and Imaging, San Carlos Clinic Hospital of Madrid, Madrid, Spain

Emilio Muñoz, Fernando Pardo-Aranda, Noelia Puértolas, Itziar Larrañaga, Judith Camps and Enrique Veloso
Hospital Universitari Mutua Terrassa, 08221 Barcelona, Spain

Faruk Karateke, Ebru Menekşe, Koray Das and Sefa Ozyazici
Numune Training and Research Hospital, Department of General Surgery, 01170 Adana, Turkey

Pelin Demirtürk
Numune Training and Research Hospital, Department of Pathology, 01170 Adana, Turkey

Suhail Aslam Khan, Edmond Boko, Haseeb Anwar Khookhar and A. H. Nasr
Department of Surgery, Our Lady of Lourdes Hospital, Drogheda, County Louth, Ireland

Sheila Woods
Department of Radiology, Our Lady of Lourdes Hospital, Drogheda, County Louth, Ireland

Shigeo Ninomiya, Kazuya Sonoda, Hidefumi Shiroshita, Toshio Bandoh and Tsuyoshi Arita
Department of Surgery, Arita Gastrointestinal Hospital, 1-2-6 Maki, Oita 870-0294, Japan

Kazuhito Yajima, Tatsuo Kanda, Ryo Tanaka, Yu Sato, Takashi Ishikawa, Shin-ichi Kosugi and Katsuyoshi Hatakeyama
Division of Digestive and General Surgery, Niigata University Graduate School of Medical and Dental Sciences, 1-757 Asahimachi-dori, Niigata 951-8510, Japan

Tadayuki Honda
Advanced Disaster Medical and Emergency Critical Care Center, Niigata University Medical and Dental Hospital, 1-754 Asahimachi-dori, Niigata 951-8520, Japan

V. Stohlner, N. A. Chatzizacharias, M. Parthasarathy and T. Groot-Wassink
Department of Surgery, Ipswich Hospital, Ipswich, Suffolk IP4 5PD, UK

Paul E. Kaloostian and James Fred Harrington
Department of Neurosurgery, The University of New Mexico, MSC 10 5615, Albuquerque, NM 87131-0001, USA

Marc Barry
Department of Pathology, The University of New Mexico, MSC 10 5615, Albuquerque, NM 87131-0001, USA

Kristel De Vogelaere and Georges Delvaux
Department of Abdominal Surgery, UZ Brussel, Laarbeeklaan 101, 1090 Brussels, Belgium

Vanessa Meert
Department of Pathology, OLV Aalst, Moorselbaan 163, 9300 Aalst, Belgium

Frederik Vandenbroucke
Department of Radiology, UZ Brussel, Laarbeeklaan 101, 1090 Brussels, Belgium

Anne Hoorens
Department of Pathology, UZ Brussel, Laarbeeklaan 101, 1090 Brussels, Belgium

Andrew T. Schlussel
Department of General Surgery, Tripler Army Medical Center, 1 Jarrett White Road, Honolulu, HI 96859, USA

Aaron B. Fowler
University of Utah, School of Medicine, 30 North 1900 East, Salt Lake City, UT 84132, USA

Herbert K. Chinn
Department of Urology, Queens Medical Center, 1329 Lusitana Street, Suite 108, Honolulu, HI 96813, USA

Linda L. Wong
Department of Surgery, University of Hawaii School of Medicine, 550 South Beretania Street, Suite 403, Honolulu, HI 96813, USA

Ikuo Watanobe, Yuzuru Ito, Eigo Akimoto, Yuuki Sekine, Yurie Haruyama, Kota Amemiya, Fumihiro Kawano, Shohei Fujita, Satoshi Omori, Shozo Miyano, Taijiro Kosaka, Michio Machida, Toshiaki Kitabatake and Kuniaki Kojima
Department of General Surgery, Juntendo University Nerima Hospital, 3-1-10 Takanodai, Nerima, Tokyo 177-8521, Japan

Asumi Sakaguchi, Kanako Ogura and Toshiharu Matsumoto
Department of Diagnostic Pathology, Juntendo University Nerima Hospital, 3-1-10 Takanodai, Nerima, Tokyo 177-8521, Japan

Kwang-Kuk Park and Song-I Yang
Department of Surgery, Kosin University College of Medicine, 34 Amnam-dong, Seo-gu, Busan 602-703, Republic of Korea

Alexander Giakoustidis
Department of HPB Surgery, Royal London Hospital, London, UK

Thomas Goulopoulos, Aristidis Kainantidis and Dimitrios Giakoustidis
Department of Surgery, European Interbalkan Medical Centre, Thessaloniki, Greece

Anastasios Boutis
Department of Oncology, "Theagenion" Anti-Cancer Hospital, Thessaloniki, Greece

George Kavvadias
Department of Anesthesiology, European Interbalkan Medical Centre, Thessaloniki, Greece

Thomas Zaraboukas
Department of Pathology, European Interbalkan Medical Centre, Thessaloniki, Greece

Dimitrios Giakoustidis
Division of Transplant Surgery, Department of Surgery, Medical School, Aristotle University of Thessaloniki, Thessaloniki, Greece

Yalin Iscan, Bora Karip, Yetkin Ozcabi, Birol Ağca and Kemal Memisoglu
General Surgery, Fatih Sultan Mehmet Eğitim ve Araştırma Hastanesi, İçerenköy, 34752, İstanbul, Turkey

Yesim Alahdab
Gastroenterology, Fatih Sultan Mehmet Eğitim ve Araştırma Hastanesi, İçerenköy, 34752, İstanbul, Turkey

Georgios Lianos, Konstantinos Vlachos, Nikolaos Papakonstantinou, Christos Katsios, Georgios Baltogiannis and Dimitrios Godevenos
Division of Surgery, University Hospital of Ioannina, St. Niarchou Avenue, 45110 Ioannina, Greece

İhsan Yıldız, Yavuz Savaş Koca and Sezayi Kantar
Department of General Surgery, Suleyman Demirel University Medical School, Isparta, Turkey

S. Popeskou and D. Christoforidis
Department of Surgery, Lugano Regional Hospital, Switzerland

M. Gavillet
Department of Hematology, University Hospital of Lausanne, Switzerland

N. Demartines
Department of Surgery, University Hospital of Lausanne, Switzerland

D. Christoforidis
University Hospital of Lausanne, Switzerland

Maykong Leepalao
Department of General Surgery, Marshfield Clinic, Marshfield, WI 54449, USA

Jessica Wernberg
Department of Surgical Oncology, Marshfield Clinic, Marshfield, WI 54449, USA

Gokhan Cipe, Fatma Umit Malya, Mustafa Hasbahceci, Yeliz Emine Ersoy, Oguzhan Karatepe and MahmutMuslumanoglu
Bezmialem Vakıf University, Department of General Surgery, 34093 Istanbul, Turkey

Jai P. Singh, Heena Rajdeo, Kalyani Bhuta and John A. Savino
Department of Surgery, Westchester Medical Center, New York Medical College, Valhalla, NY 10595, USA

Ashish Lal Shrestha
Department of General Surgery, United Mission Hospital, Tansen, Palpa, Nepal

Girishma Shrestha
Department of Pathology, Patan Academy of Health Sciences, Lagankhel, Kathmandu, Nepal

Enver Kunduz, Huseyin Bektasoglu, Samet Yigman and Huseyin Akbulut
Department of General Surgery, Faculty of Medicine, Bezmialem Vakif University, Istanbul, Turkey

Rachel Mathis and Joshua Stodghill
Department of Surgery, Inova Fairfax Hospital, Fairfax, VA, USA

Timothy Shaver and George Younan
Virginia Surgery Associates, Fairfax, VA, USA

Aroub Alkaaki, Basma Abdulhadi, Murad Aljiffry, Mohammed Nassif and Ashraf A. Maghrabi
Department of Surgery, Faculty of Medicine, King Abdulaziz University, Jeddah, Saudi Arabia

Haneen Al-Maghrabi
Department of Pathology, King Faisal Specialist Hospital and Research Center, Jeddah, Saudi Arabia

George Younan, Max Schumm, Fadwa Ali and Kathleen K. Christians
Division of Surgical Oncology, Department of Surgery, Milwaukee, WI, USA

Makoto Tomatsu, Jun Isogaki, Takahiro Watanabe, Kiyoshige Yajima, Takuya Okumura, Kimihiro Yamashita, Kenji Suzuki and Akihiro Kawabe
Department of Surgery, Fujinomiya City General Hospital, 3-1 Nishiki-cho, Fujinomiya, Shizuoka 418-0076, Japan

Akira Komiyama
Department of Diagnostic Pathology, Fujinomiya City General Hospital, 3-1 Nishiki-cho, Fujinomiya, Shizuoka 418-0076, Japan

Seiichi Hirota
Department of Surgical Pathology, Hyogo College of Medicine, 1-1 Mukogawa-cho, Nishinomiya, Hyogo 663-8501, Japan

Paolo Panaccio, Michele Fiordaliso, Domenica Testa, Mariangela Battilana and Roberto Cotellese
Department of Medical and Oral Sciences and Biotechnologies, "G. d'Annunzio" University, Chieti, Italy

Lorenzo Mazzola and Federico Selvaggi
General Surgery Unit, Renzetti Hospital, Lanciano, Italy

Yoshifumi Nakayama, Nobutaka Matayoshi, Masaki Akiyama, Yusuke Sawatsubashi, Jun Nagata and Keiji Hirata
Department of Surgery 1, University of Occupational and Environmental Health, 1-1 Iseigaoka, Yahata-nishi-ku, Kitakyushu 807-8555, Japan

Yoshifumi Nakayama, Masaki Akiyama, Yusuke Sawatsubashi and Jun Nagata
Department of Gastroenterological and General Surgery, Wakamatsu Hospital of University of Occupational and Environmental Health, 1-17-1 Hamamachi, Wakamatsu-ku, Kitakyushu 808-0024, Japan

Masanori Hisaoka
Department of Pathology and Oncology, School of Medicine, University of Occupational and Environmental Health, 1-1 Iseigaoka, Yahata-nishi-ku, Kitakyushu 807-8555, Japan

Lynn Model and Cathy Anne Burnweit
Nicklaus Children's Hospital, Miami, FL, USA

Barış Özcan and Alihan Gürkan
Department of General Surgery, Medstar Antalya Hospital, Antalya, Turkey

Metin Çevener
Department of Radiology, Medstar Antalya Hospital, Antalya, Turkey

Ayşegül Kargı and Mustafa Özdoğan
Department of Medical Oncology, Medstar Antalya Hospital, Antalya, Turkey

Paddy Ssentongo
Center for Neural Engineering, Department of Engineering, Science and Mechanics, Pennsylvania State University, University Park, PA, USA

Mark Egan
Department of Pathology, Eastern Regional Hospital, Koforidua, Ghana

Temitope E. Arkorful, Theodore Dorvlo and Forster Amponsah-Manu
Department of Surgery, Eastern Regional Hospital, Koforidua, Ghana

Oneka Scott
Ministry of Public Health, 1 Brickdam, Georgetown, Guyana

John S. Oh
Department of Surgery, Penn State Hershey College of Medicine and Milton S. Hershey Medical Center, Hershey, PA, USA

Jessica S. Crystal
Rutgers Robert Wood Johnson Medical School, New Brunswick, NJ, USA

Kristin Korderas and David Schwartzberg
Monmouth Medical Center, Long Branch, NJ, USA

Steven C. Tizio, Min Zheng and Glenn Parker
Jersey Shore University Medical Center, Neptune, NJ, USA

Meryem Rais, Hafsa Chahdi, Abderrahmane Albouzidi and Mohamed Oukabli
Department of Pathology, Faculty of Medicine and Pharmacy and Mohammed V Military Hospital, Mohammed V University, Rabat, Morocco

Mohammed Elfahssi
Department of Digestive Surgery, Faculty of Medicine and Pharmacy and Mohammed V Military Hospital, Mohammed V University, Rabat, Morocco

Kyle Szymanski, Estrellita Ontiveros, James S. Burdick, Daniel Davis and Steven G. Leeds
Division of Minimally Invasive Surgery, Baylor University Medical Center at Dallas, Dallas, TX 75246, USA

James S. Burdick
Department of Gastroenterology, Baylor University Medical Center at Dallas, Dallas, TX 75246, USA

Daniel Davis
Division of Bariatric Surgery, Baylor University Medical Center at Dallas, Dallas, TX 75246, USA

J. W. O'Brien, R. Tyler and A.M. Harris
Department of Laparoscopic and Upper Gastro-Intestinal Surgery, Hinchingbrooke Healthcare NHS Trust, Hinchingbrooke Park, Huntingdon PE29 6NT, UK

S. Shaukat
Department of Gastroenterology, Hinchingbrooke Healthcare NHS Trust, Hinchingbrooke Park, Huntingdon PE29 6NT, UK

Yuki Yamasaki, Tomoya Tsukada, Tatsuya Aoki, Yusuke Haba, Katsuhisa Hirano, Toshifumi Watanabe, Masahide Kaji and Koichi Shimizu
Department of Surgery, Toyama Prefectural Central Hospital, 2-2-78 Nishinagae, Toyama, Toyama 930-0975, Japan

O. S. Balogun, A. O. Osinowo, M. O. Afolayan and A. A. Adesanya
General Surgery Unit, Department of Surgery, Faculty of Clinical Sciences, College of Medicine, University of Lagos, PMB 12003, Idi Araba, Lagos, Nigeria

Seyed Mohammad Reza Nejatollahi
The Division ofHepatobiliary and Organ Transplantation, TaleghaniHospital, Shahid Beheshti University of Medical Sciences, Tehran, Iran

Omid Etemad
Shahid Beheshti University of Medical Sciences, Tehran, Iran

Kazuhito Yajima, Yoshiaki Iwasaki, Ken Yuu, Ryouki Oohinata, Misato Amaki, Yoshinori Kohira, Souichiro Natsume, Satoshi Ishiyama and Keiichi Takahashi
Department of Surgery, Tokyo Metropolitan Cancer and Infectious Diseases Center, Komagome Hospital, 3-18-22 Honkomagome, Bunkyo-ku, Tokyo 113-8677, Japan

Bradley Sherman
Department of Surgery, OhioHealth Doctors Hospital, 5100 West Broad Street, Columbus, OH 43228, USA

Mark Arnold
Division of Colon and Rectal Surgery, Wexner Medical Center,)e Ohio State University, N737 Doan Hall, 410 West 10th Avenue, Columbus, OH 43210, USA

Savaş Bayrak, Hasan Bektaş, Ekrem Çakar and Şükrü Çolak
Department of General Surgery, Istanbul Training and Research Hospital, Istanbul, Turkey

Necdet Derici
Private Ataköy Hospital, Istanbul, Turkey

Ali Bohlok, Fikri Bouazza, Melody El-Khoury, Deborah Repullo and Vincent Donckier
Service de Chirurgie, Institut Jules Bordet, Université Libre de Bruxelles (ULB), Bruxelles, Belgium

Thierry De Grez
Service de Gastroentérologie, CHR Sambre et Meuse, Namur, Belgium

Roland De Wind
Service d'Anatomie Pathologique, Institut Jules Bordet, Université Libre de Bruxelles (ULB), Bruxelles, Belgium

Jun-wen Qu, Gui-yang Wang, Zhi-qing Yuan and Ke-wei Li
Department of Biliary-Pancreatic Surgery, Renji Hospital, School of Medicine, Shanghai Jiao Tong University, No. 160, Pujian Road, Pudong New Area, Shanghai 200127, China

Caroline E. Sheppard and DanielW. Birch
Department of Medicine, Division of Gastroenterology, Zeidler Ledcor Centre, University of Alberta, Edmonton, AB, Canada T6G 2X8

Richdeep Gill
Rm3656WestWing, Peter LougheedHospital, 3500 26th Avenue NE, Calgary, AB, Canada T1Y 6J4.

Index

www.ingramcontent.com/pod-product-compliance
Lightning Source LLC
Chambersburg PA
CBHW080516200326
41458CB00012B/4224